The Management of the Menopause & Post-Menopausal Years

Edited by Stuart Campbell

The Management of the Menopause & Post-Menopausal Years

The Proceedings of the International Symposium held in London 24–26 November 1975 Arranged by the Institute of Obstetrics and Gynaecology, The University of London

MTP

Published in the UK by
MTP Press Limited
St Leonard's House,
Lancaster,
England

First published 1976

ISBN 0 85200147 9

Typeset in Great Britain by
The Lancashire Typesetting Co. Ltd, Bolton
and printed by R. & R. Clark Ltd, Edinburgh

Contents

SECTION C

PSYCHOLOGICAL ASPECTS

Chairman: C. H. Naylor

SECTION D

LIPID METABOLISM *Chairman: T. M. Coltart*

SECTION E

CALCIUM METABOLISM

Chairman: G. V. P. Chamberlain

Part 2: Cancer *Chairman: R. B. K. Rickford*

SECTION I

THERAPEUTIC PROBLEMS

Chairman: J. C. McClure Browne

SECTION J

MANAGEMENT OF THE MENOPAUSE

Chairman: J. W. W. Studd

List of Contributors

Dr J. M. Aitken,
Consultant Physician,
Essex County Hospital,
Lexden Road,
Colchester,
Essex, CO3 3NB

Dr M. Aylward,
Clinical Research Consultant,
Cefn Cottage,
Cefn Coed,
Merthyr Tydfil
Glam., CF48 2PH

Dr C. Barbara Ballinger,
Lecturer in Psychiatry,
Ninewells Hospital and
Medical School,
Dundee, DD2 1UB

Mr R. J. Beard,
Consultant Obstetrician and
Gynaecologist,
Royal Sussex County Hospital,
Eastern Road,
Brighton,
Sussex, BN2 5BE

Professor R. W. Beard,
Department of Obstetrics and
Gynaecology,
St Mary's Hospital,
Paddington,
London, W2 1PG

Dr C. H. Bolton,
Lecturer in Biochemistry,
Department of Medicine,
Bristol Royal Infirmary,
Bristol, BS2 8HW

Professor J. Bonnar,
Department of Obstetrics and
Gynaecology,
Trinity College Medical School,
University of Dublin,
Rotunda Hospital,
Dublin, 1

Professor J. C. M. Browne,
Institute of Obstetrics and
Gynaecology,
Hammersmith Hospital,
Du Cane Road,
London, W12 0HS

Mr S. Campbell,
Senior Lecturer,
Institute of Obstetrics and
Gynaecology,
Queen Charlotte's Hospital for
Women,
Goldhawk Road,
London, W6 0XG

Mr G. V. P. Chamberlain,
Consultant Obstetrician and
Gynaecologist,
Queen Charlotte's Hospital for
Women,
Goldhawk Road,
London, W6 0XG

Dr Margaret E. Christie Brown,
Consultant Psychotherapist,
Chelsea Hospital for Women,
Dovehouse Street,
London, S.W.3

Mr T. M. Coltart,
Senior Lecturer,
Guy's Hospital Medical School,
London, SE1 9RT

Professor I. D. Cooke,
Department of Obstetrics and
Gynaecology,
Jessop Hospital for Women,
Sheffield, S3 7RE

Dr Jean K. M. Coope,
General Practitioner,
Group Practice Centre,
Bollington,
Nr Macclesfield,
Cheshire

Mrs Wendy Cooper,
Author and Journalist,
32 Vesey Road,
Sutton Coldfield,
Warwickshire

Mr E. Cope,
Consultant Obstetrician and
Gynaecologist,
85 Banbury Road,
Oxford, OX2 6LG

Mr I. L. Craft,
Senior Lecturer,
Institute of Obstetrics and
Gynaecology,
Queen Charlotte's Hospital for
Women,
Goldhawk Road,
London, W6 0XG

Mr A. E. Crompton,
Consultant Obstetrician and
Gynaecologist,
St James's Hospital,
Leeds, LS9 7TF

Professor C. E. Dent,
Department of Human Metabolism,
University College Hospital
Medical School,
University Street,
London, WC1E 6JJ

Professor C. J. Dewhurst,
Institute of Obstetrics and
Gynaecology,
Queen Charlotte's Hospital for
Women,
Goldhawk Road,
London, W6 0XG

Dr K. Fotherby,
Reader in Biochemistry,
Royal Postgraduate Medical School,
Hammersmith Hospital,
Du Cane Road,
London, W12 0HS

Dr L. Goldman,
Medical Correspondent,
Mill Green,
29 Dartnell Park Road,
West Byfleet,
Surrey

Mr H. Gordon,
Senior Lecturer,
Institute of Obstetrics and
Gynaecology,
Hammersmith Hospital,
Du Cane Road,
London, W12 0HS

Dr C. B. Hammond,
Associate Professor,
Duke University Centre,
North Carolina,
U.S.A.

Mr R. F. Harrison,
Lecturer,
Institute of Obstetrics and Gynaecology,
Queen Charlotte's Hospital for Women,
Goldhawk Road,
London, W6 0XG

Dr H. S. Jacobs,
Senior Lecturer in Gynaecological Endocrinology,
St Mary's Hospital Medical School,
Paddington,
London, W2 1PG

Dr L. J. B. Jaszmann,
Head, Department of Obstetrics and Gynaecology,
Regional Protestant Hospital,
Bennekom,
Netherlands

Dr M. Dorothea Kerr,
Clinical Assistant Professor of Psychiatry,
Cornell University Medical College,
New York, N.Y. 10021,
U.S.A.

Professor C. Lauritzen,
Frauenklinik,
Universität Ulm,
79 Ulm/Donau,
Prittwitzstr. 43,
Germany

Mr T. L. T. Lewis,
Consultant Obstetrician and Gynaecologist,
Queen Charlotte's Hospital for Women,
Goldhawk Road,
London, W6 0XG

Mr J. Malvern,
Consultant Obstetrician and Gynaecologist,
Queen Charlotte's Hospital for Women,
Goldhawk Road,
London, W6 0XG

Dr R. Marks,
Senior Lecturer,
Department of Medicine,
The Welsh National School of Medicine,
Heath Park,
Cardiff, CF4 4XN

Dr Audrey Midwinter,
Senior Lecturer,
Department of Obstetrics and Gynaecology,
Bristol Royal Infirmary,
Bristol, BS2 8HW

Professor N. F. Morris,
Department of Obstetrics and Gynaecology,
New Charing Cross Hospital,
Fulham Palace Road,
London, W.6

Dr M. A. F. Murray,
Research Biochemist,
St Mary's Hospital Medical School,
Paddington,
London, W2 1PG

Mr C. H. Naylor,
Consultant Obstetrician and Gynaecologist,
Central Middlesex Hospital,
Park Royal,
London, N.W.10

Professor M. F. Oliver,
Reader in Medicine and Consultant Physician, Department of Cardiology and Medicine, The Royal Infirmary, Edinburgh, EH3 9YW

Mr J. L. Osborne,
Lecturer, Institute of Obstetrics and Gynaecology, Queen Charlotte's Hospital for Women, Goldhawk Road, London, W6 0XG

Dr L. Poller,
Consultant Haematologist, University Hospital of South Manchester, Manchester, M20 8LR

Dr T. Pyörälä,
Lecturer in Obstetrics and Gynaecology, Central Hospital of Middle Finland, 40620 Jyväsklä 62, Finland

Professor L. Rauramo,
Department of Obstetrics and Gynaecology, University Central Hospital of Turku, 20520 Turku 52, Finland

Mr R. B. K. Rickford,
Consultant Obstetrician and Gynaecologist, Chelsea Hospital for Women, Dovehouse Street, London, S.W.3

Professor R. A. Sellwood,
Department of Surgery, University Hospital of South Manchester, Manchester, M20 8LR

Dr P. Shahrad,
Clinical Research Assistant, Department of Medicine, The Welsh National School of Medicine, Heath Park, Cardiff, CF4 4XN

Mr P. J. B. Smith,
Consultant Urologist, St Martin's Hospital, Midford Road, Bath, BA2 5RP

Mr J. W. W. Studd,
Consultant Obstetrician and Gynaecologist, King's College Hospital, Denmark Hill, London, SE5 9RS

Professor R. W. Taylor,
Department of Obstetrics and Gynaecology, St Thomas's Hospital, Lambeth Palace Road, London, SE1 7EH

Foreword

Despite the fact that the average woman spends one third of her life after the menopause, medical research has been devoted almost entirely to the reproductive period of her life span. This is perhaps not surprising in our youth-orientated society and yet there is increasing evidence that properly applied and supervised hormonal therapy could alleviate many of the severe physical symptoms which are associated with the ovarian menopause and that in the long term other aspects of physical deterioration could be modified. This lack of scientific research has made it difficult to assess which symptoms are due to the altered hormonal status of the post-menopausal period and which are due to the normal process of ageing, or the various psychological pressures which build up around most women in the fourth and fifth decades of life.

In America doctors have been treating the 'menopausal syndrome' with estrogens for over 30 years, but in the United Kingdom gynaecologists and family doctors have been reticent to prescribe these steroid preparations. As a consequence, they have been labelled reactionary by the media and while there may be some truth in this, it should be remembered that the hazards associated with synthetic estrogens in the contraceptive pill were first brought to light by British epidemiological surveys. The American experience has been none too reassuring and an apparent alliance between feminist movements and certain gynaecological interests has produced the 'feminine for ever' cult which implies that estrogens should be prescribed from the menopause to the grave. This specious therapeutic approach to therapy has unfortunately not been accompanied by adequate epidemiological and follow-up studies and now from the U.S.A. there is evidence of a major reappraisal of hormone replacement therapy due to the finding in two poorly-documented retrospective studies[1, 2] that there may be an association between post-menopausal estrogens and endometrial cancer. This syndrome of therapeutic overkill followed by over-reaction can only be prevented by a deep understanding of the psychological, hormonal and other pathophysiological changes of the post-menopause, knowledge of the cellular metabolic effects of the steroid hormones and clinical evaluation of such effects by well designed prospective scientific studies. We are at the moment a long way from this but there are now many workers throughout the world who are bringing science to the menopause. It was for this reason that the Institute of Obstetrics and Gynaecology decided to hold this international multidisciplinary meeting to discuss present clinical and scientific knowledge and indicate into which areas future research should be directed. We planned the conference with several basic questions in mind:

(1) What short and long term psychological and physical changes can be related to the loss of ovarian function associated with the menopause, and to what extent do these changes contribute to morbidity and ill health in the post-menopausal population.

(2) What effects do exogenous 'synthetic' and 'natural' estrogens or indeed any other pharmacological agents have on these changes.

(3) What other metabolic effects can be produced by exogenous estrogens and in what respect do any of these effects represent a risk to the patient's health.

(4) In the light of present day knowledge what is the recommended management of the post-menopausal patient with—or without—symptoms.

Needless to say no simple clear answer can be given to any of the above questions at this moment. Nevertheless, all the speakers at the meeting gave clear and comprehensive expositions on present day knowledge and we hope that this collection of their papers will be of interest to all doctors dealing with the varied problems facing the post-menopausal woman. Most of the speakers are actively engaged in research but all have avoided giving the 'narrow view' and commendably have placed their work in the broader context of present day knowledge. There is inevitably, as in any large symposium, some overlap in the areas covered by the speakers, but we believe this has been kept to a minimum. The reader with specialized interest however, would be wise to read in regions which are outside his field, for there are 'pearls' hidden in the most unlikely places; for example under Management of the Menopause, Dr Charles Hammond gives a masterly summary of post-menopausal endocrinological changes.

We have included all the end-of-session discussions as they were lively and provocative and we hope that our attention to syntax has not detracted from the spontaneity of the exchanges.

The publication of symposia is of most value when publication is rapid for in that way the latest information and research can quickly be disseminated to a wide audience; MTP are to be congratulated on publishing this volume within five months of the symposium, thus fulfilling a pre-conference promise. Rapid publication, however, is impossible without the cooperation of the participants and I thank all of them for promptly providing us with their scripts.

This conference was inspired by Professor Dewhurst, who has taken a keen interest in our own research and indeed in all aspects of the menopause for many years. We are also indebted to Ayerst Laboratories Ltd., Schering Chemicals Ltd., Syntex Pharmaceuticals Ltd., and Abbott Laboratories Ltd., without whose financial help it would have been impossible to mount a conference of this size. In this time of financial stringency it is a pleasure to acknowledge the invaluable support the pharmaceutical industry gives to academic medicine in this country.

Stuart Campbell March 1976

References

1. Smith, D. C., Prentice, R., Thompson, D. J. and Herrmann, W. L. (1975). Association of exogenous estrogen and endometrial carcinoma. *N. Engl. J. Med.*, **293**, 1164
2. Ziel, H. K. and Finkle, W. D. (1975). Increased risk of endometrial carcinoma among users of conjugated estrogens. *N. Engl. J. Med.*, **293**, 1167

Section A

EPIDEMIOLOGY

Chairman: N. F. MORRIS

I

A woman's view of the menopause

Wendy Cooper

There's been a wild rumour, current for a few thousand years, that the female mind is illogical. Obviously you will not expect *me* to confirm that. But I have to admit where the menopause is concerned women's views, if not illogical, can at least be strangely ambivalent. With one part of her mind a woman may positively welcome the onset of infertility and the end of risk of pregnancy, while simultaneously at a deeper level she may feel threatened, diminished and devalued.

Women's views on the menopause are, of course, subject to many influences—to memories of her mother's menopause experience—to her own experience—to contemporary attitudes her husband's—her doctor's and not least these days to what she may learn from the media. But there is another factor also involved. We may like to consider today that science has banished superstition, emancipation overcome prejudice, and that women are well on the way to being liberated (whatever that may mean). But no-one has yet found how to liberate any evolving organism, let alone a woman, from the bonds of cultural and genetic endowment. So, despite logic and liberation, I believe women still show signs of atavistic response to the menopause.

Old attitudes

Before we examine contemporary attitudes, therefore, I want briefly to look back to see how original attitudes to the menopause arose. Although until this century the process of ovarian failure was not understood, we must assume the onset of infertility was recognized and almost certainly welcomed by women in the past as the only relief then known from constant pregnancies. The price that had to be paid—the adverse train of events, the accelerated ageing, the degenerative changes, which we now know to be linked to estrogen deficiency, were *not* recognized. In fact until very recently they were accepted as a normal and inevitable part of ageing in a woman. But there was still a recognized price the menopause exacted—it brought a sudden and drastic drop in status—the menopausal woman was relegated, as it were, to the fourth division. Not only did the menopause mean that a woman was usually considered no longer sexually interesting, but since she could no longer produce sons, it also further diminished her value as a wife.

One can imagine clear elements of personal tragedy in this for the individual woman, but it has to be said that to society and to men it was of little importance. A man might get through several wives in the course of a lifetime. He could go on enjoying sexual adventures and fathering children right into old age.

Its unimportance to men and the fact that so few women lived to reach the menopause, let alone survive long beyond it, meant that it received little social or medical attention. It was what we would call today a 'non-event', a negative thing—the end to fertility—the absence of the monthly issue of blood. And it is here that we must look for old attitudes to the menopause—menopause mythology is inextricably linked to that of menstruations[1, 2], but assuming the negative, the opposite interpretation.

Because of the coincidence of the 28-day cycle, the moon was widely believed to trigger menstruation, and just as an example of how long old superstitions can survive, as recently as 1938, American medical students could still read in an authoritative textbook on obstetrics 'over 71% of women menstruate every 28 days and the majority during the new moon'.

But it is beliefs regarding the *purpose* of menstruation which are important. It was widely held to be a form of purging in which women were relieved of evil humours and toxic substances. This not only led to women being segregated during this 'dangerous' time, but to the belief that menstruating women had devastating effects on quite ordinary things. In his book *Natural History*, Pliny refers to menstruating women turning wine sour, seed sterile and even withering the grass on which they sat. As recently as 1878 the *British Medical Journal*, no less, was still perpetuating this with reports of two hams being spoiled because they had been cured by menstruating women. In my book *No Change*[3] I was able to quote 1974 newspaper reports of women complaining that flowers worn as a corsage faded faster during menstruation.

The other view put forward by Hippocrates, who was at least groping toward the relationship with reproduction, insisted that the menstrual flow was the nourishment which fed the child. Pliny went further believing it was the actual substance from which the child was formed.

But either way, the menopause, the opposite to menstruation, had to be a bad thing. It either meant a woman was no longer getting rid of her evil humours and they were building up inside her, which led to the old fears of madness at the menopause, *or* it meant she no longer produced the substance of life. Either way she was diminished—she was no longer a real woman. Margaret Mead in her book, Male and Female, strongly makes the point that in primitive societies pre-pubertal girls and post-menopausal women were treated as men; she adds that the older women no longer had to observe modest behaviour and could use obscene language 'as freely or more freely than any man'.

So you see, the loss of femininity after the menopause, and the change to a neuter or masculine state, is not just something dreamed up 20 years ago by a British-born gynaecologist called Robert Wilson[4] to justify hormone replacement therapy. It is something deeply enshrined and emphasized by old attitudes and old superstitions, and something still deeply felt by many women, particularly those whose status and satisfaction in life has almost entirely derived from their maternal and domestic role.

Modern attitudes

Today a woman accepts how much things have changed. With her conscious and reasoning mind she accepts that her usefulness is no longer measured by her fertility, and that in our present over-crowded world infertility may even be a virtue. Living to the new time-scale, which in the developed world gives her a life expectancy of almost 80, she accepts that at 50 she is still relatively young. She accepts that far from being ready for the discard heap, far from being encouraged or even permitted to go into a gentle decline and wield nothing more vigorous than a crochet hook, the chances are she will be facing the most challenging and demanding time of her life within the family or within a career. She has learned to accept and appreciate her own sexuality and is not prepared to opt out of her sexual role. Indeed with fear of pregnancy gone and with children gone too, she can often need more than ever the satisfaction and comfort of closer sexual ties. Yet at this very time, she may find herself with the onset of menopause, beset by crippling loss of confidence and deep fears of sexual inadequacy and of mental and emotional instability. In all this I believe there are echoes of atavistic memory at work. Unfortunately these irrational fears are too often confirmed by rational experience. On all sides there is evidence of menopausal women who do suffer from depression, do lose confidence in themselves, and suffer from the wretched vaginal atrophy, which brings in its train falling libido and the very sexual inadequacy they dreaded.

In 1969 the International Health Foundation carried out the only major survey I have discovered into woman's attitudes to the menopause[5]. Some 2000 women between the ages of 46 and 55 were questioned in Belgium, France, Great Britain, Italy and West Germany—a sort of Menopausal Common Market. Some fascinating cultural differences were thrown up and I am glad to say that British women in proverbial stiff-upper lip tradition emerged as the most stoical and optimistic. The women of Belgium and Italy were the most gloomy, and in particular twice as many of them thought the menopause marked not only the start of old age, but the end of attractiveness to men. While the most common symptoms were flushes, tiredness, nervousness, sweating, headaches, insomnia, depression, irritability, joint and muscle pains, dizziness, palpitations and formication, in that order, it is interesting that the symptoms women were most worried about and for which they most desperately wanted help were very different. Right at the top was depression, followed by faulty memory, overweight, brittle bones and painful sexual relations. A very recent survey by Syntex in this country showed very similar results—the symptoms women worried about most were again headed by depression, followed by insomnia, headaches, fatigue, loss of libido, loss of confidence, irritability and dyspareunia. My own letters from women show much the same, confirming that they worry most about those symptoms which spill over to affect the family and their marriage. I would like to quote from just one of more than 5000 on my files. It is not by any means the most harrowing and I've chosen it because the writer is clearly well balanced and sensible. She writes:

> 'Like a lot of women I have a doctor who seems to feel that Librium is the answer to all female ailments at this time. From having a happy married life and being an ordinary individual, over the last three and a half years I have become an anxious, irritable, moody, introspective *thing*. Because of continual irritation in the vagina, intercourse has become a memory and when my husband and I went together to see our family doctor we were told, "There is nothing I can do about it."
>
> I have a wonderful husband but the feelings of frustration loom larger than life at times. At 53 sex is not the vital thing it was when we were 22, but it is still there and the discomfort amounting to real pain, and the lack of help from the doctor whom I thought could help, has meant our sense of humour like our relationship has become very

strained. I find it hard to believe that the present "me" is the same woman who used to sing over the housework and enjoy family and friends. I wouldn't have believed the "change" could be just that—transformation is a better word.'

Doctors tell me that they do not get many women presenting with vaginal atrophy. I can only say I get dozens of letters mentioning painful intercourse and often admitting they are too shy to mention this to their doctor. Obviously this is part of the trouble. My generation of women are inhibited about discussing these things but I do feel when a woman presents with other menopause symptoms, perhaps by asking the *right* questions, the doctor would often uncover this hidden problem. Its particularly distressing that when a woman does screw up courage to ask for help, that she can still be told 'nothing can be done'. Vaginal atrophy, like hot flushes, responds readily and rapidly to oral estrogen—even for that matter to local estrogen.

Depression is the other symptom which recurs time and again in letters to me from menopausal women, particularly following hysterectomy. As you know, British work has confirmed depression to be four times as common in women following removal of ovaries as it is even in women who have had other major surgery[6]. It is also more severe and of longer duration. I know this is a complicated subject and that some women may have been depressive types with the menopause emphasizing this existing tendency. I accept too that some middle-aged depression can be rooted in the life-situation—in children having left home—the busy husband—the woman lonely or lacking a purpose in life. But before assuming the need for anti-depressants or even psychiatric treatment, particularly where other menopause symptoms exist, I believe estrogen replacement should first be tried. I am delighted to see that later today we shall be hearing about this in more detail both from Dr Aylward[7] and Dr Kerr.

Other so-called psychological symptoms, once believed to be 'all in the mind' have also proved to respond to HRT. These are very frequently mentioned in letters to me from career women. One such letter, from a woman well into the post-menopause, stated that she held a highly responsible post and was currently experiencing great difficulties with her job and impaired efficiency due to a growing sense of confusion—when I looked at the bottom of the letter it was signed 'Barbara'! Well, this Barbara was the assistant head of a large comprehensive school in the Midlands, who had been put on Premarin following a hysterectomy some years before while working in America. She wrote, 'I was absolutely fine physically and mentally until I came back to England where to my horror my own doctor insisted I come off the treatment. I soon became aware of hot flushes and more gradually of growing confusion, lack of confidence, loss of memory and inability to concentrate. Needless to say I have been back to my doctor but he adamantly refuses to renew the prescription.'

Finally to get HRT again Barbara was driven to change her doctor. She is now back on Premarin and reports she is once again thriving. But as you know women hate changing their doctors. The fact that they are so often prepared to do so if it is the only way to obtain this treatment indicates the strong motivation and the entirely new attitude to the menopause. Once women know an effective medical treatment exists for the menopause, once they realize they don't now have to 'put up with it', they are no longer prepared to suffer themselves or see their families, jobs and marriages suffer. The International Health Foundation Survey would appear to confirm this—out of the 86% of women who said they suffered during the menopause, only 53% knew any effective medical treatment existed—the percentage who sought the treatment was virtually the same, 52%.

Luckily for the human race, women are both stoical and philosophical . . . what can't be cured must be endured and until recently that was their attitude to the menopause. But no longer. Now they are beginning to know that HRT exists, to be aware of its benefits, understand the logic. What is more, they realize they face not just a few years without estrogen, but perhaps a third of a life-time in which the ravages of estrogen deficiency can show up in brittle bones, vaginal atrophy, increased risk of depression, increased risk of heart disease and in generally accelerated ageing.

Within the last few weeks two major women's organizations, the National Council of Women and the Women's Institutes, have indicated their intention of putting forward resolutions calling for wider availability of HRT. Other women have already taken the practical step of setting up a free advisory service, Women's Health Care, whose aim is to inform women about Hormone Replacement and about the availability in their area. In the same way that women made it clear they wanted the right to anaesthesia in childbirth and later to the contraceptive pill, even in the face of traditional medical caution, so women now are indicating strongly that they want wider availability of HRT.

Women are grateful to modern medicine and have good cause to be, most especially for the knowledge which has already granted them a greater quantity of life. Now their concern and I am sure yours, must be with the quality of that life. That surely means giving them the choice at the menopause if they need it and if they want it, of proper hormonal support.

References

1. Crawfurd, R. (1915). Of superstitions concerning menstruation. *Proc. Roy. Soc. Med.*, **9**, 49

2. Frazer, J. G. (1963). *The Golden Bough* (MacMillan)
3. Cooper, W. (1975). *No Change, A Biological Revolution for Women* (Hutchinsons)
4. Wilson, R. A. and Wilson, T. A. (1963). The fate of the non-treated menopausal woman. *J. Am. Geriatrics Soc.*, **11**, 347
5. International Health Foundation (1969). *Workshop Meeting on The Menopause:* I.H.F., Geneva
6. Richards, D. M. (1973). A post-hysterectomy syndrome. *Lancet*, **ii**, 430
7. Aylward, M. (1973). Plasma tryptophan levels and mental depression in post-menopausal subjects: effects of oral piperazine-estrone-sulphate. *IRCS. Med. Sci. International Research Communications System* (73–7) 3–5–11

2

Epidemiology of the climacteric syndrome

L. J. Benedek Jaszmann

Introduction

Research in the medical field is traditionally more concerned with pathology than with normality. This certainly holds for the subject of this symposium.

During recent decades clear changes have taken place in the second half of the lives of women in the Netherlands and in other western countries. The gradual increase in lifespan of the population has resulted in a life expectancy of 77 years.

Because of the change in population structure, geriatrics and allied problems have received a good deal of attention. However, an important phase in the life of women, the transition from childbearing age to the stage beyond, has been relatively neglected. Many medical men have considered the treatment of women in this phase of life to be sufficient if it is consisted of a sedative and a few encouraging words. More active treatment is advocated in some quarters nowadays; a more preventative approach to symptoms and complaints resulting from estrogen deficiencies during the years of transition is even propagated.

Times have changed; women have adopted a different role in society and the doctor is now consulted about complaints which used to remain untreated or used to be treated by self-medication. Simultaneously, the number of the women in this transitional age group has increased.

Recent epidemiological data are necessary to decide whether the traditional conservative attitudes concerning the climacteric years can be maintained or whether there is a need for intensification of treatment.

Altogether there are reasons enough to pay much attention to this group of the population.

A study in the Netherlands

A few years ago a population survey was done in Ede, a partly urbanized rural community in the Netherlands, which had at that time 66 000 inhabitants. Following careful and intensive preparation and motivation of the whole population by lectures, press publicity, etc. a questionnaire was mailed to all women between the ages of 40 and 60: 6628 women. The response rate was high, 71%[1].

The age at menopause

One of the aspects of our basic research was concerned with the age at the menopause. Based on the data supplied by those subjects who had never undergone surgery of the uterus and/or ovaries, the following conclusions could be drawn.

(1) The age at menopause is approximately normally distributed and the mean age was found to be 51·4; the standard deviation 3·8 years. This study found 269 women who had undergone an artificial (surgical) menopause, 6·4% of the total survey sample with a mean age of 45·5 years (Figure 2.1).

(2) The age at menopause appeared to be independent of environmental factors, education or physical type. No effect could be demonstrated of age at menarche, number of pregnancies or age at last pregnancy. A significant difference was found between women who were married or had at one time

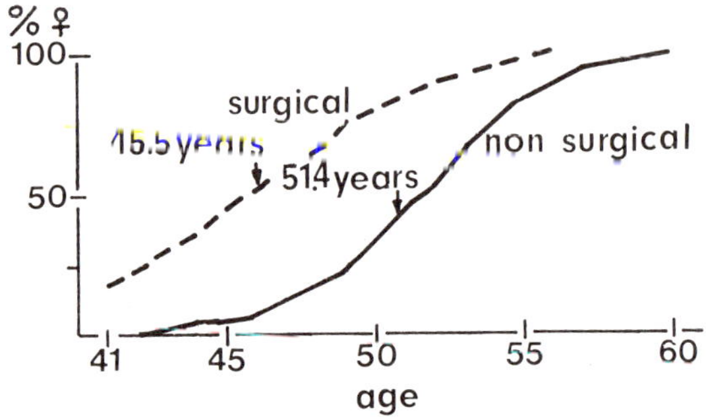

Figure 2.1 Frequency distribution of age at menopause. ——— non-surgical groups; - - - - - - surgical groups

been married and those who had never been married. The mean ages at menopause for these groups were respectively 51·4 and 50·3 years.

The definition of menopause and climacteric period

First, we would like to draw attention to some definitions concerned with the periods of middle-aged woman.

The definition *menopause* has an importance because in the literature we often find this synonymous with climacteric. The term 'menopause' is only a mile stone, the last bleeding from the uterus and this must be considered as the counterpart of the first blood loss from the uterus called 'menarche'.

The *climacteric period* is a phase of life when woman changes, mentally and physically from sexual maturity to old age (Figure 2.2).

The period preceding the menopause we call *pre-menopause* and not only from theoretical but also from practical considerations; the years following the menopause belong to the *post-menopause*.

We often use also the term 'perimenopausal' mostly for clinical purposes, for the few years prior to and the last year following the menopause.

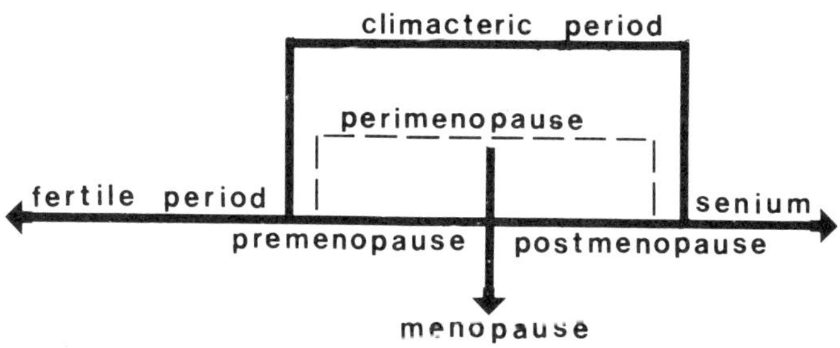

Figure 2.2 The climacteric period

The duration of reproductive stage and final pregnancy

The investigation of the duration of the reproductive stage and the age at the final pregnancy of climacteric women was made within the framework of our research of the problems surrounding the middle-aged woman.

The mean duration of the reproductive stage (menopause minus menarche) was found to be a good 37 years. The oldest (post-menopause) group of women participating in the survey yielded a mean duration of 35·4 years ($n = 1056$). Table 2.1 shows the frequency distribution for the post-menopausal group of the age at last pregnancy in our material. However, the reproductive frequency of women of the younger generation appeared to decrease over the age of 30 in the Netherlands.

Table 2.1 Age at last pregnancy in the postmenopausal group

Age at last pregnancy	*Percentage*
25 years or less	5
26–30	10
31–35	22
36–40	39
41–45	21
46 and over	3
total number 1056	100

From a practical point of view it is valid to consider whether the prolonged reproductive stage influences the actual fertile span of women.

Figure 2.3 shows the menstrual pattern in women who had not undergone surgical treatment. Although the pre-menopause is characterized by infertility and an increase in anovulatory cycles, we found no changes in the menstrual pattern in 50%, between 46 and 48 years; it can not be excluded that these menstrual patterns are also subject to a secular shift with an increasing possibility of pregnancy during the pre-menopause. Better nutritional

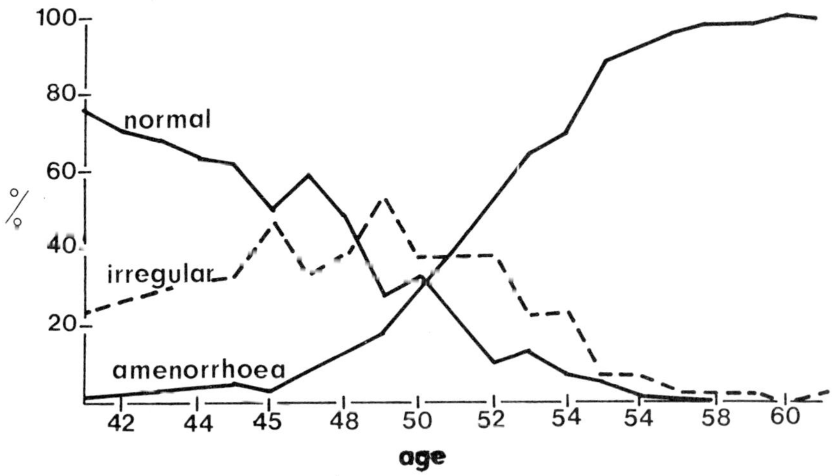

Figure 2.3 Menstrual pattern in women who had not undergone surgical treatment

habits and medical care, better social and economic conditions, application of steroid hormone therapy for gynaecological complaints and other factors have probably caused women to menstruate until a later age than previously.

The more every-day problems of a prolonged reproductive period concern the pre-menopausal years.

Analysis of the symptoms/complaints of the climacteric woman

The normal symptoms of this phase can be divided into

(1) genital symptoms, and
(2) extragenital symptoms

The *genital symptoms* are very well known from normal menses via a changed pattern of menstruation, accompanied by infertility to cessation of uterine bleeding, and post-menopausal genital atrophy. The cause of these changes is entirely *hormonal* and can be seen *in every woman*. In contrast, the *extragenital symptoms* of this phase of life *do not* necessarily *occur in all women* and the causes are *neurovegetative, psychosomatic and hormonal*.

Genital symptoms, the changes in the menstrual pattern, are in general regarded by women as 'normal' and are only mentioned as a complaint when the bleedings are abnormally heavy or frequent. Extragenital symptoms, however, differing in intensity and frequency from one woman to another, are often regarded as unpleasant symptoms and so as 'complaints'.

The menstrual pattern was taken as the basis for further analysis of complaints. Most studies into climacteric complaints describe the frequency of such symptoms in relation to the chronological age at which they occur. This, however, seems inappropriate for there is, as Figure 2.3 showed, a wide variety in the chronological ages at which the menopause takes place.

A much better insight is obtained when the symptoms or complaints are studied in relation to the so-called 'biological age'. Our definition of the biological age is dependent on the pattern of menstruation, the menopause, and the time which has passed since then. Accordingly, the menopausal complaints of the respondents were studied when the women were grouped as shown in Table 2.2.

It will be obvious that a 'typical climacteric complaint' should be mentioned rarely by women in group A, relatively frequently by women in group B (and to some degree in groups C1 and C2), but less often by women in groups C3, C4 and C5. In order to provide a basis for comparison with other studies, the complaints listed were those of Blatt's Menopausal Index (BMI), 13 in all (Table 2.3), modified by Neugarten and Kraines[2].

To calculate this index 13 subjective climacteric complaints are taken into account. The severity of each complaint is expressed by a figure: 0 = no complaint, 1 = slight, 2 = moderate, 3 = marked or severe.

Table 2.2 Criteria for 'biological age' groups

Women menstruating regularly or with a menstrual pattern similar to that which they have had in the preceding years	*group A*
Women menstruating during the last 12 months, but with a pattern different from that of the preceding years	*group B*
Women whose LMP occurred between 12–24 months ago	*group C1*
LMP between 25–36 months ago	*group C2*
LMP between 37–48 months ago	*group C3*
LMP between 49–60 months ago	*group C4*
LMP between 5–10 years ago	*group C5*

LMP = last menstrual period

Table 2.3 Blatt's Menopausal Index modified by Neugarten and Kraines

Hot flushes	factor	4
Perspiration		2
Paraesthesia		2
Insomnia		2
Muscle-, joints-, bone-pain		1
Fatigue		1
Headache		1
Irritability		1
Vertigo		1
Depression		1
Short of breath		1
Palpitation		1
Psycholability		1

The severity of complaint:
0 = no complaint
1 = slight
2 = moderate
3 = marked or severe

The various complaints have been given a conversion factor, shown in Table 2.3. To calculate the index one multiplies the conversion factor of each complaint by the severity score. The sum of these is the Menopausal Index. The poor woman who suffers severely with all 13 complaints will have the maximum index: 57.

The rationale underlying this survey was that in a woman with normal ovulatory menses the hormones and the autonomic hypothalamic centre functions (neuro-hormonal system) are at equilibrium to form a functional entity. As soon as the menstrual pattern begins to deviate from the norm, a disturbance of endocrine function may be expected to exist. This will be most pronounced after cessation of the menses but in most cases nature will eventually restore a balance between the two functional systems (neuro vegetative and hormone systems).

Our findings showed that the extragenital complaints such as fatigue headache, irritability, dizziness and to a lesser degree, depression, had their highest frequency in women of group B, women whose menstrual pattern had altered within the last year (Figure 2.4). Such complaints could be regarded as psychosomatic manifestation of the beginning of a disturbance in

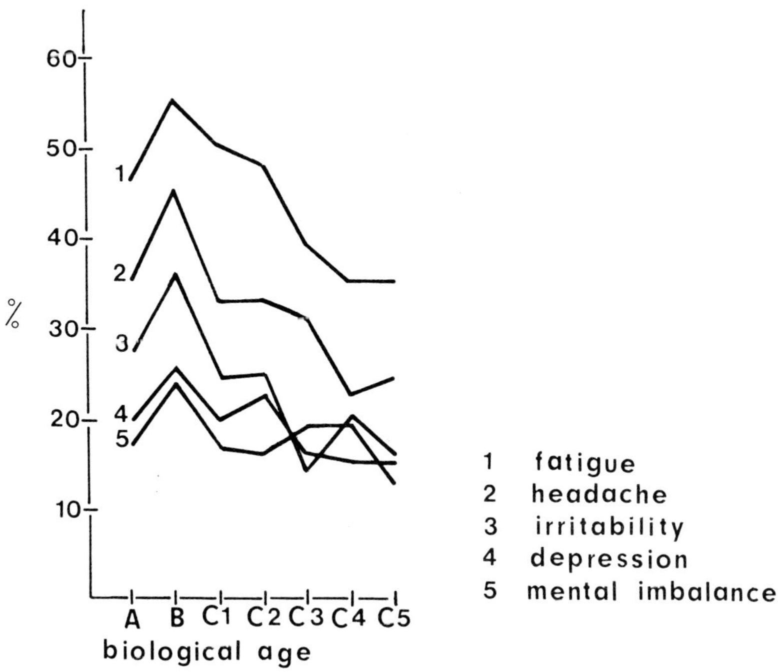

Figure 2.4 Complaints in women whose menstrual pattern had altered within 1 year

the balance between the neurovegetative and the endocrine system. In these women an ovarian function, albeit to a lesser extent, is still present.

Hot flushes, perspiration, formication and pains in the muscles and joints were all most frequently reported by women in the early post-menopause: in groups C1 and C2 (Figure 2.5). These complaints therefore, could be regarded as symptoms of a hypothalamic dysregulation and as complaints related to a decrease in endogenous estrogen production. The distribution of their frequency over the (so called), biological ages is typical for a climacteric complaint.

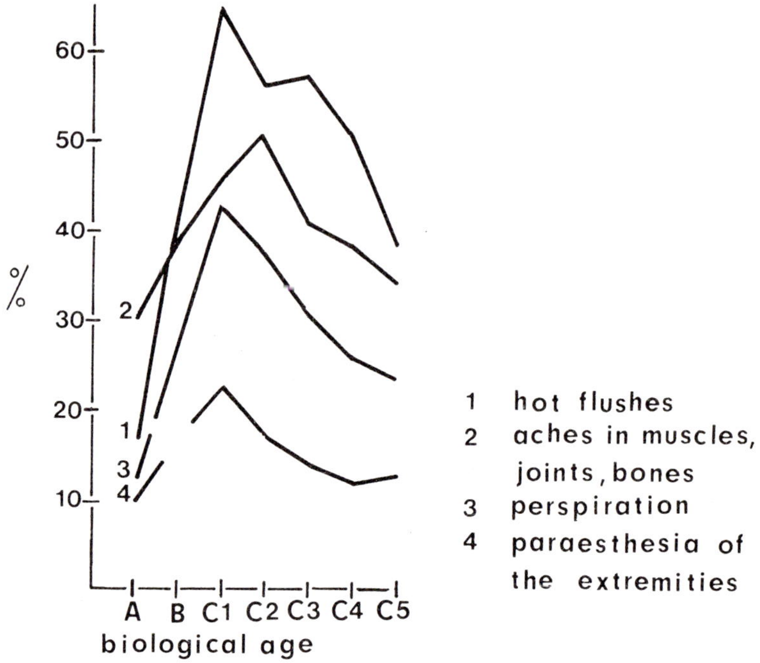

Figure 2.5 Complaints during early post-menopause

Sleeplessness, breathlessness, palpitation and mental imbalance (psycholability) did not show a peak in any one of the biological age groups (Figure 2.6). These complaints, therefore, are most probably not complaints which are peculiar to the climacteric age. Sleeplessness showed a special picture. The incidence was highest in group C4 and remained high in group C5. It seems likely, therefore, that this is a geriatric complaint rather than one of the climacteric or of the early post-menopause.

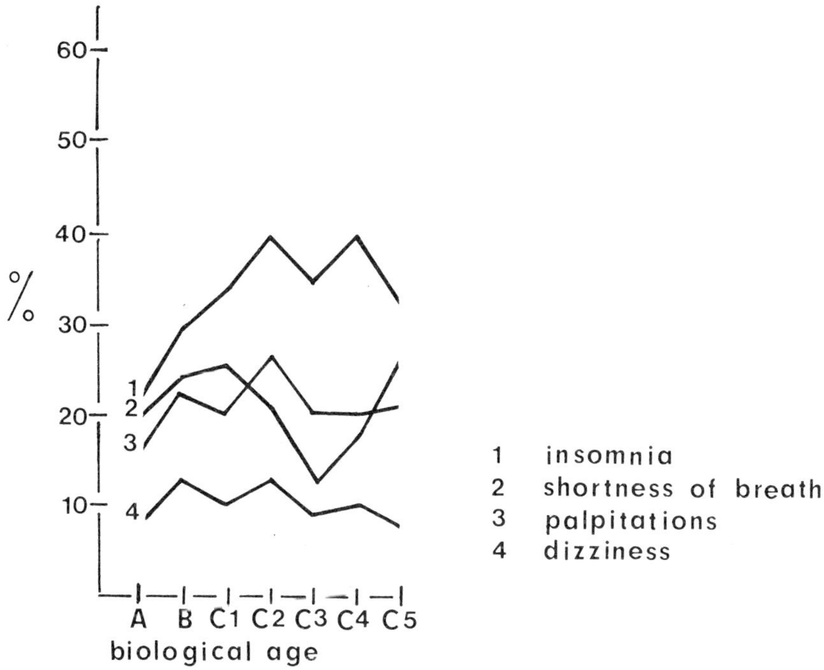

Figure 2.6 Complaints during early post-menopause

Figure 2.7 gives the median values of the BMI in the various biological age groups. Group C1 has clearly the highest index. This is partly explained by the heavy weight which is attached to hot flushes, perspiration and paraesthesia. If more weight had been given to fatigue, headache, psycholability and irritability and muscle-, joint- and bone-pains, group B would have reached a higher index—about the same as group C1.

Figure 2.8 shows that the percentage of women with more than four complaints was highest, almost 40%, in groups B, C1 and C2, and the percentage with two to four complaints was very constant, at around 45%, until some 5 years later after the menopause.

Influence of certain variables on the incidence of complaints

It is a well-known fact that the extragenital symptoms or complaints can be influenced by various factors. In no phase of life, however, is the line between what is normal and what is pathological, thinner than here. This phase of life

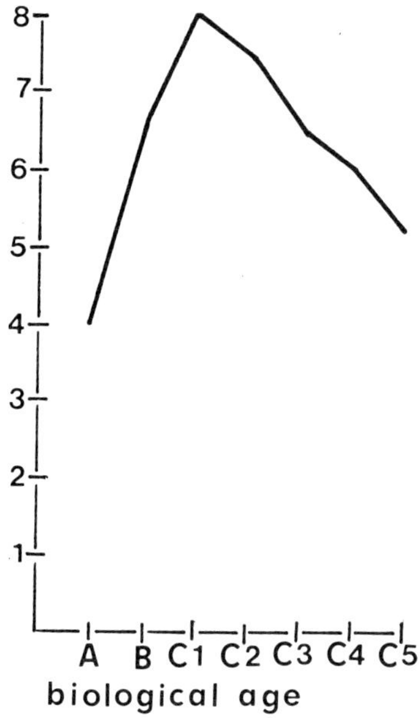

Figure 2.7 The median Blatt's Menopausal Index

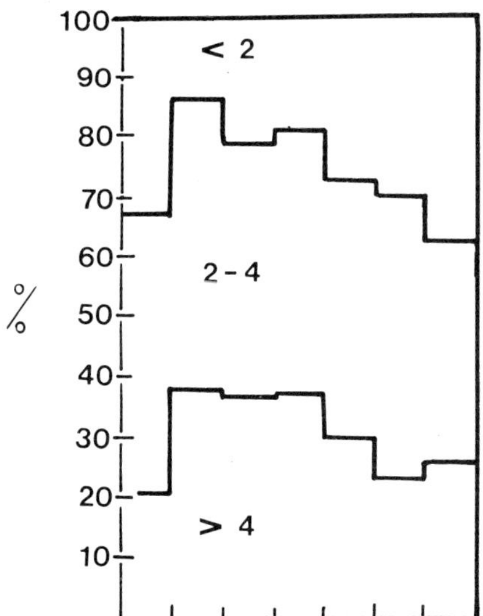

Figure 2.8 The frequency of the number of complaints per 'biological age' group

with its transformation in all its aspects makes the middle aged woman with her symptoms or complaints, a person with a typical psychosomatic entity.

The variables tested in this study were age at menarche, number of pregnancies, age at last pregnancy, income level, education, marital status and physical type. A summary of the conclusions gained is given below; more detailed data were published elsewhere[1, 3-7].

It was found that women who had a late menarche had fewer complaints than women whose menarche came early. Women who had never been pregnant had fewer complaints than women who had had one or more pregnancies. Women who had their last pregnancy after the age of 40, had fewer climacteric complaints than women whose last pregnancy occurred earlier. Women in the higher income groups had fewer complaints than women in the lower income groups. Women who had only a primary school education had more complaints than women educated to a higher standard. Physical type did not appear to be an influencing factor. Unmarried women had fewer complaints than married women.

The variables were analysed only one-dimensionally. It is clear that some variables are highly correlated, therefore one and the same difference may be found in several ways. The conclusion that fewer complaints were reported be women who were never pregnant in fact conveys to a large extent the same information as: married women appeared to have more complaints than single 'full time' working women.

The practical value of Blatt Menopausal Index

Medical literature shows a wide variety of psychic, psychosomatic, neurovegetative, endocrine, extragenital and somatic symptoms being regarded as climacteric complaints, and opinions as to the exact relationship between these and the climacteric vary from one author to another. Every list of climacteric complaints, therefore, is somewhat arbitrary when it is not based on a study of the epidemiology of complaints.

The Blatt Menopausal Index devised in 1953 and modified by Neugarten and Kraines in 1966[8] has been extremely useful in the past in evaluating climacteric complaints and, indeed, is often still used in its original form. In view of subsequent findings, however, it is perhaps not too disrespectful to suggest that the time has now come when this index should be revised.

The new index, which might be called the International Menopausal Index (IMI) would, I suggest, be linked to the so called 'biological age'.

Such an index would have two prime uses:

(1) It would be of great use in helping to objectivate the subjective psychic,

neurovegetative and psychosomatic symptoms of women, and could be a guide for therapy.

(2) It would permit a more exact registration of the results of therapy, and allow a better comparison of different estrogenic compounds.

Genital symptoms of the post-menopause

The Ede study did not deal with genital symptoms in the post-menopause. Few reliable epidemiological data relating to such symptoms are available.

van Keep[8] in his study of 2000 European women between the ages of 45 and 55, specifically asked respondents if they had experienced metrorrhagia; 17% said that they had. One-third of these women had ignored this sign of possible danger and not sought medical advice for it.

Vaginitis with discharge, one of the symptoms of estrogen deficiency most easily corrected, is, in my opinion, rather more common than has previously been supposed. This complaint, however, is surrounded by a taboo that makes it difficult for women to talk about it, although they often hesitantly admit to the existence of dyspareunia when specifically asked about it by the doctor. The same may be said for stress incontinence, which without anatomical pathology, is very easily corrected.

Closing remarks

For the last two years we have been working in a multidisciplinary research group in the University of Utrecht which is concerned with the problems of the climacteric woman.

Our research groups consists of gynaecologists, specialists for internal medicine, psychosociologists, dietists, with the cooperation of the laboratory of endocrinology, for cytological examination and the department of roentgenology.

We hope in the future to contribute some data on the middle aged woman and her interwoven complex of medical, psychological and sociological problems.

The average life expectancy for a woman of 50 years of age in most of the western countries is about 27 years. Most of these countries are so affluent that women expect, rightly so, to live these 27 years in good health, and that is the aim of our effort.

References

1. Jaszmann, L. J. B., van Lith, N. D. and Zaat, J. C. A. (1969). The age at menopause in the Netherlands. *Int. J. Fert.*, **14**, 106
2. Neugarten, B. L. and Kraines, R. J. (1966). 'Menopausal symptoms' in women of various ages. *Psychosomat. Med.*, **27**, 266

3. Jaszmann, L. J. B., van Lith, N. D. and Zaat, J. C. A. (1969). The duration of the reproductive stage and the age at final pregnancy of women in their forties and fifties. *Med. Gyn. Soc.*, **4**, 263
4. Jaszmann, L. J. B., van Lith, N. D. and Zaat, J. C. A. (1969). The perimenopausal symptoms; part A and part B. *Med. Gyn. Soc.*, **4**, 268
5. Jaszmann, L. J. B. (1972). The woman during the change. *Med. Gyn. Soc.*, **6**, 9
6. Jaszmann, L. J. B. (1973). Ageing and estrogens. In P. A. van Keep and C. Lauritzen (eds). Epidemiology of climacteric and postclimacteric complaints, pp. 22–34. (Basel: S. Karger)
7. Jaszmann, L. J. B. (1975). The value of the different parameters in the assessment of extragenital symptoms in the climacteric woman. The Fourth Int. Congr. of Psychosomat. Obst. Gyn. Tel-Aviv, Israel (Basel: S. Karger)
8. Keep, P. A. van (1970). The menopause, a study of the attitudes of women in Belgium, France, Great Britain, Italy and West Germany. International Health Foundation, Geneva.

3

Frequency and severity of menopausal symptoms

C. J. Dewhurst

This paper will seek to answer the following questions:

(1) How often do women about the time of the menopause and after suffer from vaso-motor symptoms?
(2) How severe are these symptoms?
(3) Untreated, how long are they likely to last?

Comparatively little information is available on the percentage of women about the time of the menopause and after who suffer moderate to severe vasomotor symptoms, nor on how long these symptoms last. When McKinlay and Jefferys[2–5] in 1974 reviewed the literature they were able to find only four recent studies in Western society which they considered to be free from methodological defects. McKinlay and Jefferys[1] themselves based their own study upon a questionnaire of 638 women between the ages of 45 and 54 who were living in the London area in 1964 and 1965. They found, with regard to the frequency of hot flushes, that of women who last menstruated between 3 and 12 months previously 75% reported having this symptom. In a study reported by Thompson *et al.*[5], 74% of postmenopausal women in a general practice in North-East Scotland reported having hot flushes.

Information on the duration of flushes is also obtainable in both these papers. McKinlay and Jefferys reported that of those patients whose menopause occurred 5 or more years previously 82% reported flushes lasting for more than 1 year and 26% lasting for more than 5 years. Thompson *et al.* also present data which suggest that in many instances the duration of flushing is quite prolonged. Among their patients who were still having flushes 17% had been having them for over 1 year, 50% for 2–5 years and 19% for more than 5 years; among their patients who had previously suffered from hot flushes which had now ceased 15% reported having had them for more than 1 year, 25% for 2–5 years and 19% for more than 5 years.

These figures suggest that the frequency of vasomotor symptoms during the early post-menopausal years is quite high and that they are much more prolonged than is generally believed.

The phrase 'hot flushes' is generally taken to mean a feeling of warmth passing over all of the body or part of it with the face and neck being the parts usually affected. The term itself 'hot flush' does not suggest a symptom of any severity. It may be imagined that it is embarrassing to a middle-age lady since it may well draw attention to her 'change of life' but the suggestion is often implied that flushes amount to little more than this. McKinlay and Jefferys have data which suggest this is not so. Almost half (48·5%) of the women in their survey who had ever had flushes said that they felt 'acute physical discomfort' and some had embarrassment as well. A further 20·5% of women felt embarrassment alone. The acute discomfort associated with hot flushes is worse when they occur at night. Then they are apt to produce marked sweating, the patient wakes bathed in perspiration and she may even have to get out of bed to wash or dry herself down with a towel or even to change her nightclothes. Naturally enough her sleep and her husband's is disturbed, possibly on several occasions. Night sweats, when they do occur, are almost always associated with day-time hot flushes, some patients finding the former worse than the latter and vice versa.

No similar grading of symptom severity is attempted by Thompson *et al.*[5], although they do have data which are relevant to an assessment of severity. Thus, of 90 patients reporting on the frequency of flushes, 19 (21%) said that they experienced flushes every few hours and 43 (47·7%) admitted that their flushes were less often but they occurred at least daily. 45% of patients with vasomotor symptoms consulted their doctor for relief. The percentage seeking relief from their doctor was smaller in McKinlay and Jefferys' survey[1] since only 46·7% of those patients who reported acute physical discomfort consulted the doctor about them.

Speaking as someone who has been specially interested in the management of this symptom in post-menopausal women for some years my observations are in accord with the facts presented by these two groups of investigators. I believe that hot flushes occur relatively frequently and that untreated they last many months and sometimes many years. Some patients have tried to put up with them for quite a prolonged period of time before consulting the doctor who may, or may not, be sympathetic to their requests for treatment.

We cannot be certain why many of the women in the two series quoted here did not go to see their doctor. Perhaps some experienced symptoms which, at their worst, were short-lived, perhaps others did not wish to 'make a fuss' which is a phrase one often hears in people ultimately obliged to come for medical help with this symptom. Many women believe flushes to be a natural phenomenon which they should endure. Certainly many middle-aged women are not well informed about the menopause and Allan is quoted by Thompson *et al.*[5] as saying that many such patients felt too embarrassed to consult their general practitioner or thought that it was inappropriate to seek help from him about problems of 'the change'.

If I can attempt to summarize the data which these two papers and my own experience suggest one would say that of every 100 post-menopausal women probably 75 will experience vasomotor symptoms; perhaps half of these will experience acute physical discomfort from these symptoms; a quarter to a half of the patients with symptoms will seek help from their doctor; if they are untreated the symptoms may last for between 1 and 5 years. These symptoms *can* be relieved by estrogen therapy in almost all cases and that data I have provided on the frequency, duration and severity of vasomotor symptoms does not seem to me to constitute a valid reason for withholding treatment in those moderately or more severly affected.

References

1. McKinlay, Sonja, M. and Jefferys, Margot (1974). The menopausal syndrome. *Brit. J. Prevent. Soc. Med.*, **28**, 108
2. Neugarten, B. L. and Kraines, R. J. (1965). 'Menopausal symptoms' in women of various ages. *Psychosomat. Med.*, **27**, 266
3. Prill, H. J. (1966). Die Beziehung von Erkrankungen und sozialpsychologischen Fakten zum Klimakterium. *Med. Klin.*, **61**, 1325
4. Jaszmann, L., van Lith, N. D. and Zaat, J. C. A. (1969). The perimenopausal symptoms. *Med. Gynaecol. Sociol.*, **4**, 268
5. Thompson, B., Hart, S. A. and Durno, D. (1973). Menopausal age and symptomatology in a general practice. *J. Biosocial Sci.*, **5**, 71

4

Physical changes associated with the post-menopausal years

E. Cope

Introduction

The title of my paper poses the question 'Do women age in a manner different from men and if so is this desirable and if not can we safely improve matters with the medicaments that are at present available?'

I have always drunk to the toast *vive la difference* and it seems logical that we should, if possible, *préserve la difference*. I think it is interesting that in the Oxford French Dictionary the verb *préserver* is illustrated by the phrase *Dieu vous préserve de ce malheur*, or God preserve you from this misfortune and now that He has given it to women to live so much longer, has He also provided the wherewithal to protect them from the misfortunes of the menopause, the physical changes of which range from loss of libido to the Dowager's hump?

There are those who regard libido as psychogenic but most consider that there is a large physical element and some who regard this as the very stuff of life. Byron in Don Juan says that 'her climacteric teased her like her teens' and I have seen many women with atrophic vaginitis whose libido has become so excessive presumably from clitoral irritation that life is one long frustration and yet intercourse has not been possible due to contraction and dyspareunia and yet both these symptoms have been resolved to the mutual satisfaction of husband and wife with simple hormone therapy.

Cessation of periods and loss of fertility

Two of the most important physical changes are the cessation of periods and the loss of fertility.

There is not much written history about the menopause but in the Talmud, which is the Hebraic equivalent of our common law, it states that if a woman misses three periods she is old but that if her periods restart she is young.

In Genesis it is recorded that Sarah conceived at an advanced age 'when it had ceased to be with her in the manner of women' and furthermore she is said to have been irritable, cantankerous and to have nagged old Abraham—symptoms commonly ascribed to the menopause so that when God announced the forthcoming birth of Isaac, Abraham fell upon his face and laughed and said 'Shall Sarah, that is 90 years old, bear?' In fairness to Sarah, she had recently been sufficiently attractive to be taken by Abimelech, King of Gerar, who obviously knew a mature women when he saw one. Furthermore, 10 years after the return from Egypt when she was still barren and seemingly old, Sarah instructed Abraham to go unto Hagar, her maidservant, and said that 'It may be that I may obtain children by her'. Abraham went unto Hagar and she bore Ishmael. Sarah adopted Ishmael and promptly conceived.

This illustrates the difficulty in defining the menopause.

Woman is the only creature who ceases to ovulate at a relatively young age though some laboratory animals go into permanent estrous in captivity.

It is true that fertility in animals diminishes with age but many an elderly mare has produced a foal that has fetched a high price in the ring.

The word 'menopause' was first used in 1872 and means simply the cessation of periods. The word 'climacteric' is Greek for the rung of a ladder and has been used for centuries to denote high points in the life-span, the significant ages being the odd multiples of 7 and 9. Of these the multiple of 7 by 7 is the most important and is the one with which we are concerned. Its use has been debased to cover approximately a 5-year span during which the overt symptoms of the change of life become manifest.

The reason for ovarian failure is not clearly understood but it is reasonable to suppose that the ovary simply runs out of eggs and the rate of run down is shown in Table 4.1. This run down does not appear to be related either to the age of the menarche or to parity and during the last four years fertility is rapidly reduced (Figure 4.1) and anovulatory cycles become increasingly common.

It is not possible to predict the exact menopause for any particular woman nor to assure a woman whose periods have ceased for some months that she is infertile without doing serial levels of luteinizing hormone (LH) and

Table 4.1 Effect of maternal age on number of oocytes

Age (yr)	*No. of cases*	*No. of oocytes*
Birth	7	733 000
4–10	5	499 200
11–17	5	389 300
18–24	7	161 800
25–31	11	62 500
32–38	8	80 200
39–45	7	10 900

From Block, E. (1952). *Acta Anat.*, **14**, 108

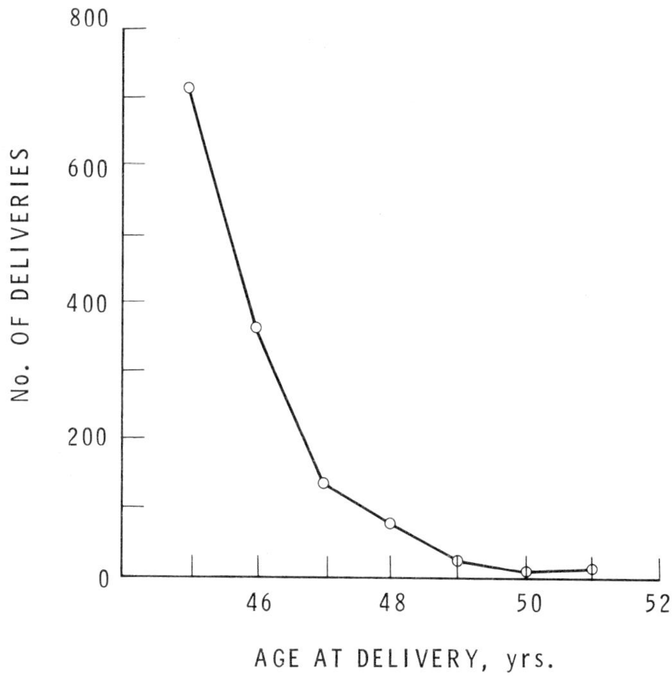

Figure 4.1 Deliveries in women aged more than 44 years—England and Wales, 1967

preferably also follicle stimulating (FSH) as these hormones are released in a pulsatile manner. One particular source of error would be a single reading at the time of luteinizing surge before ovulation which could be misinterpreted as a menopausal level for this gonadotrophin.

The oldest documented birth is reported in the Guinness Book of Records[1] as a daughter born on 18th October, 1956 to Ruth Alice Kistler at the age of 57 years 129 days, therefore care must be taken when advising a woman as to when it would be safe to stop the contraceptive pill or other form of birth controls.

The male menopause

Some form of male menopause occurs in some men though androgen excretion in diminishing quantities continues until death. Fertility and orgasm continue for most men until an advanced age and male impotence occurs in only 25% of Americans at the age of 70. (Figure 4.2). Orgasm at that age continues to occur at fortnightly intervals or half an orgasm a week! (Figure 4.3). Women at that age are not fertile but it would be quite wrong to assume that they are impotent particularly if they are taking estrogen replacement therapy. Therefore it would be unwise for a gynaecologist not to fashion a functional vagina in the repair of a prolapse in a woman over 70 whether married or otherwise.

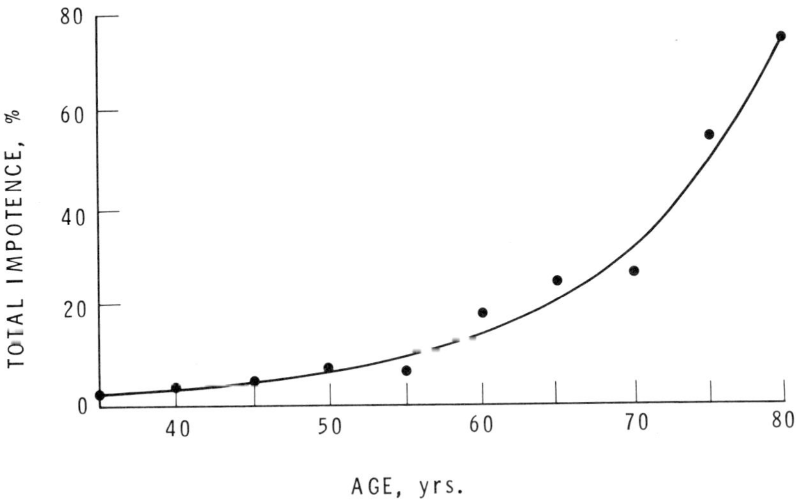

Figure 4.2 Accumulating frequency of impotence in relation to age (redrawn from Kinsey, Pomeroy and Martin, 1948)[15]

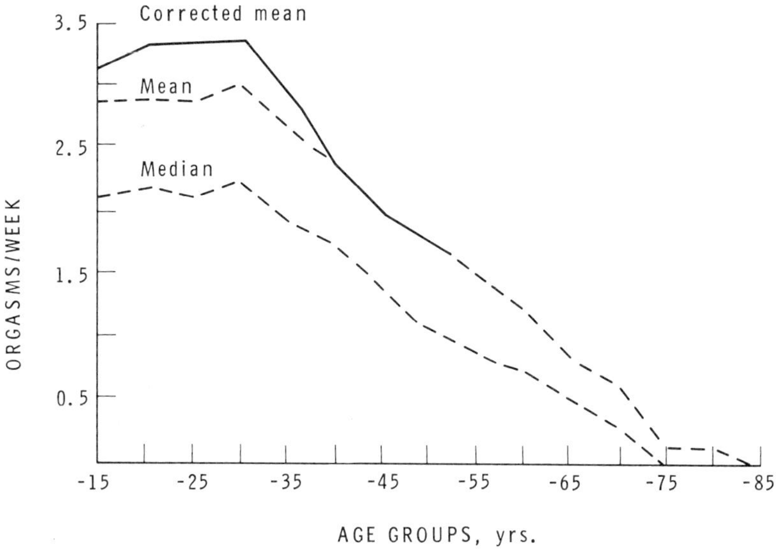

Figure 4.3 Total frequency of orgasm in relation to age in men (redrawn from Kinsey, Pomeroy and Martin, 1948)[15]

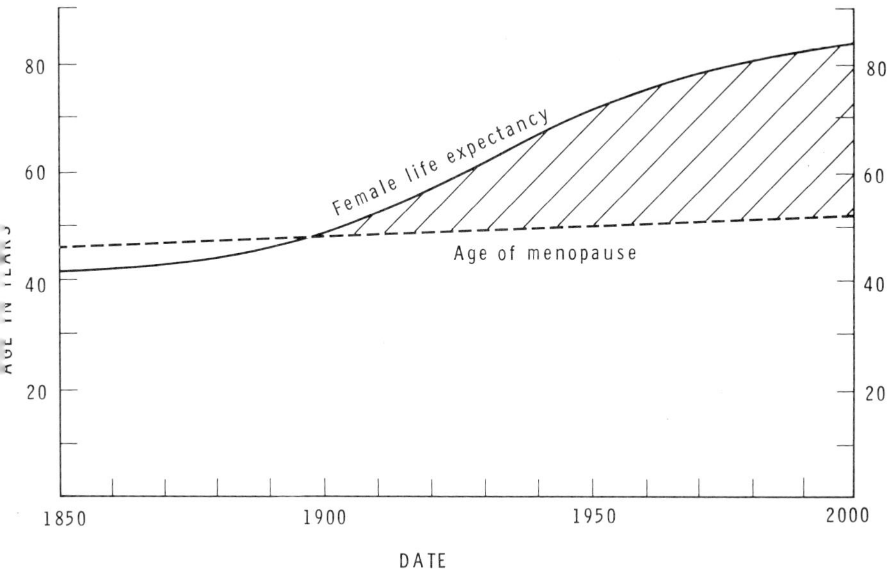

Figure 4.4 Female life expectancy

The menopause did not provide a major social problem until recent times as it was only in this century that the average life-span of women reached 45 years, (Figure 4.4), and the widower merely sought a younger bride or, if his wife survived, sought solace elsewhere as necessary.

For those women who did survive, Richardson[2] in his book *The Menopause—A Neglected Crisis* writes 'The menopause was a negative event of no importance in the life of the community. So, when a woman's usefulness was seen to be ended, she ceased to be a woman'. Shakespeare summed it up as follows: 'A man loves the meat in his youth that he cannot endure in his age'.

Disorders related to estrogen deficiency

Joint and muscle pains

In addition to the list of possible disorders (Table 4.2) should be added joint and muscle pains. This is a common and troublesome feature of the menopause that has received little investigation. These pains probably reflect a reduction in muscular strength with probably a reduced ability to disperse the build up in muscle of lactic acid after exercise, with an associated laxity of the ligamentous structures that bind the skeleton. These pains are not likely to be associated with osteoporosis as the response to estrogen is often dramatic occurring within two weeks, long before there can be any significant change in bone absorption and unlikely also to be related to the altered levels of plasma calcium that are a feature of the change in mineral metabolism.

Table 4.2 Disorders related to estrogen deficiency

Definite	Hot Flushes Atrophic Vaginitis
Possible	Hypertension Coronary Heart Disease Raised Serum Lipids Osteoporosis Urethral Syndrome Skin, Hair and Breast Changes Psychiatric Problems Psychosexual Problems

Vasomotor symptoms

Doisy and others[3] in 1930 finally prepared crystalline ovarian hormone from the urine of pregnant women and three main estrogens have been shown to be active in the human, the most important being estradiol-17β. Estrone which is inactive, can be converted mainly in the liver to estradiol-17β. This is important as the ovaries of many post-menopausal women continue to produce estrone in high quantity though in others the level is low. This can easily be demonstrated by taking samples from the ovarian veins at the time of operation.

It is a reasonable hypothesis that menopausal women with a high or low steady state of estrone are free of flushes and therefore if long term hormone replacement therapy is to be recommended for all women the estrogen levels should be assayed in those who are free of vasomotor symptoms.

The precise mechanism of these symptoms is not known but it is of interest that women who have marked pre-menstrual changes commonly in

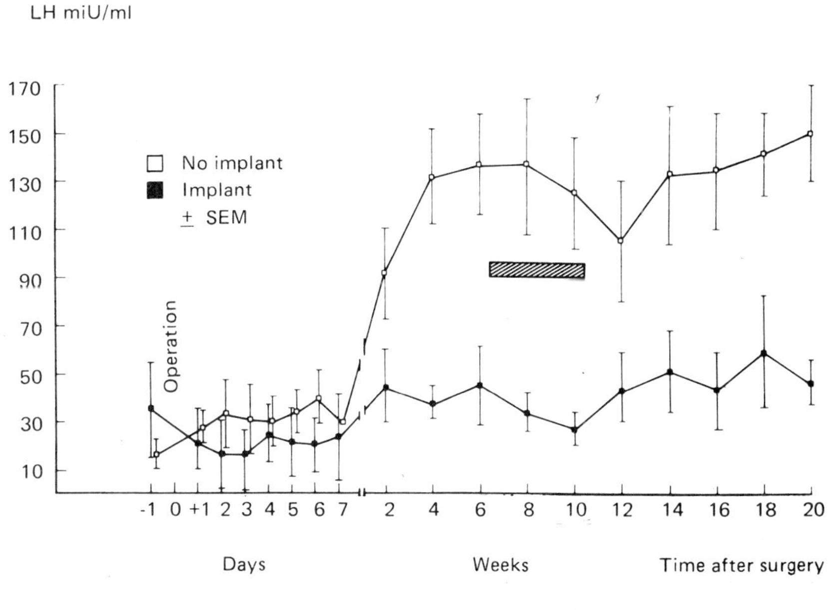

Figure 4.5 Plasma LH values after hysterectomy and removal of ovaries with estradiol implant compared with those without implant[4]

later life suffer the most from flushes and night sweats and there would appear to be a very delicately balanced relationship between feedback from the ovaries and the activity of the hypothalamus and pituitary in this group of women. It also seems probable that this element of their autonomic nervous system is particularly labile. However, there is no direct relationship established between vasomotor symptoms and gonadotrophin levels. In castrated women the rise in gonadotrophins is quite sudden (Figures 4.5 and 4.6), but can be controlled by an implant of estradiol benzoate 100 mg and these patients are free of vasomotor symptoms. (Figure 4.7)[5]. The absorption from these pellets produces a relatively steady level of estrogen. In the natural menopause many women show a marked fluctuation of estrogen production and it would appear that this fluctuation is important in the production of vasomotor symptoms. It is interesting that in phaeochromocytoma flushes occur in association with fluctuating levels of adrenalin, histamine and bradykinin and it is reasonable to postulate that the fluctuating

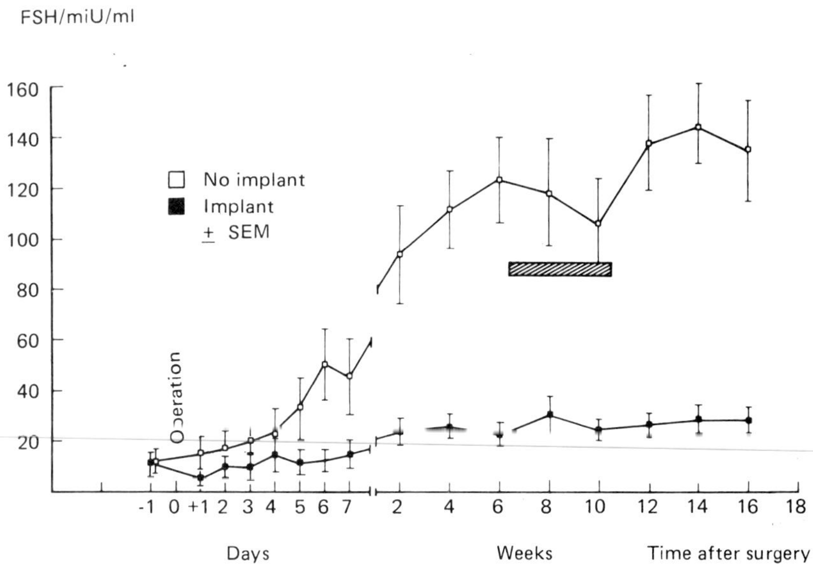

Figure 4.6 Plasma FSH values after hysterectomy and removal of ovaries with estradiol implant compared with those without[4].

estrogen of the menopausal woman with vasomotor symptoms is associated with fluctuations of one or more of these substances.

In treatment, therefore, it is important to maintain a sufficient and steady level of estrogen. Fortunately this is possible by giving a single daily oral dose as the estrogen receptors in tissue cells bind the estrogen very powerfully and release is slow and steady. The precise dose will obviously vary from one patient to another.

Atrophic vaginitis and the urethral syndrome

These conditions should be considered together as the vulva, lower part of the vagina, urethra and trigone are embryologically similar and respond in the same manner both to estrogen deprivation and replacement. The discomforts, disability and management of atrophic vaginitis are well known. Unfortunately less has been said about the effect of estrogen deprivation on

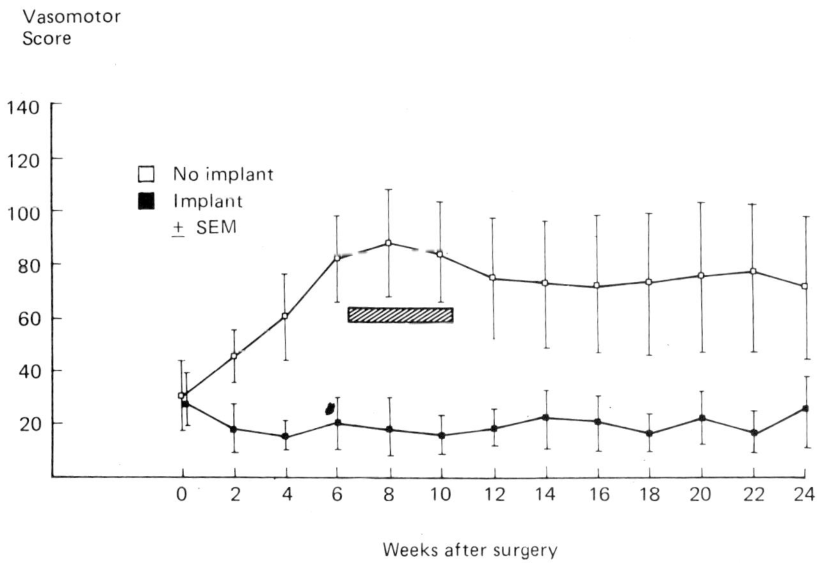

Figure 4.7 Vasomotor scores after hysterectomy and removal of ovaries with estradiol implant compared with those without[5]

the bladder and urethral mucosa. The symptom of urge incontinence, though quite characteristic, is nevertheless confused far too often with stress incontinence which results in unnecessary and unsuccessful operations that may even aggravate the condition.

There are numerous aetiologies of urge incontinence one of which is estrogen deprivation. We have cystoscoped many of these patients before and after estrogen therapy and have seen trigonitis disappear along with the patient's complaint. It would be wrong to over simplify this complex condition but equally wrong to forget one very useful remedy.

Cardiovascular system

The relationship between cardiovascular disease and the menopause is still somewhat tenuous. Nevertheless some significance must be attached to the fact that in non-smoking women before the menopause, coronary heart disease is extremely rare whereas after the menopause the incidence approaches that of men. The American workers Parrish *et al.*[6] have demonstrated that in women castrated before the age of 40 and in women who have had a premature menopause, coronary heart disease increased though serious atherosclerosis does not appear for about 14 years. Furthermore there is an association between plasma cholesterol concentration and estrogen secretion. Plasma cholesterol is lowest at mid-cycle when estrogen secretion is maximal and following bilateral oophorectomy or in the post-menopause the levels of cholesterol, lipoproteins and triglycerides rise. Estrogen administered to these patients markedly reduces the level of cholesterol but does not appear to affect the triglycerides. There is a great deal of scope here for long term prospective studies in menopausal clinics. This should be done in conjunction with studies of the clotting mechanisms in relation to hormone replacement therapy in order to compare the apparent protection against atherosclerosis with the possible risk of thromboembolism, low though this is likely to be with the natural estrogens.

Skin and connective tissues

In addition to the genital tract estrogens affect other target tissues which at puberty include the breasts, body form, skin, subcutaneous tissues, pubic and axillary hair. At the menopause deprivation causes a negative nitrogen balance with diminution of muscle which is replaced by fibrous tissue. The epidermis becomes thin and sub-cutaneous fat atrophies with loss of elasticity. This particularly affects the breasts which atrophy and lose their shape. The importance of this can be seen in the demand for plastic surgery and the enormous sale of specially contoured brassières.

Psychiatric problems

I include this under physical changes because it is increasingly apparent that endogenous depression and possibly other psychiatric ailments have a physical background. This can be seen in the response of depression to a variety of drugs. There also seems to be little doubt that in post-menopausal women estrogen increases the level of free tryptophan and in our own work, as yet unpublished, estrogen replacement therapy has a beneficial effect in a significant number of patients though it would be wrong to infer that it can be used in place of accepted methods of treatment but rather as a useful adjunct.

Osteoporosis

Albright[7] and his co-workers in 1941 showed the relationship between the menopause and osteoporosis in a series of crush fractures of the vertebrae and ever since then the mineral metabolists have blown as hot and cold as their patients about estrogen and osteoporosis. This is due to a number of factors of which two are outstanding.

The first has been the pedantic necessity to equate the estrogen effects exactly with the changes in calcium phosphorous homeostasis.

Now that it is generally accepted that the changes in the third metacarpal correlate well with the rest of the skeleton and can be used as an index of bone resorption and absorption and now that we also have specialized tools like radioimmunoassay, auto-analysis, photon absorptiometry, atomic absorption spectrophotometry, it has become possible to do prospective studies. Those of Aitken *et al.*[9] and Gallagher *et al.*[10] (Figure 4.8) indicate that bone resorption is related to estrogen deficiency in castrated women. By plotting the cortical area of a cross section of long bone against the total area of the cross section, Gallagher *et al.* have shown that the cortical area to total area ratio falls progressively from the age of 50 in women whereas comparable data in men show that the bone loss is less and starts at least 10 years later. The effect of this is shown quite dramatically in Figure 4.9 which demonstrates the high incidence of fractures in women compared with men. It will be seen in this diagram that by the age of 70 fractures are five times as common in women as they are in men in Malmo, Oxford and Dundee[11, 12].

In their prospective study, Gallagher *et al.*[10] (Figure 4.8) showed a significant rise in fasting plasma and urine calcium after removal of the ovaries without any corresponding change after simple hysterectomy. There was also a rise in urinary hydroxyproline which verifies the likelihood that the rise in fasting plasma and urine calcium was due to an increase in bone

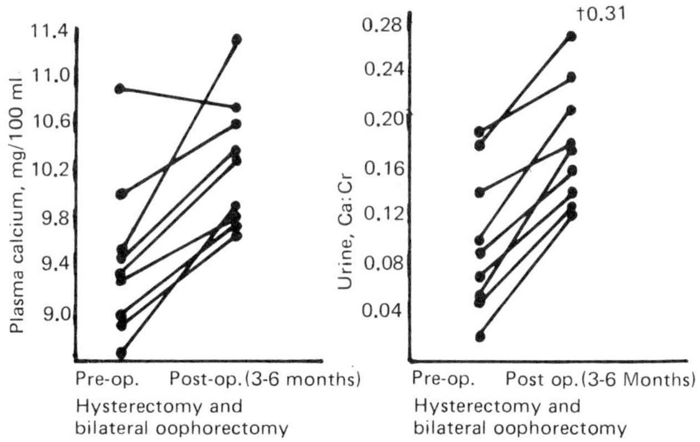

Figure 4.8 Effect of oophorectomy on plasma and urine calcium[10]

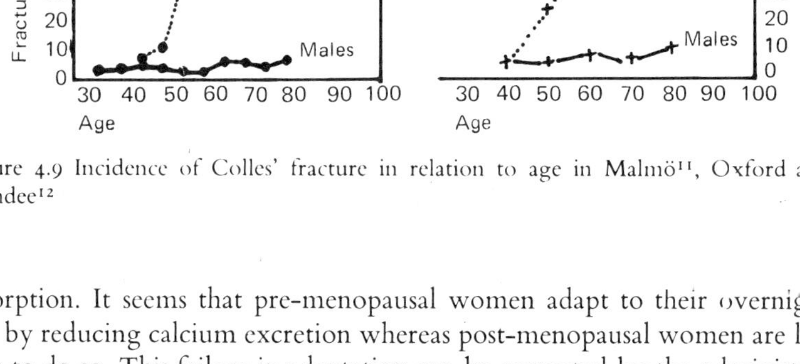

Figure 4.9 Incidence of Colles' fracture in relation to age in Malmö[11], Oxford and Dundee[12]

resorption. It seems that pre-menopausal women adapt to their overnight fast by reducing calcium excretion whereas post-menopausal women are less able to do so. This failure in adaptation can be corrected by the administration of ethinyl estradiol 0·05 mg daily to the post-menopausal women. The same workers have resolved the problem of the imprecise relationship between the biochemical changes and osteotrophic response by their ingenious hypothesis that estrogen reduces the sensitivity of bone to parathyroid hormone, a hypothesis which has withstood their rigorous testing and should be accepted until it can be disproved.

The second act of faith that is required is to accept the work of Cannigia and his co-workers[8] on the intestinal absorption of calcium after treatment with oral estrogen-gestogen. It is difficult to separate the two factors of bone resorption due to estrogen deprivation and the failure of gut absorption of calcium.. If we accept the work of Cannigia in which the presentation of estrogen improved absorption of calcium we do not at the same time have to disprove the theory that estrogen protects bone against parathyroid hormone. In fact, the two can be shown to be quite consistent one with the other.

If calcium is, in fact, lost at the rate of approximately 1% per year after the menopause[14] and the preservation of bone structure in the post-menopausal woman is as estrogen-dependant as we have suggested then this is one of the most potent arguments in favour of long term hormone replacement therapy.

Conclusion

In 1850 Monsieur Colombat De L'Isère gave the following advice in his Hygiene Rules Relative to the Change of Life:

> 'Compelled to yield to the power of time, women now cease to exist as the species, and henceforward live only for themselves. Their features are stamped with the impress of age, and their genital organs are sealed with the signet of sterility. The first advice they ought to receive is to reject all sorts of drugs and receipts that are loudly proclaimed by ignorance and puffed by charlatanism. They ought not to sleep upon feather beds, nor in any bed that is too soft and too warm, for such are attended with the disadvantage of exciting the generative organs, which should henceforth, be left, as far as possible, in a state of inaction.
>
> It is the dictate of prudence to avoid all such circumstances as might awaken any erotic thoughts in the mind, such as the spectacle of lascivious figures and the reading of passionate novels.'[13]

Monsieur Colombat De L'Isère led contemporary thought in France at a time when fashion resided in Paris. Ideas have modified only slowly since then and many consider that hormone replacement therapy for menopausal women is either dangerous or more than we can at present afford. It should be pointed out that we are living in a youth-orientated sex-drenched society which gives free contraception and encourages the social mores described in Tennessee Williams' *Cat on a Hot Tin Roof* and yet has too little sympathy for the post-menopausal woman with aching joints, Colles' fractures, femoral pins and stenosed burning vaginae.

Would it not be better in the Autumn of their lives to give these women some prospect of an Indian Summer of happiness rather than a Winter of discontent?

References

1. *The Guinness Book of Records.* (1974). Ed. N. D. McWhirter and R. A. McWhirter, (London: Guinness Superlatives Ltd.)
2. Richardson, R. G. (1973). *The Menopause—a Neglected Crisis.* (Queensborough: Abbott Laboratories)
3. Doisy, E. A., Veler, C. D. and Thayer, S. A. (1930). The preparation of the crystalline ovarian hormone from the urine of pregnant women. *J. Biol. Chem.*, **86,** 499
4. Hunter, D. J. S., Nuffield Department of Obs. and Gynae., John Radcliffe Hospital, Oxford. Personal Communication
5. *Ibid.*
6. Parrish, H. M., Carr, C. A., Hall, D. G. and King, T. M. (1967). Time interval from castration in premenopausal women to development of excessive coronary atherosclerosis. *Amer. J. Obstet. Gynec.*, **99,** 155
7. Albright, F., Smith, P. H., and Richardson, A. M. (1941). Post-menopausal osteoporosis—its clinical features. *J. Amer. Med. Ass.*, **116,** 2465
8. Caniggia, A., Gennari, C., Borrello, G., Bencini, M., Cesari, L., Poggi, C. and Escobar, S. (1970). Intestinal absorption of Ca-47 after treatment with oral oestrogen-gestogens in senile osteoporosis. *Brit. Med. J.*, **4,** 30
9. Aitken, J. M., Hart, D. M. and Lindsay, R. (1973). Oetrogen replacement therapy for prevention of osteoporosis after oophorectomy. *Brit. Med. J.*, **3,** 515
10. Gallagher, J. C. and Nordin, B. E. C. (1973). Oestrogens and calcium metabolism. Ageing and estrogens. *Frontiers Hormone Res.*, Vol 2, pp 98–117. (Basel: Karger)
11. Alffram, P. A. (1964). An epidemologic study of cervical and trochanteric fractures of the femur in an urban population. *Acta Orthop. Scand. Suppl.* 65
12. Knowelden, J., Buhr, A. J. and Dunbar, O. (1964). Incidence of fractures in persons over 35 years of age. *Brit. J. Prev. Soc. Med.*, **18,** 130
13. Ricci, J. V. (1945). *100 Years of Gynecology.* (Philadelphia: Blakeston Company), p. 532
14. Nordin, B. E. C., Horsman, A., Aaron, J. and Gallagher, J. C. (1975). Post-menopausal bone loss. *Curr. Med. Res. Obin.*, **3,** Suppl 3, 28
15. Kinsey, A. C., Pomeroy, W. B. and Martin, C. E. (1948). *Sexual Behaviour in the Human Male.* (Philadelphia and London: W. & B. Saunders)

Discussion on Section A:

Epidemiology

Chairman: *Professor N. F. Morris*

Mr E. S. Saunders (Gynaecologist, London): For the last 35 years, I have done special research on the menopause and the climacteric, and have propagated the use of hormone replacement therapy. However, 35 years ago I was speaking to stone, and no one listened. It is the height of my satisfaction to be present today at the Symposium, and the organizers are to be congratulated in arranging it, and in proving that the profession, particularly in this country, now realizes the importance of this phase of a woman's life. The suffering of women in this age group has been neglected for much too long, and has not really been taken seriously.

The standard of this symposium proves how the profession has awakened. Over the past 5 to 10 years remarkable changes have taken place, as is proved by the various papers published in different countries, and by different congresses. One further point. The gerontologists have realized that the menopause, or the climacteric, is an important geriatric phase, and now consider hormonal treatment as a geriatric tool.

Mr R. J. Beard (Gynaecologist, Brighton): Is there any connection between the severity of short-term symptoms, and the severity of long-term estrogen deficiency symptoms, such as osteoporosis?

Mr E. Cope (Gynaecologist, Oxford): I take it that the questioner is asking whether the woman who has very severe flushes is more likely to develop osteoporosis. I do not know the answer to that, and it is likely to take us another 15 years to find it out.

Dr N. G. Mussalli (Gynaecologist, Welwyn Garden City): Could Dr Jaszmann say something about the effect of nutritional factors on the menopause. I know that the menopause in animals is largely due to nutritional deficiency, and occurs when the teeth fall out.

Dr L. J. B. Jaszmann (Gynaecologist, Netherlands): Not only nutritional factors, but other factors, in all Western countries, influence the middle age of a woman.

A hundred years ago the menopause was at about 40 years of age, and in recent decades it has been as late as 51. Nutrition, and other factors must have an influence on the menopausal age in Western countries.

Professor C. J. Dewhurst (Gynaecologist, London): If that is so, then there is a curious contrast in that the same nutritional factors lower the age of the menarche and raise the age of the menopause. It seems odd that that should happen, and I do not quite see how it does, but it would appear to be so.

Mr C. A. R. Lamont (Gynaecologist, Portsmouth): What exactly is the mechanism of vaso-motor instability on estrogen withdrawal?

Professor C. J. Dewhurst: To be truthful, I do not know that it has been clarified. It is possibly related to the raised FSH and LH levels, and certainly a reduction in these is associated with a relief of the symptoms. But, it must be more complicated than that. It is not some very simple cause-and-effect relationship so far as FSH and LH are concerned. I believe Mr Campbell will be discussing some hormonal parameters in relation to hot flushes later.

Mr E. Cope: Women well past and well before the menopause appear not to be troubled with flushes. The symptoms appear to exist in a mid-band of estrogen level. If patients are given estrogen therapy, they must be taken above that band if their flushes are to be cured, or else they must be left below the band. Fluctuating estrogen levels within that band appear to be associated with flushes. How that directly affects adrenaline, histamine, and other substances which influence the autonomic nervous system has not as yet been worked out.

Dr M. L. Snaith (Rheumatologist, London): I am particularly interested in musculo skeletal symptoms, arthritis and arthralgia associated with the menopause. It is one of the areas where an interdisciplinary approach to a problem is needed. I would be particularly interested to hear whether any of the members of the panel have applied themselves to the type, nature, and response to treatment, of the rheumatic symptoms associated with the menopause.

Mr E. Cope: We have no results at all as yet, and it will take quite a long time, but we are looking into it.

Ms Wendy Cooper (Author and Journalist, Birmingham): Mine is not a scientific comment, but an impression based on letters that I get and cases that I have come across in the course of four years of research. Sometimes a certain type of menopausal arthritis appears to improve with HRT. Currently there is a case in the Westminster Hospital of a woman with a degenerative neck who is in appalling pain if she does not take estrogen; she has just had a mastectomy, and there was a problem of whether to put her back on the estrogen replacement, or whether to keep her off it. The doctors have finally decided to put her back on estrogen replacement, and the painful neck condition is once more under control.

Professor N. F. Norris (Chairman): I take it that the questioner is distinguishing between rheumatoid arthritis and osteoarthritis. So far as rheumatoid arthritis is concerned, we really do not know.

Professor C. J. Dewhurst: May I add further comment, which arises directly from what Wendy Cooper has just said. I suppose that this is what we shall try to get at over the next few days. There has been a great deal of impression in this field—

so many patients *seem* to do better. However, there has been a minimum of very careful, controlled trials in which hormones have been compared with something else, a placebo of some sort. I do not believe that anybody knows the answer to this question, because I do not believe that this particular comparison has been properly made.

Professor N. F. Norris: That is a very important statement.

Mr S. Campbell (Gynaecologist, London): We have some information on joint pains in a placebo trial, which will be presented during the afternoon's session.

Mr J. McQueen (Gynaecologist, London): Have epidemiological investigations shown any relation between taking oral contraceptives and the age of the menopause? The theory that the menopause occurs when the ovary exhausts itself of ova would suggest that if ova are saved up by preventing ovulation, the menopause might perhaps be delayed.

Professor C. J. Dewhurst: I would have difficulty in answering the question in a factual manner, but I believe that no such relationship has been shown. There is no significant delay in menopausal age in women who are on the pill. This is easy to understand if one accepts that it is not essential to have ovulation to waste a vast number of eggs in an ovary. Far more wastage of eggs takes place before puberty than ever happens after puberty. At birth a woman can have 2 million eggs in her ovary, and perhaps a quarter of a million at puberty, so a large number have disappeared by the process of low-grade FSH–LH stimulation. I think that this sort of stimulation, short of ovulation, continues even in patients who are on the pill.

Anonymous (written question): Why are hot flushes generally confined to the face and upper half of the body?

Mrs Wendy Cooper: I do not think that that is the case. Judging from the experiences of many women whom I meet, and talk to, and their letters, I gather that this can be a great wave of heat over the whole body, and certainly with night sweats the whole body is bathed in perspiration. Perhaps the gynaecologists could confirm that.

Professor C. J. Dewhurst: I would agree. I do not think that they are limited to the upper part of the body. They may be, but equally they may not. They may be over the whole of the body surface.

Mr E. Cope: Different women flush differently. Perspiration affects the whole body. Blushing affects the neck, chest and face more than the trunk, and it affects the hands also, but that is to be expected. Those areas of the skin are rather more delicately under the control of the autonomic nervous system.

Professor N. F. Morris: We have had a very good morning, which has emphasized how much more we require to find out. To conclude the session, may I take one trite, and perhaps rather obvious comment.

When we are 25, the idea of people having intercourse over the age of 50 strikes us as being mildly indecent and unpleasant. But in general, if practitioners are honest, we have given far too little consideration to the idea of maintaining sexual intercourse in our patients as a therapeutic exercise, as, to some extent, a prevention against various disorders, psychological and otherwise. Part of the discussion has emphasized that we can do more in maintaining this part of their lives, to probably very good effect.

Section B

ENDOCRINOLOGY

Part I

Chairman: R. W. BEARD

5

Endocrine changes associated with the menopause and post-menopausal years

I. D. Cooke

The basic feature of the menopause is that the primordial follicle and its derivatives, the granulosa cells and the surrounding theca cells degenerate or fail to react to endogenous gonadotrophins. The granulosa cells in the pre-menopausal ovary are capable of producing estrogens from acetate (Figure 5.1) the most rudimentary steroid precursor, but tend to accumulate progesterone and 17α hydroxyprogesterone. The theca cells tend to produce the androgens, dehydroepiandrosterone, and particularly testosterone and androstenedione from progesterone, and continue the biosynthetic pathway to estradiol and estrone. Both granulosa and theca cells working synergistically produce steroids maximally. The stromal cells produce the androgens androstenedione, testosterone and dehydroepiandrosterone in the normal pre-menopausal ovary and this process continues in the post-menopausal ovary.

Ovarian vein blood obtained from an ovary with a pre-ovulatory follicle contains all the steroids seen in the biosynthetic pathway showing that different 'compartments' contribute to ovarian steroid secretion (Table 5.1). It is worth noting that much more estradiol than estrone is secreted, and that substantial amounts of androstenedione and testosterone may be found. The androstenedione levels fluctuate during the menstrual cycle and a pre-ovulatory rise of some days' duration occurs, as may have been anticipated since McDonald *et al.*[1] showed it to be the principal precursor of estrone in the pre-menopausal woman.

As pituitary gonadotrophins are primarily controlled by feedback of ovarian steroids to the hypothalamus, failing ovarian steroid production

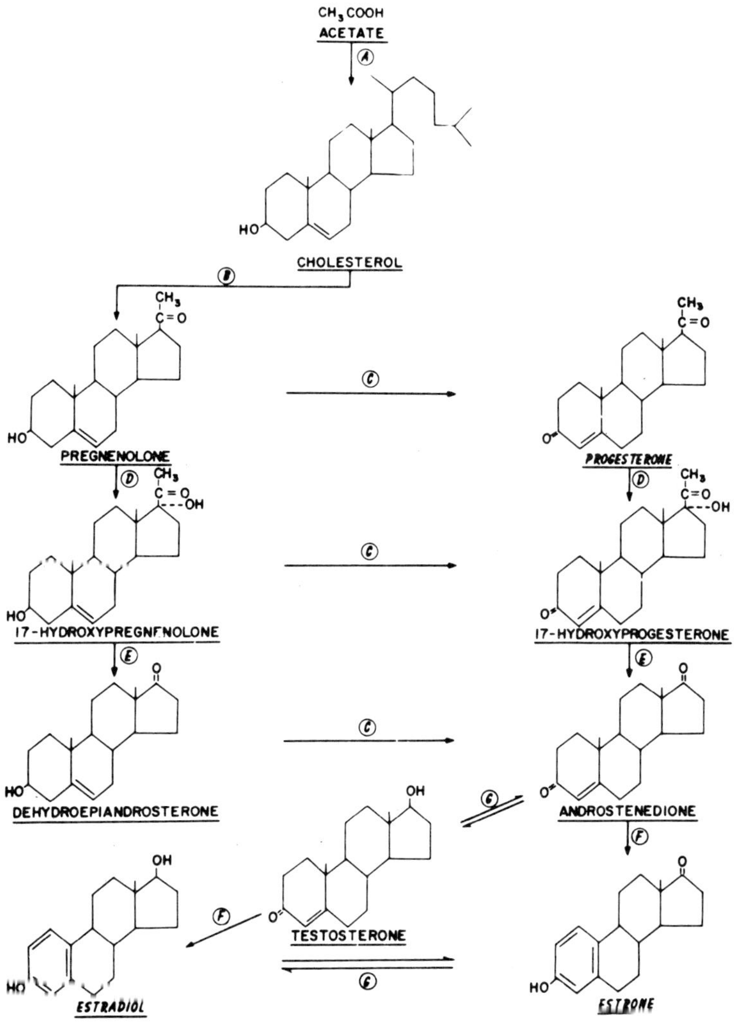

Figure 5.1 Steroid pathway for estrogen synthesis from acetate (with permission from Smith, O. W. and Ryan, K. J. (1962). *Am. J. Obstet. Gynecol.*, **84**, 141)

results in excessive hypothalamo-pituitary responses as shown by the urinary excretion studies of Adamopoulos *et al.*[2] The low urinary estrogen excretion is noteworthy, particularly the lower estradiol, relatively higher estrone and

Table 5.1 Plasma steroids in a 34-year old patient, gravida 3, para 3, dated 12 days post-menstrual

		Ovarian plasma	
Steroid	*Peripheral plasma* (μg/100 ml)	*Right* (μg/100 ml)	*Left** (μg/100 ml)
Progesterone	0·149	0·393	1·550
17α-Hydroxyprogesterone	< 2·000	< 2·000	4·437
20α-Hydroxy-4-pregnene-3-one	0·276	0·040	0·108
20β-Hydroxy-4-pregnene-3-one	0·011	0·015	0·024
Androstenedione	0·683	8·520	8·852
Testosterone	0·083	0·190	0·242
Dehydroepiandrosterone	1·861	3·956	4·236
Estrone	0·038	0·071	0·172
Estradiol	0·125	0·359	1·760

* Ovary containing the ripe follicle.
(With permission from Mikhail, G. *Clin. Obstet. Gynecol.*, **10**, 29, 1967)

the peripheral metabolite estriol in the pre-menopausal patient (Figure 5.2). The 24-hour excretion of FSH and of LH may fluctuate enormously, and this has obvious clinical implications in attempting to make a diagnosis; clearly a number of specimens on separate occasions are necessary.

Blood production rates of estrone and estradiol[3] are shown in Figure 5.3, together with their precursors, and the relative production rates of the two estrogens in the post-menopausal and cycling woman are apparent. It emphasizes again the change in product from estradiol to estrone at the menopause. However plasma estrone levels may not even be the best index of post-menopausal estrogen levels, as estrone sulphate with its very much longer half life my have greater biological significance, particularly as it can be derived from precursor androstenedione[4].

Judd *et al.*[5] have assayed testosterone and androstenedione levels in ovarian and peripheral vein plasma in post-menopausal women, and noted a 15-fold and 4-fold excess respectively in ovarian over peripheral vein levels, demonstrating that the post-menopausal ovary contributes significantly to peripheral androgen levels (Figure 5.4). On the other hand estradiol and estrone concentrations are barely 2-fold greater in the ovarian vein than in a peripheral vein, indicating that the post-menopausal ovary contributes very little to estrone and estradiol levels in the peripheral circulation and hence as excretory products. The effects of oophorectomy on peripheral

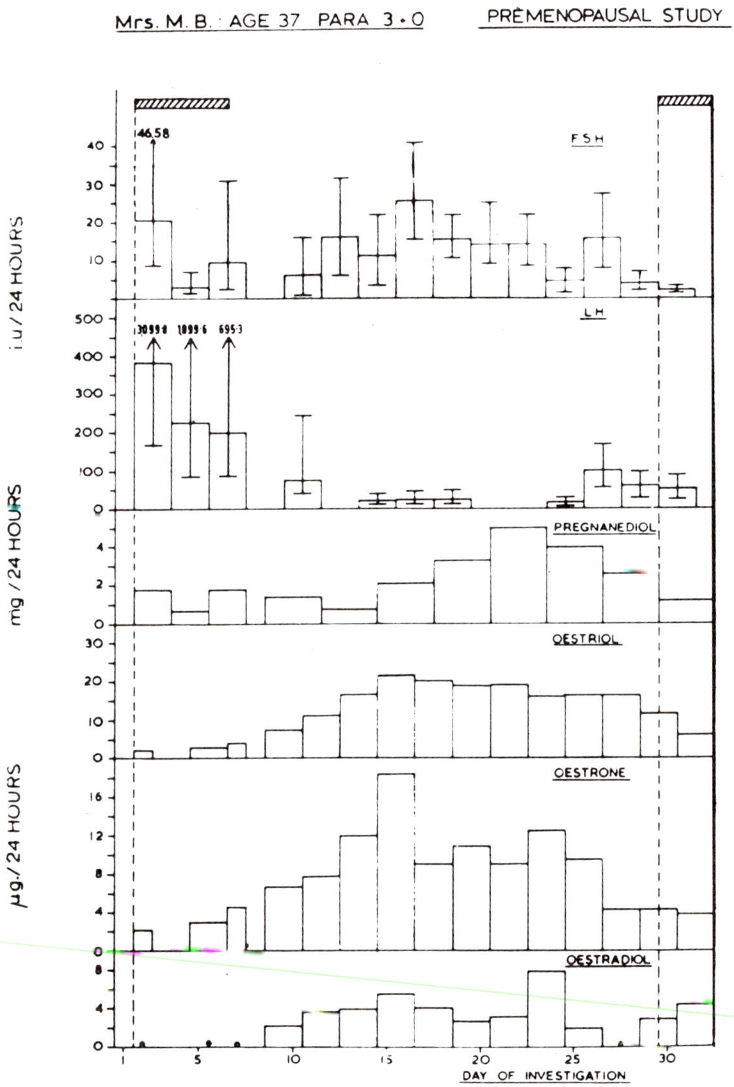

Figure 5.2 Hormone excretion in a pre-menopausal subject (± 2 SD) (with permission from Adamopoulos, D. A., Loraine, J. A. and Dove, G. A. (1971). *J. Obstet. Gynaecol. Br. Commonlth.*, **78**, 62)

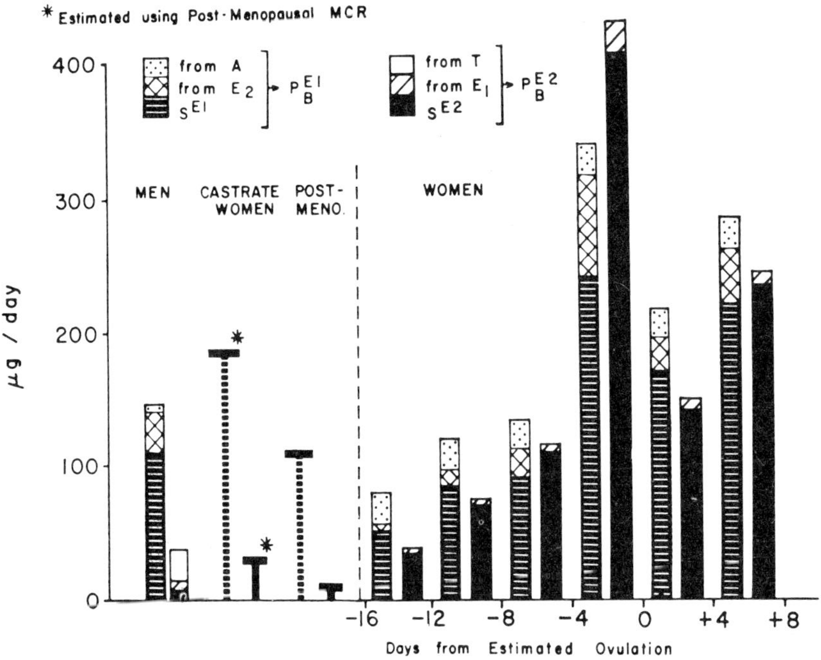

Figure 5.3 Blood production rates (P_B) for estrone (E_1) and estradiol (E_2). On the left of the dotted line is the blood production rate in post-menopausal women and the capped lines show production rates only, no secretion rates or precursor contributions are shown. On the right of the dotted line are the blood production rates in normal women calculated from plasma concentrations obtained throughout the cycle and from metabolic clearance rates measured in the follicular and luteal phases. The peak of plasma LH is taken as day 0, negative numbers refer to follicular phase, positive to luteal. The height of each bar represents P_B with the subdivisions showing secretion rates (S) and contributions from precursors according to the legends (with permission from Baird, D. T. Horton, R., Longcope, C. and Tait, J. F. (1969). *Rec. Progr. Horm. Res.*, **25**, 611)

levels of testosterone and androstenedione were demonstrated by Judd *et al.*[6] in patients with endometrial carcinoma, some before, and some after the menopause (Figure 5.5). They showed that testosterone and androstenedione levels fell to about half in pre-menopausal patients after oophorectomy, although androstenedione levels were of course much higher; this fall must represent the ovarian contribution. The ovarian contribution to androstenedione levels in the post-menopausal patient is much less, and as about 50% of testosterone is converted to androstenedione this fall in androstenedione alone would account for most of the reduction in testosterone. The metabolic

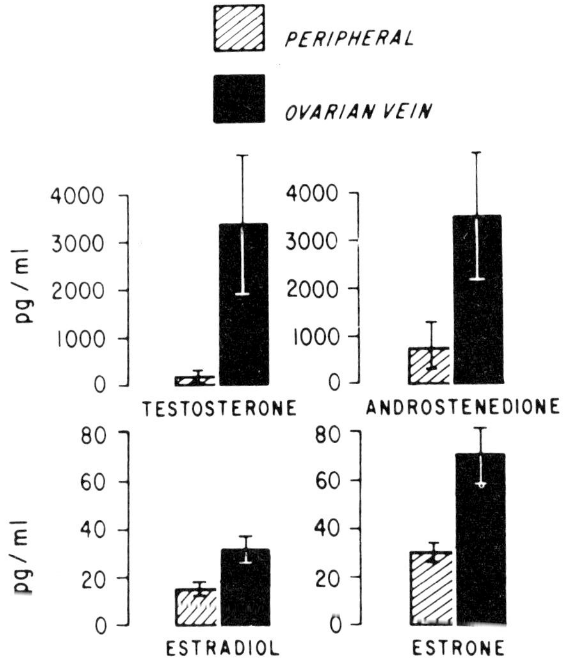

Figure 5.4 Peripheral and ovarian vein plasma concentrations of testosterone and androstenedione in post-menopausal women (with permission from Judd, H. L., Judd, G. E., Lucas, W. E. and Yen, S. S. C. (1974). *J. Clin. Endocrinol. Metab.*, **39**, 1020).

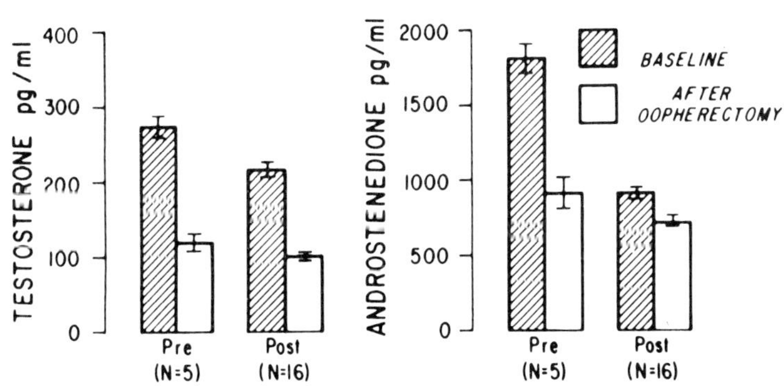

Figure 5.5 Plasma concentrations of testosterone and androstenedione before and after oophorectomy in groups of pre- and post-menopausal women (with permission from Judd, H. L., Lucas, W. E. and Yen, S. S. C. (1974). *Am. J. Obstet. Gynecol.*, **118**, 793)

clearance rate, at least for androstenedione is somewhat reduced after oophorectomy but even without ovaries it may be seen that the post-menopausal woman continues to secrete substantial amounts of androstenedione and lesser amounts of testosterone. Thus in the post-menopausal patient about 40 μg per day of estrone is excreted and virtually none of it is secreted by the ovary, almost all of it is derived from androstenedione. The androstenedione is secreted largely from the adrenal gland and conversion occurs peripherally, that is outside the ovary. This site is likely to be adipose tissue[4], and such a suggestion would support the clinical observation that carcinoma of the corpus uteri tends to be found in obese women and the observation of de Waard *et al.*[7] that the repeated finding of estrogenic vaginal smears was more likely in obese patients.

The plasma estradiol and LH levels from our laboratory may be seen in Figure 5.6 for comparison with Figure 5.7, where in spite of a pre-ovulatory

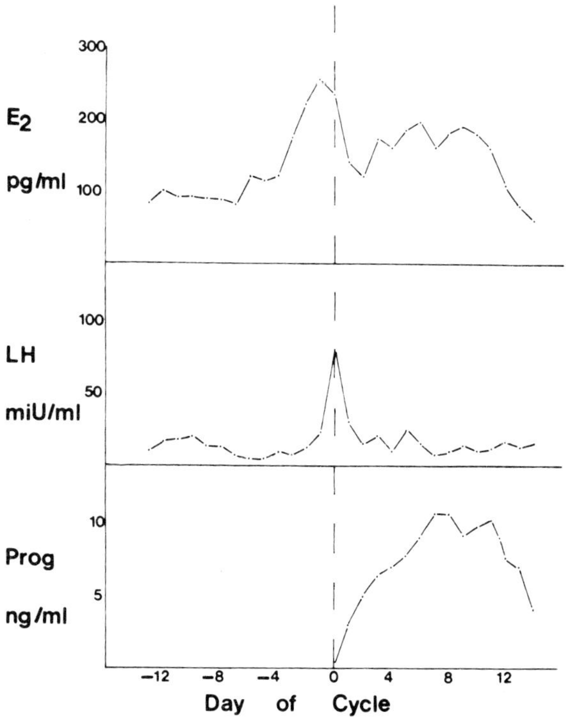

Figure 5.6 Plasma estradiol, luteinizing hormone and progesterone throughout a menstrual cycle in a normal woman.

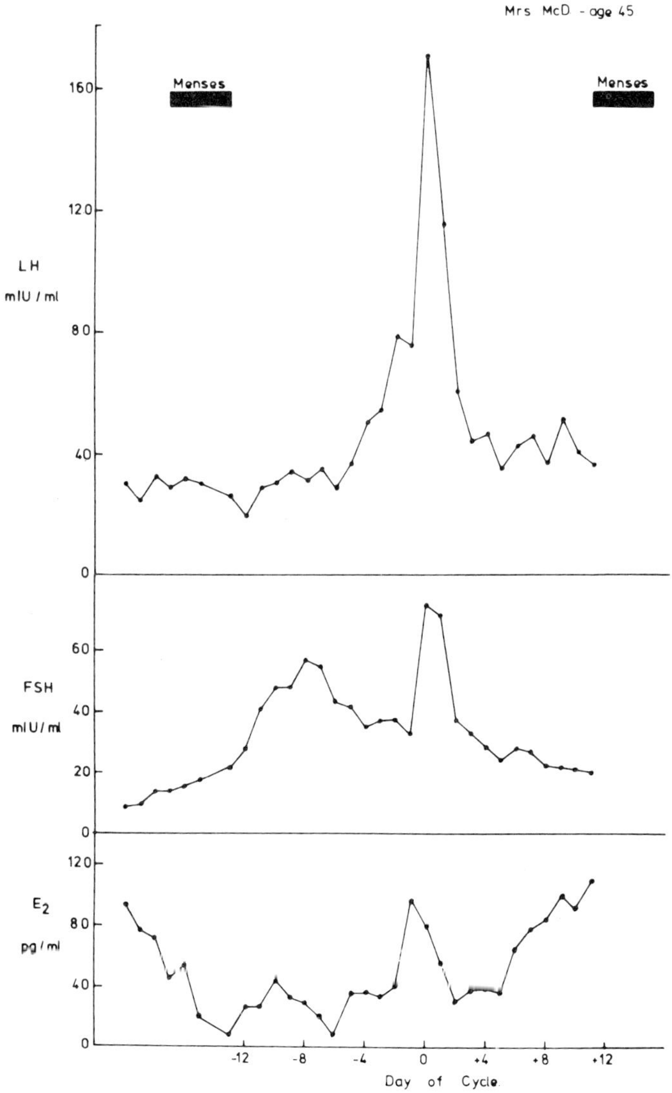

Figure 5.7 Plasma luteinizing hormone, follicle stimulating hormone and estradiol throughout a menstrual cycle in an infertile subject, presumably pre-menopausal (with permission from Cooke, I. D., Anderton, K. J., Lenton, E. and Burton, M. (1976). *Postgrad. Med. J.* (in press))

estradiol peak and an LH surge the estradiol levels are derived from a failing follicle and require an excessive FSH and LH stimulus. A more acute progression may be seen in Figure 5.8, where there was a rapid exhaustion of the ovarian response and an excessive rise of FSH and LH characteristic of the menopausal stituation associated in this patient with the emergence of hot flushes. A surgically induced (Figure 5.9) or a radiation menopause (Figure 5.10) also gives rise to acute FSH and LH increases on the same time scale[8].

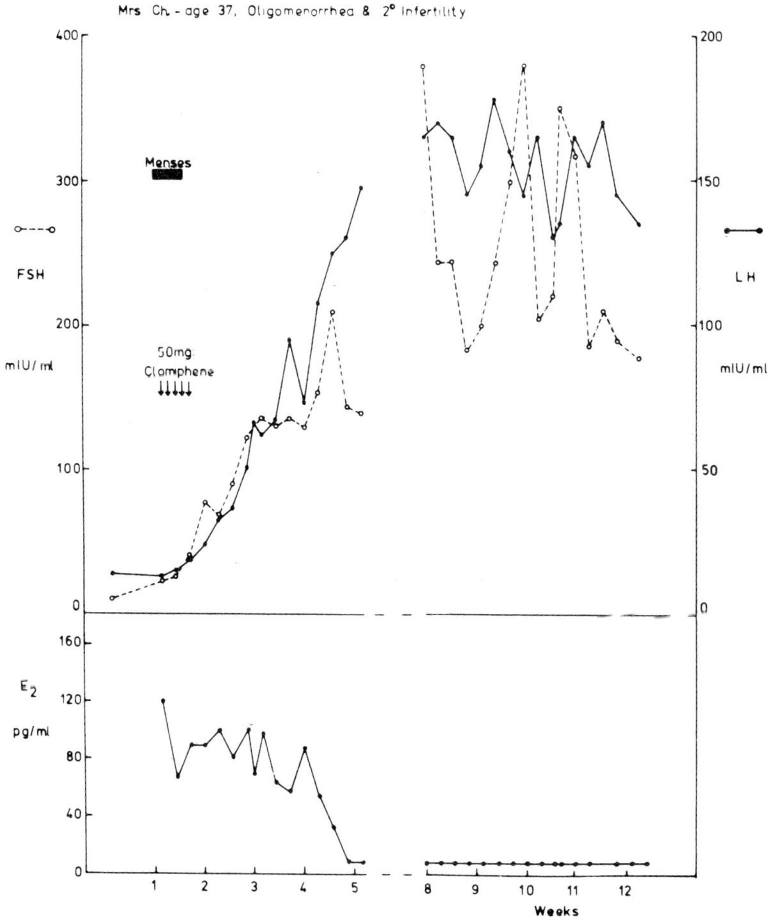

Figure 5.8 An acute transition from pre-menopausal to menopausal levels of follicle stimulating hormone, luteinizing hormone and estradiol associated with clomiphene treatment (with permission from Cooke, I. D., Anderton, K. J., Lenton, E. and Burton M. (1976). *Postgrad. Med. J.* (in press))

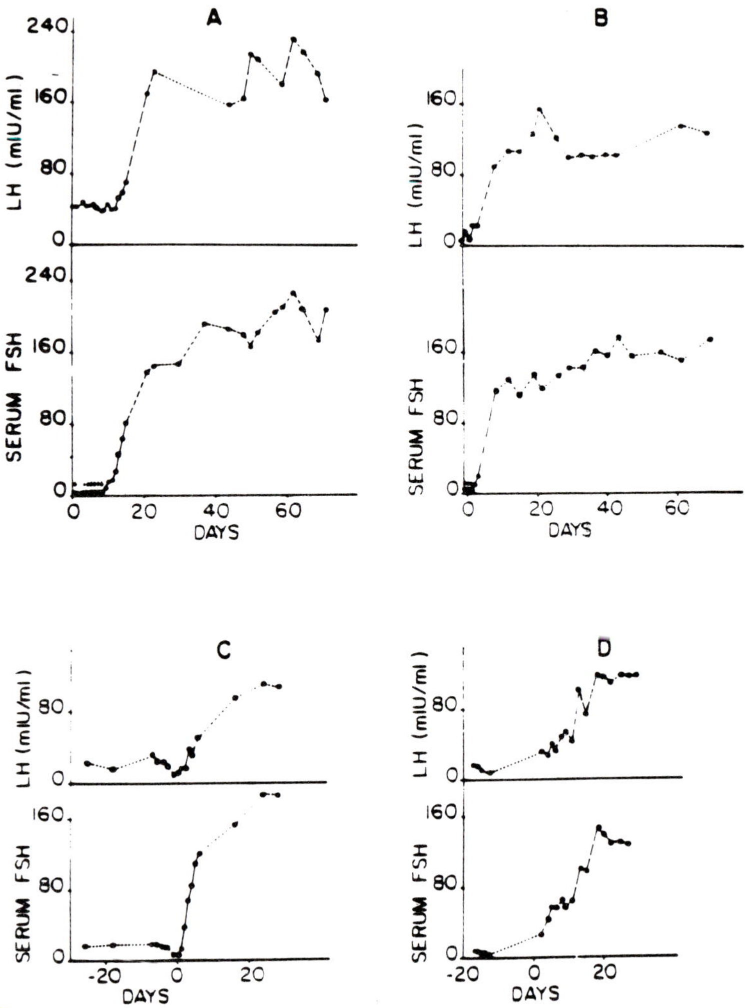

Figure 5.9 Serum gonadotrophin concentrations following oophorectomy (day 0) in four women. Subject A had been pregnant prior to oophorectomy, the other three subjects had been cycling regularly (with permission from Ostergard, D. R., Parlow, A. F. and Townsend, D. E. (1970). *J. Clin. Endocrinol. Metab.*, **31**, 43)

The hypothalamus and pituitary continue to function normally, i.e. excessively, in the absence of normal circulating estrogen levels. However, in addition to the daily fluctuation of gonadotrophin excretion there is

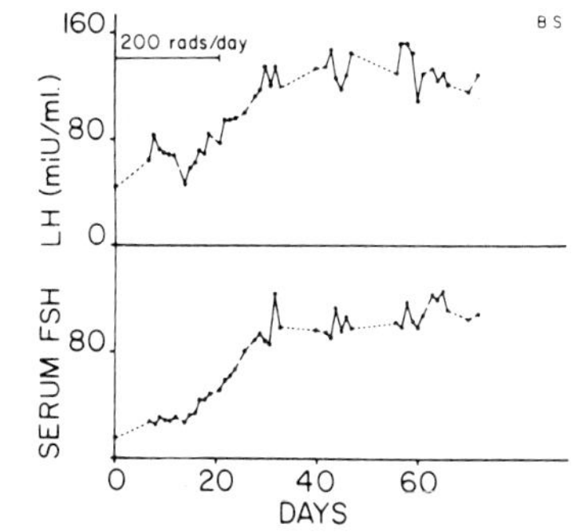

Figure 5.10 Effect of ovarian irradiation on serum gonadotrophins. Irradiation was begun on day 0 (with permission from Ostergard, D. R., Parlow, A. F. and Townsend, D. E. (1970). *J. Clin. Endocrinol. Metab.*, **31**, 43)

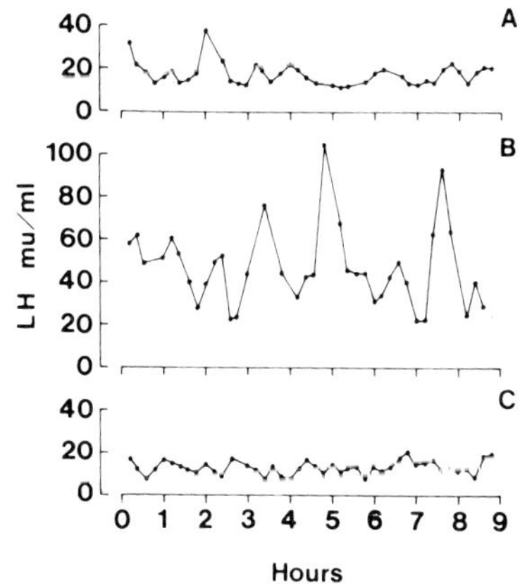

Figure 5.11 Episodic release of plasma luteinizing hormone shown by 15-min sampling. The profiles were obtained at (A) mid-follicular phase (B) pre-ovulatory phase and (C) mid-luteal phase (with permission from Lenton, E. and Cooke, I. D. (1974). *Clinics Obstet Gynaecol.*, **1**, 313, London: Saunders)

episodic pituitary release of FSH and to a much greater extent LH into the peripheral circulation. This is a normal function in the pre-menopausal woman (Figure 5.11) and may be seen in the post-menopausal one in the resting or LHRH stimulated state, indeed it is not suppressed by short-term intravenous estradiol infusions (Figure 5.12). It is apparent therefore that the

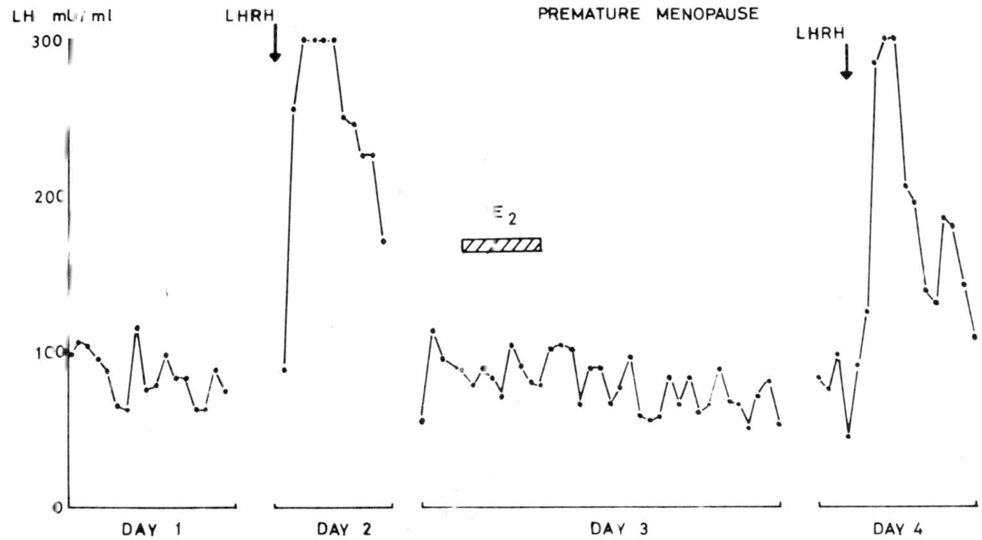

Figure 5.12 Fifteen minute episodic release of luteinizing hormone in a subject with a premature menopause. On day 2 an LHRH stimulation test (100 μg i.v.) was undertaken after basal observation on day 1; on day 3 a 3-hour intravenous infusion of estradiol was given such that levels of estradiol comparable to the normal pre-ovulatory phase were achieved. On day 4 the LHRH test was repeated

caution expressed about interpretation of urinary gonadotrophin data applies even more strongly to plasma data, where multiple samples are essential. Rebar *et al.*[9] have calculated the secretion rate of pituitary LH and have confirmed its episodic nature, and Seyler and Reichlin[10] have suggested that LHRH is also released episodically in the post-menopausal state.

Once the pituitary gonadotrophins have been allowed to rise, for example 2–3 weeks after acute cessation of ovarian function or more gradually in the physiological situation, it is much more difficult to suppress them requiring much higher doses of steroids. McPherson *et al.*[11] have shown that the efficacy of a level of estrogen or a dose of progesterone is dependent on the time after castration that it is administered, and this may have implications for replacement therapy at the time of operative removal of the ovaries. It seems that the hypothalamus changes its sensitivity when deprived of estrogen. On the other hand, to remove the ovaries at operation in a patient of over 40 years because they are not producing estrogen is also inappropriate, as apart from a small estrone or estradiol contribution, the ovarian stroma is producing significant quantities of the estrogenic precursors, androstenedione and testosterone.

Finally McLennan and McLennan[12] showed that about 40% of women maintain moderately estrogenized vaginal smears until they are over the age of 75. Such patients surely have adequate endogenous estrogen and should they not be identified before either surgical castration or replacement therapy are undertaken? Indiscriminate replacement therapy has no place in the management of these patients; we need much more extensive and careful research to define its role.

Acknowledgements

Grateful thanks are due to Mrs V. Y. E. Pryor for typing the manuscript and to the Department of Medical Illustration, Sheffield Area Health Authority (Teaching) for the photography. Permission to reproduce the Figures and the Table is acknowledged individually in each legend. The data for Fig. 12 were obtained from unpublished work of Adams, M., Singleton, G., Lenton, E. and Cooke, I. D.

References

1. McDonald, P. C., Rombaut, R. P. and Siiteri, P. K. (1967). Plasma precursors of estrogen I. Estimates of conversion of plasma 4-androstenedione to estrone in normal males and non-pregnant normal, castrate and adrenalectomized females. *J. Clin. Endocrinol. Metab.*, **27**, 1103
2. Adamopoulos, D. A., Loraine, J. A. and Dove, G. A. (1971). Endocrinological studies in women approaching the menopause. *J. Obstet. Gynaecol. Br. Cmnwlth.*, **78**, 62

3. Baird, D. T., Horton, R., Longcope, C. and Tait, J. F. (1969). Steroid dynamics under steady-state conditions. In: E. B. Astwood (ed.) *Recent Progress in Hormone Research*, **25,** 611–655 (New York: Academic Press)
4. Grodin, J. M., Siiteri, P. K. and MacDonald, P. C. (1973). Source of estrogen production in post-menopausal women. *J. Clin. Endocrinol. Metab.*, **36,** 207
5. Judd, H. L., Judd, G. E., Lucas, W. E. and Yen, S. S. C. (1974). Endocrine function of the postmenopausal ovary: Concentration of androgens and estrogens in ovarian and peripheral vein blood. *J. Clin. Endocrinol. Metab.*, **39,** 1020
6. Judd, H. L., Lucas, W. E. and Yen, S. S. C. (1974). Effect of oophorectomy on circulating testosterone and androstenedione levels in patients with endometrial cancer. *Am. J. Obstet. Gynecol.*, **118,** 793
7. de Waard, F., Pot, H., Tonckens-Nanniga, N. E., Baanders-van Halewijn, E. A. and Thijssen, J. H. H. (1972). Longitudinal studies on the phenomenon of postmenopausal estrogen production. *Acta Cytol. (Balt)*, **16,** 273
8. Ostergard, D. R., Parlow, A. F. and Townsend, D. E. (1970). Acute effect of castration on serum FSH and LH in the adult woman *J. Clin. Endocrinol. Metab.*, **31,** 43
9. Rebar, R., Perlman, D., Naftolin, F. and Yen, S. S. C. (1973). The estimation of pituitary lutenizing hormone secretion *J. Clin. Endocrinol. Metab.*, **37,** 917
10. Seyler, L. E. Jr and Reichlin, S. (1973). Luteinizing hormone-releasing factor (LRF) in plasma of postmenopausal women. *J. Clin. Endocrinol. Metab.*, **37,** 197
11. McPherson, J. C. III, Costoff, A. and Mahesh, V. B. (1975). Influence of estrogen–progesterone combinations on gonadotrophin secretion in castrate female rats. *Endocrinology*, **97,** 771
12. McLennan, M. T and McLennan, C. E. (1971). Estrogenic status of menstruating and menopausal women assessed by cervico-vaginal smears. *Obstet Gynaecol.*, **37,** 325

6

Intensive steroid and protein hormone profiles on post-menopausal women experiencing hot flushes, and a group of controls

S. Campbell

Post-menopausal women tend to be regarded in scientific studies as a homogeneous group and there is little information, certainly as far as plasma hormones are concerned, on comparative data between patients with and without vasomotor symptoms. Furthermore, we are unaware of any data on changes in plasma levels of steroid or protein hormones in such patients over a period of 24 hours and most studies have tended to regard values from single samples as representative of a whole 24-hour period. For this reason we present here 24-hour plasma steroid and protein hormone profiles on seven post-menopausal women with hot flushes and four age-matched controls who had no vasomotor symptoms. It was hoped to determine if any differences in the 24-hour profile could be observed between flushing and non-flushing patients and to discover whether or not any correlation could be established between changes in a particular hormone and the occurrence of a hot flush.

Patients and methods

All patients studied were at least 6 months post-menopausal. The four non-flushing patients had a mean age of 50·8 years and were a mean of 1 year post-menopause. The seven flushing patients were themselves divided into two groups; four were closely matched with the four non-flushing patients in age, the mean age being 51·5 years, and the mean number of years post-menopause 1·2. Three flushing patients were slightly older, the mean age being 55·7 years and the mean number of years post-menopause 6·3, but on analysis their results were not significantly different from those of the younger flushing patients and all patients with vasomotor symptoms have been grouped together in this analysis.

The patients were admitted to hospital for a period of 36 hours and blood was removed at 2-hour intervals through an in-dwelling intravenous canula from 08.00 until 08.00 hours the following morning. Blood was centrifuged soon after withdrawal and the plasma or serum refrigerated at −4 °C until analysis. The assays undertaken, techniques, sensitivity and reproducibility are summarized in Table 6.1. Some of the estriol results were below the level of sensitivity, (i.e. 10 pg/ml) but the results have been plotted for the sake of completeness.

Table 6.1 24-hour profile study

Hormone	*Assay method*	*Sensitivity*	*Coefficient of variation (%)*	
			Intra-assay	*Inter-assay*
Estradiol Estrone Estriol	Liquid phase RIA[1]	10 pg/ml	8	16
Androstenedione Testosterone	Liquid phase RIA[2]	0·2 ng/ml	8	16
FSH LH	Double antibody RIA[3]	0·5 ml U/ml	5	10
Prolactin		2 ng/ml	5	10
Growth hormone		1 ng/ml	5	10

1. Modification of: Emment, Y., Collins, W. P. and Sommerville, I. F. (1972). Radioimmunoassay of oestrone and oestradiol in human plasma. *Acta Endocrinol.* (*Copenhagen*), **69**, 567
2. Collins, W. P., Mansfield, M. D., Alladina, N. S. and Sommerville, I. F. (1972). *Steroid Biochem.*, **3**, 333
3. Modification of: Biswas, S., Hindocha, P. and Dewhurst, C. J. (1972). *J. Endocrinol.*, **54**, 251

Results and discussion

Steroid Hormones

PLASMA ESTROGENS: *Estrone* (Figure 6.1)

Two non-flushing patients had sustained high levels of plasma estrone (means 136·8 and 81·0 pg/ml) equivalent to pre-menstrual luteal phase levels.

The patient with the highest levels was 55 years old and was 18 months post-menopause. The remaining two non-flushing patients had low levels (means 27·6 and 28·2 pg/ml) indistinguishable from those of the seven

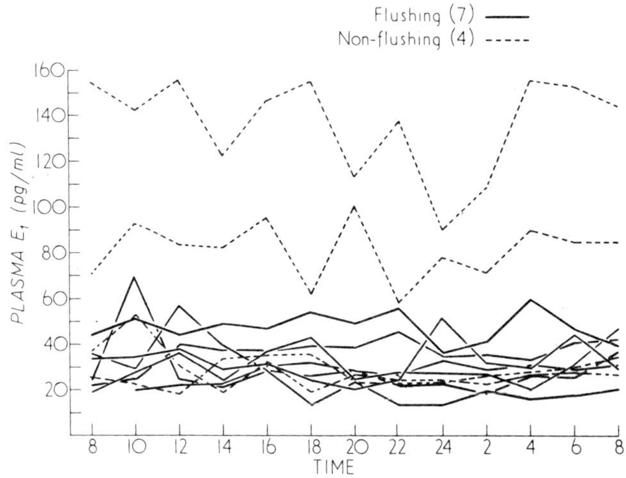

Figure 6.1 Individual 2-hour plasma estrone values in flushing and non-flushing patients

flushing patients (mean 32·2 pg/ml) although small peaks were found in these patients extending as high as 70 pg/ml.

To determine if there was a diurnal variation in plasma estrone levels, each 2-hourly value was calculated as a percentage of the mean of all the R.I.A. values for each patient; both flushing and non-flushing patients showed a similar diurnal rhythm with peaks at 10.00 and 16.00 hours, and a fall between 18.00 and 02.00 hours. (Figure 6.2).

ESTRADIOL (Figure 6.3)

The two non-flushing patients who had elevated levels of estrone also had high sustained levels of estradiol (means 144 and 100 pg/ml) while the remaining two non-flushing patients had low levels (means 19·2 and 15·6 pg/ml) similar to those of the 7 flushing patients (mean 18·6 pg/ml). The flushing patients however showed very sharp surges of plasma estradiol at 08·00–10.00, 16.00 and 00.00 hours.

ESTRIOL (Figure 6.4)

Levels of plasma estriol in non-flushing and flushing patients were consistently low with 95% of all values below 20 pg/ml. No distinction could be detected between flushing and non-flushing patients.

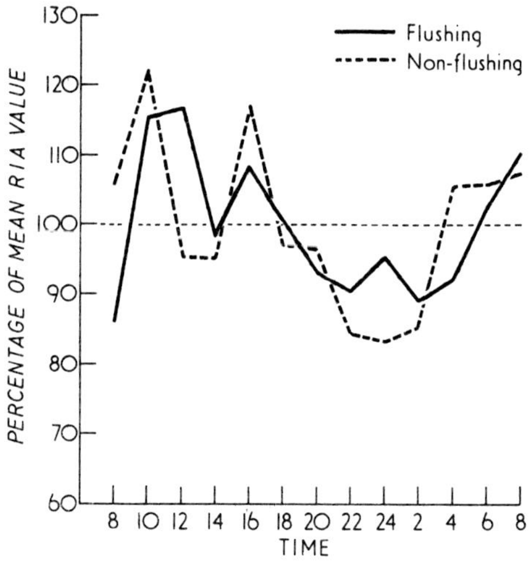

Figure 6.2 Diurnal variation in plasma estrone in flushing and non-flushing patients. Each 2-hour value is expressed as a percentage of the mean RIA value for each patient

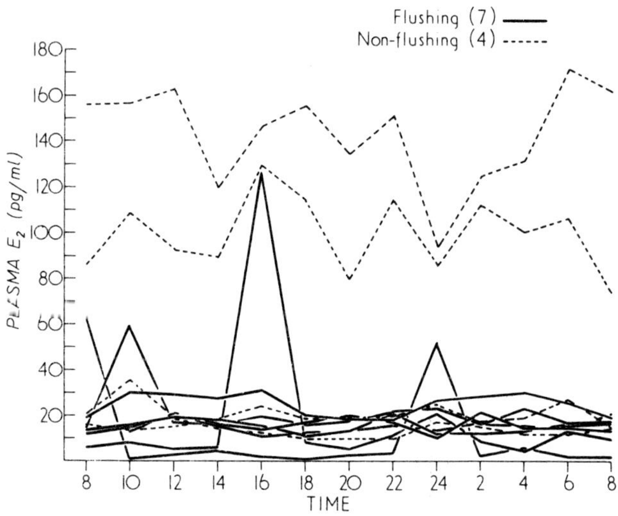

Figure 6.3 Individual 2-hour plasma estradiol values in flushing and non-flushing patients

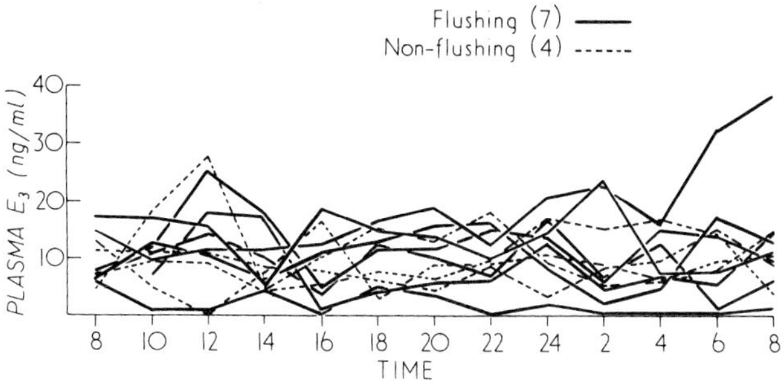

Figure 6.4 Individual 2-hour plasma estriol values in flushing and non-flushing patients

PLASMA ANDROSTENEDIONE (Figure 6.5)

Plasma androstenedione values showed a well marked diurnal variation indicating that the adrenal is the principal source of this steroid in the post-menopausal woman. In non-flushing patients levels varied from a mean of 270 ng/100 ml at 08.00 hours to 180 ng/100 ml at midnight, while in flushing patients the mean values were 224 ng and 134 ng at these times (Figure 6.6). Statistically significant differences in androstenedione levels were observed at 04.00, 10.00, 12.00, 16.00, 18.00 and 22.00 hours.

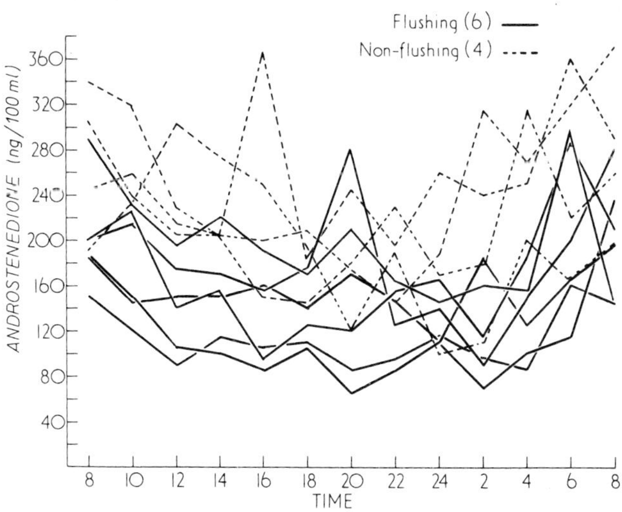

Figure 6.5 Individual 2-hour plasma androstenedione values in flushing and non-flushing patients

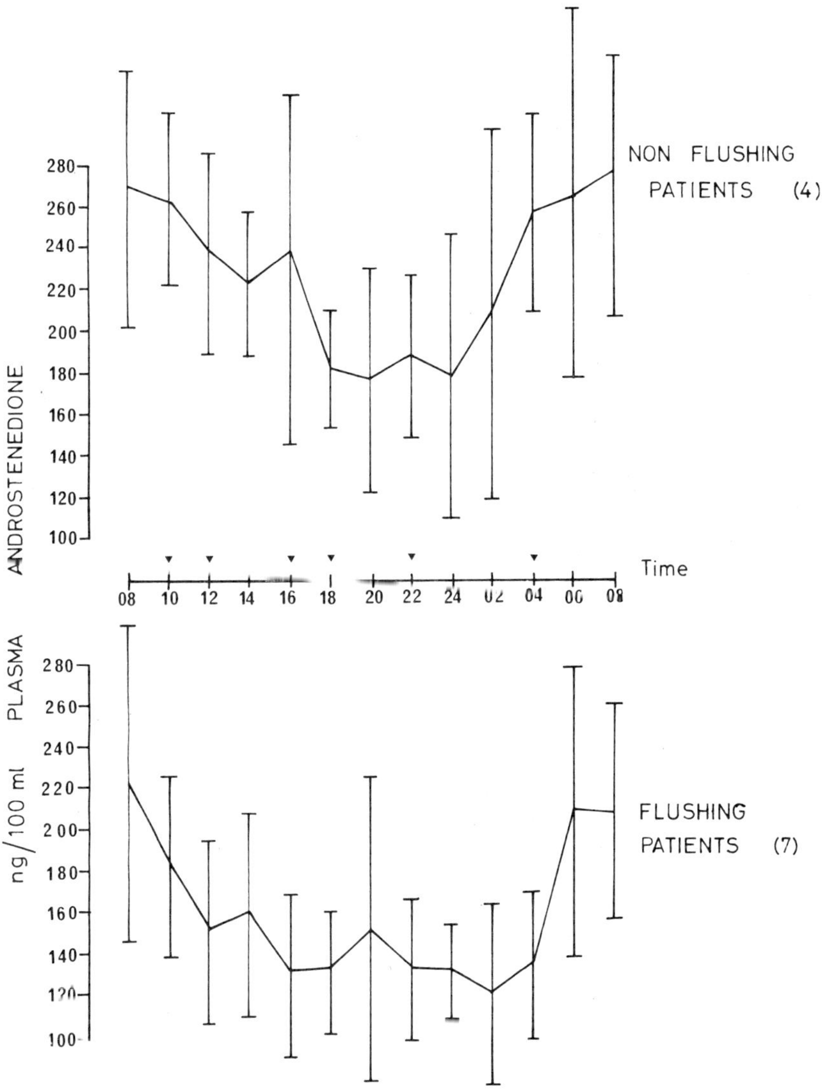

Figure 6.6 Mean plasma androstenedione levels (plus or minus standard deviations) for each 2-hourly interval in flushing and non-flushing patients. ▼ indicates a statistically significant difference between flushing and non-flushing patients

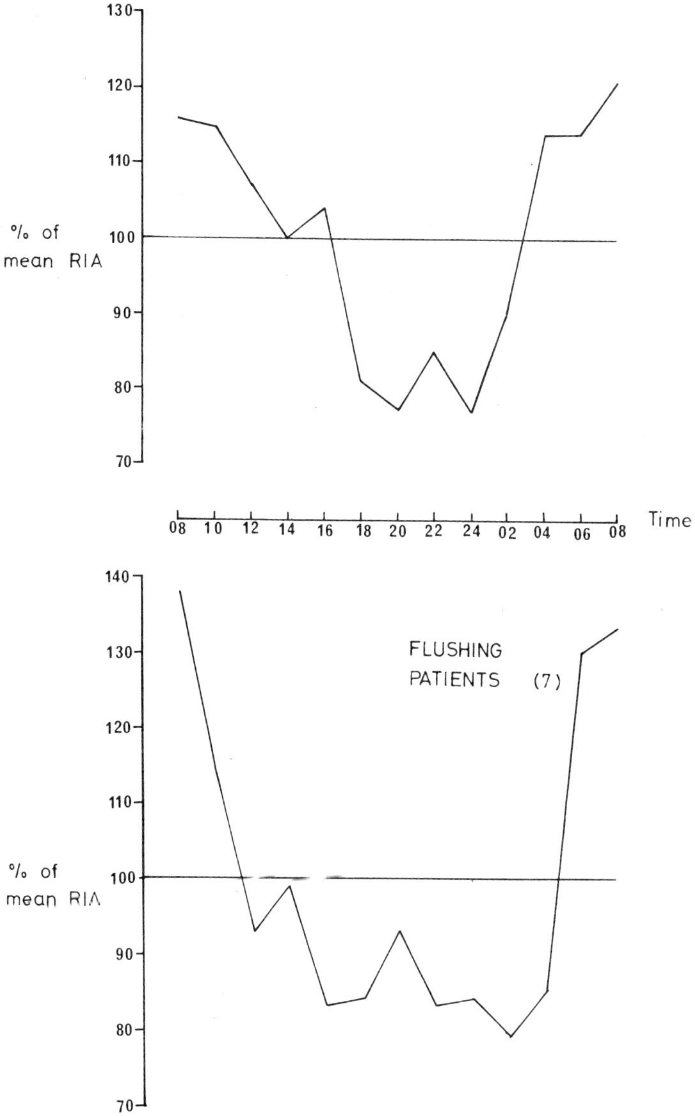

Figure 6.7 Diurnal variation in plasma androstenedione in flushing and non-flushing patients. Each 2-hour value is expressed as a percentage of the mean RIA value for each patient

The diurnal variation was again determined for each patient by calculating each 2-hourly value as a percentage of the mean R.I.A. value (Figure 6.7). There was a difference in the pattern of the diurnal variation between non-flushing and flushing patients; in the former group, plasma androstenedione values did not fall below the mean until 17.00 hours while flushing patients showed a more precipitate fall below the mean at 11.00 hours.

Thus, even the two non-flushing patients with low levels of estrone had relatively high levels of androstenedione when compared with flushing patients and it is possible in the former that local conversion of androstenedione to estrone in the hypothalamus may account for their greater vasomotor stability.

PLASMA TESTOSTERONE (Figure 6.8)

No significant difference was observed in the plasma testosterone levels between non-flushing and flushing patients. When the 2-hourly values were plotted as a percentage of the mean R.I.A. value, a definite diurnal rhythm was observed which was similar for non-flushing and flushing patients (Figure 6.9).

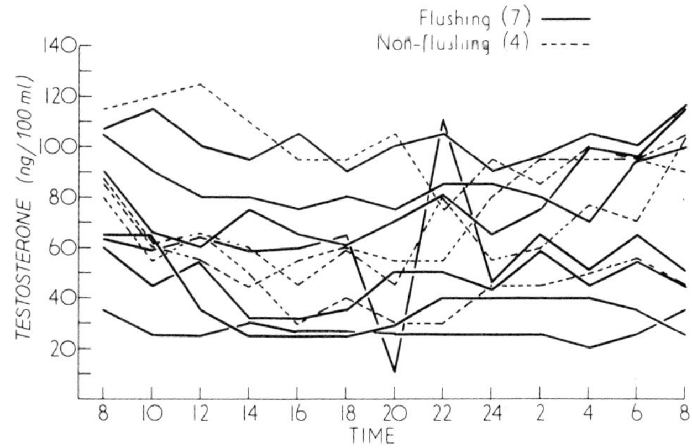

Figure 6.8 Individual 2-hour plasma testosterone values in flushing and non-flushing patients

Protein hormones

SERUM FSH (Figure 6.10)

The patients with the highest estrone and estradiol values had the lowest FSH values, suggesting a negative feedback mechanism of FSH release in

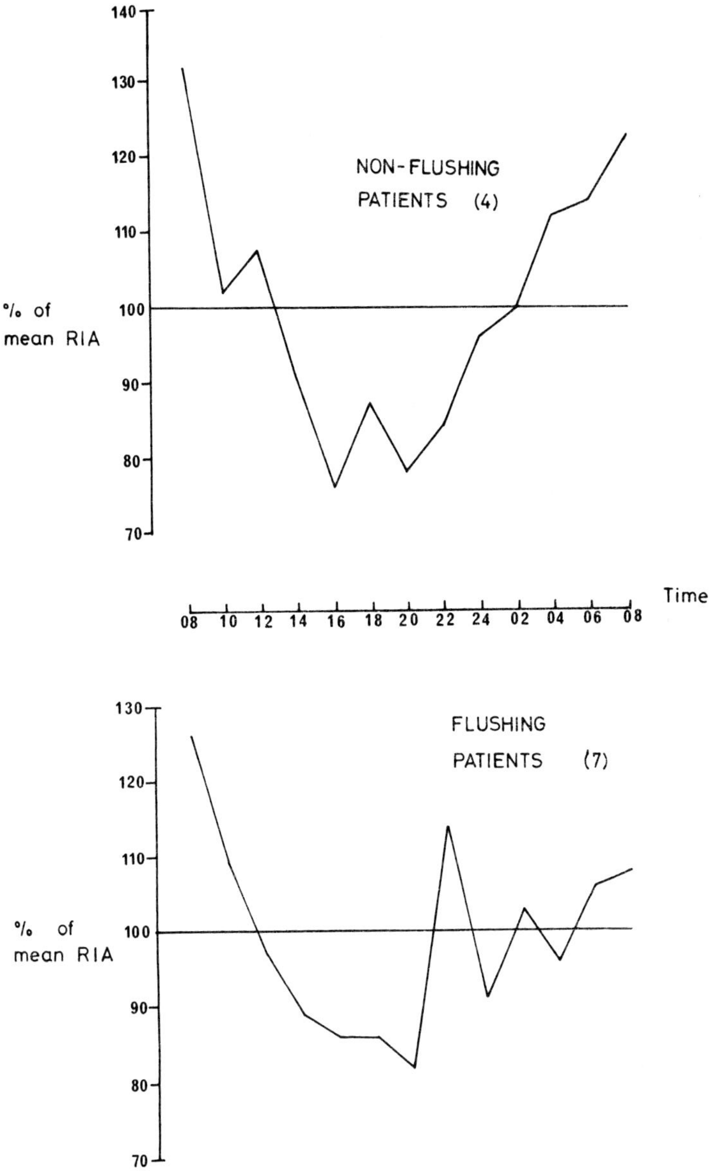

Figure 6.9 Diurnal variation in plasma testosterone in flushing and non-flushing patients. Each 2-hour value is expressed as a percentage of the mean RIA value for each patient

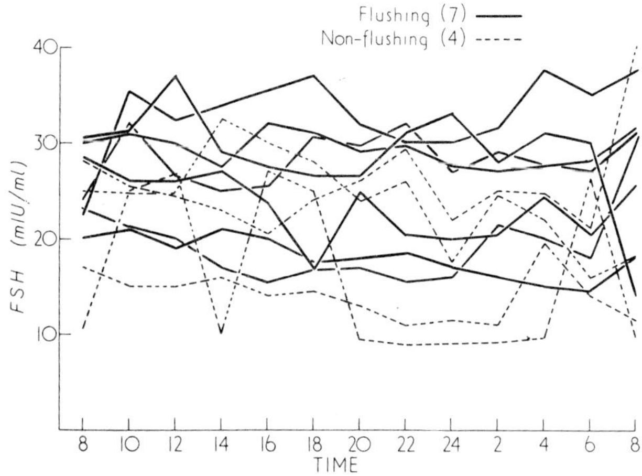

Figure 6.10 Individual 2-hour plasma FSH values in flushing and non-flushing patients

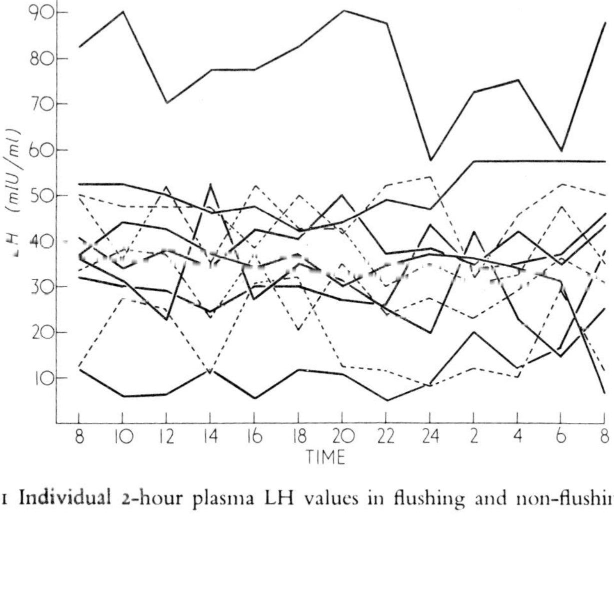

Figure 6.11 Individual 2-hour plasma LH values in flushing and non-flushing patients

the post-menopausal patient. Nevertheless there was marked fluctuation of FSH levels and the distinction between the high and low estrogen status patients was less distinct than with plasma estrogens. The two non-flushing patients with low estrogen levels had FSH values which were indistinguishable from those of the flushing patients.

SERUM LH (Figure 6.11)

This was a disappointing parameter of estrogen status. The two patients with the lowest LH vaues were flushing patients with low plasma estrogen levels and no differences were observed between flushing and non-flushing patients.

PLASMA PROLACTIN (Figure 6.12)

Results were available for the eight closely age matched flushing and non-flushing patients and no differences were observed between the two groups. The typical surge of plasma prolactin associated with deep sleep was observed at 00.00 and 02.00 hours.

PLASMA GROWTH HORMONE (Figure 6.13)

No differences in base-line values were observed between flushing and non-flushing patients, though the flushing patients tended to have higher surges of plasma growth hormone; the timing of these surges was more variable than with prolactin, but again most were associated with deep sleep.

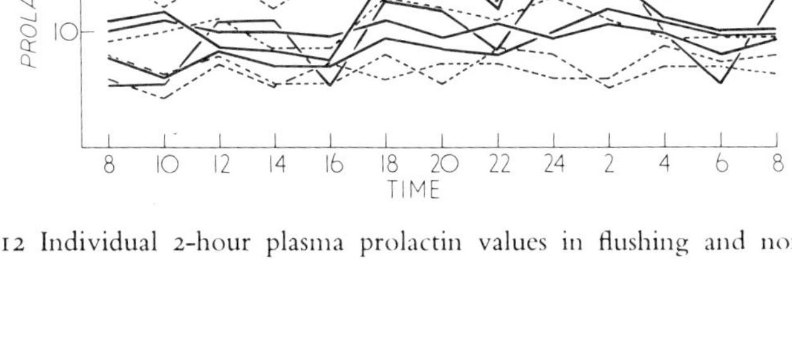

Figure 6.12 Individual 2-hour plasma prolactin values in flushing and non-flushing patients

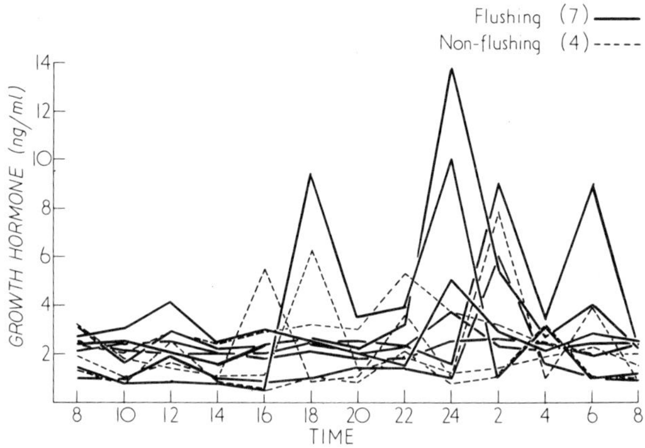

Figure 6.13 Individual 2-hour plasma GH values in flushing and non-flushing patients

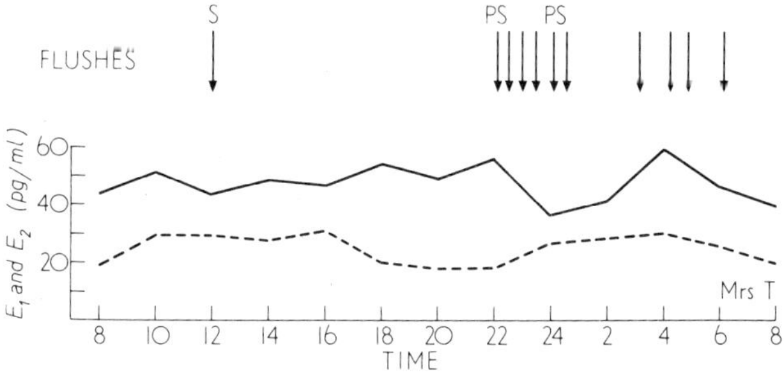

Figure 6.14 Time relationship between 2-hour plasma estrone/estradiol values and the occurrence of hot flushes (Mrs T)

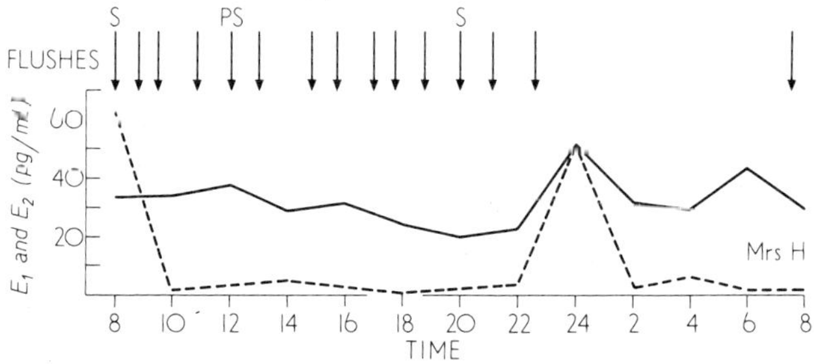

Figure 6.15 Time relationship between 2-hour plasma estrone/estradiol values and the occurrence of hot flushes (Mrs H)

Individual profiles

The hormone profile of each patient with vasomotor symptoms was studied to ascertain if there was an association between particular levels of plasma hormones and the occurrence of a hot flush. Examples from two typical cases are described below.

PLASMA ESTRONE AND ESTRADIOL

With Mrs T (Figure 6.14), flushes appeared to occur with falling E_1 values except at 04.00 hours when they occurred in spite of rising levels. With Mrs H (Figure 6.15) a flush occurred during sample taking at 08.00 hours in the presence of a high estradiol level. Following this, however, flushes appeared to occur with falling or low E_1 and E_2 levels and stop when the levels rose (e.g. 00.00 hours).

PLASMA ANDROSTENEDIONE

With Mrs T (Figure 6.16), there was demonstrated an almost perfect relationship between falling androstenedione levels and hot flushes. In Figure 6.17, however, it can be seen that with Mrs H plasma androstenedione levels show a less perfect relationship, the lowest of the values being unassociated with vasomotor symptoms.

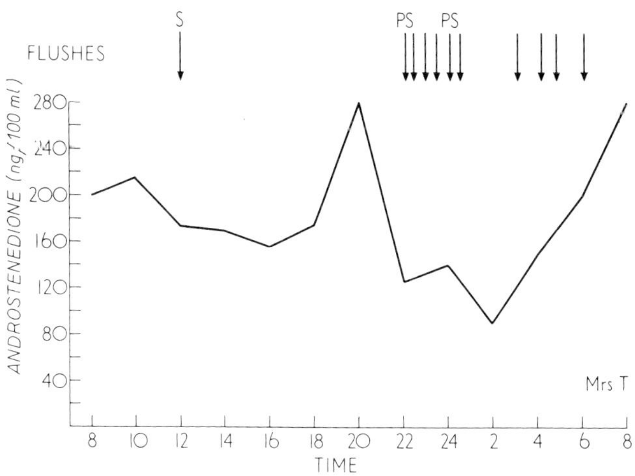

Figure 6.16 Time relationship between 2-hour plasma androstenedione values and the occurrence of hot flushes (Mrs T)

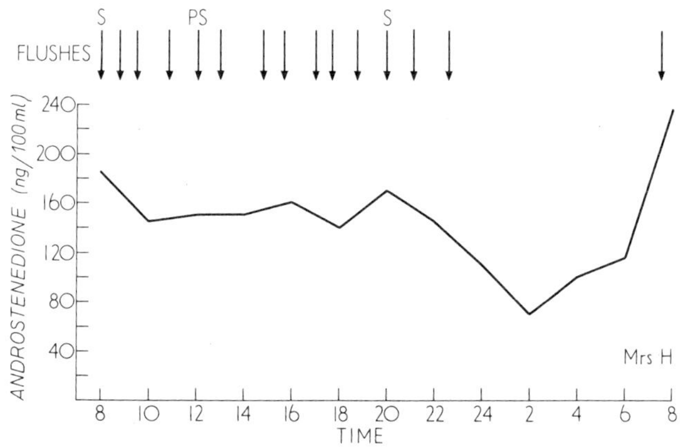

Figure 6.17 Time relationship between 2-hour plasma androstenedione values and the occurrence of hot flushes (Mrs H)

The conclusion therefore is that correlation between hot flushes and falling or low levels of plasma estrogens or androstenedione was not sufficiently close to prove a causal relationship. No other steroid or protein hormone showed any relationship between particular values and vasomotor symptoms.

Summary

24-hour steroid and protein hormone assay studies were performed on seven post-menopausal flushing women and four age-matched non-flushing controls. Blood samples were taken at 2-hourly intervals. Two non-flushing women had high sustained levels of E_1 and E_2; all the flushing and two non-flushing patients had low levels of E_1 and E_2 but sharp peaks were observed especially in flushing patients which in the case of estradiol were up to twelve times basal values. Both plasma androstenedione and testosterone showed a well marked diurnal variation suggesting that these hormones are mainly derived from the adrenal. Plasma androstenedione levels were significantly higher in non-flushing than in flushing women and the latter group showed a somewhat different diurnal rhythm, the fall below the mean R.I.A. value occurring some 6 hours earlier than that in flushing patients. Plasma testosterone levels were similar in both groups. Serum FSH values were lowest in those patients with the highest plasma estrogen levels, suggesting a negative feedback control of FSH release, but LH levels were a poor guide to estrogen status. There was no difference in plasma prolactin levels between flushing and non-flushing patients, but the surges of growth hormone appear to be higher in flushing patients. In individual cases the best correlation between hormone levels and hot flushes was demonstrated by estrogen and androstenedione but the relationship was not sufficiently close to suggest that it was causal.

Lest it be thought that this study was merely an academic exercise, I would like to close with two clinical observations. Some post-menopausal women appear to produce sustained and significant amounts of estrogen and it is therefore important that the estrogen status of patients without vasomotor symptoms should be assessed before contemplating hormone replacement therapy or unacceptably high levels will be obtained. Secondly, in view of the sharp surges of plasma estrone and estradiol levels observed in this study, it is clear that single samples are not always representative of the true estrogen status of the patient.

Acknowledgement

This chapter, presented by S. Campbell, was written jointly by Campbell, S., Breeson, A. J., Kitchin, Yvonne, Fergusson, I. K. and Biswas, S.

Discussion on Section B:

Endocrinology (Part 1)

Chairman: *Professor R. W. Beard*

Professor C. Lauritzen (Gynaecologist, University of Ulm): First I want to congratulate both speakers for their splendid presentations. We have done some similar studies, the last one from a more practical viewpoint, since we have given exogenous estrogens to castrated women, measured their estrogen levels, and registered the complaints of the patients. We administered to castrated patients with very low estrogen levels, estradiol benzoate injections, which have an effect lasting for 3–5 days after which the level of the estrogens decreases. When the level fell below 40 picograms of estrone and 20 pg estradiol/ml plasma, patients experienced hot flushes, fatigue, irritability, and the symptoms that Dr Jaszmann has shown. In another study we proceeded in a slightly different manner, giving a preparation of estradiol valerate, 20 drops for a week, then 15 drops for a week, then 10 drops, then 5, and so on, and we had similar results. At similar levels of estrone and estradiol to those previously mentioned, first fatigue, headache and irritability appeared and some days later, the hot flushes and sweating appeared. These two groups of complaints may correspond to different estrogen levels.

The same thing was noticed with the patient who had been post-menopausal or castrated for a long time and had a very low level of estrogens. When she is first given estrogens, she will have hot flushes at the beginning of the treatment. As the level of estrogen rises further, however, the hot flushes will disappear, and when the estrogen levels fall again the hot flushes will re-appear. The same applies to Turner's Syndrome. A particular level of estrogen is not necessarily correlated with the appearance of hot flushes and other symptoms, but the process of decreasing or increasing the levels causes the instability of the hypothalamic vasomotor centres.

One last comment. We have measured the releasing hormone LRH. The data are provisional because, as everybody knows, these investigations are difficult to carry out at present. However, we have found that the levels of releasing hormone LRH are between 0 and 20 in pg/ml in pre-menopausal women, and in post-menopausal women the levels increase to 30, 40 or 50 pg/ml, but we found no correlation between the peaks of releasing hormone and the peaks of LH.

Professor R. W. Beard: Two chairman's comments on the papers. Professor Cooke admirably covered what is known about the hormonal profiles in menopausal patients, and he also looked at the physiology. It seems to me that we must regard the menopause as physiological, and hopefully start to relate some of the changes in hormone profiles to what is actually happening in the organs themselves—that is in the ovaries, in the adrenal, and in the pituitary end organs.

The comment on Mr Campbell's paper, we have again a convincing comparison between women with and without symptoms, and looking at the 24-hour profiles, it certainly seems that the symptoms are hormonally related. But there is the paradox, as he pointed out, of individual cases where there are quite marked fluctuations, and yet no improvement in the symptoms when the steroids were raised. I would suggest that perhaps we should be looking also at end-organ sensitivity to these changing hormonal levels.

Mr E. S. Saunders (Gynaecologist, London): The ovaries in post-menopausal women, although they do not produce estrogens, produce testosterone, which is then converted, possibly by the subcutaneous fat, into estradiol. That would serve to support the theory held by some gynaecologists that there is no good reason to remove both ovaries as a routine from a patient undergoing hysterectomy. Some explain the removal as preventing possible malignant changes in the ovaries. But the incidence of malignancy is so small—between 2 and 5%—that there is no reason for castrating these women.

Professor I. D. Cooke (Gynaecologist, Sheffield): That is an appropriate comment although I cannot agree that the risk of malignancy is from 2 to 5%; I think it is more of the order of about 1 in 3000. I take the point that when deciding on the removal of the ovaries at hysterectomy this risk should be counter-balanced by the fact that they do have some physiological function. I am not sure, nevertheless, that the argument is proven just yet.

Mr E. S. Saunders: Have any differences been found in the hormone secretion of the ovaries after a simple hysterectomy in the younger woman? I sometimes notice typical menopausal symptoms after a hysterectomy, and I myself have suggested that every woman who has a hysterectomy should be given an implant of estradiol. That suggestion has been taken up by Professor Stallworthy of Oxford, and by other gynaecologists.

Professor I. D. Cooke: We ourselves have not been measuring estrogen production after simple hysterectomy but there are quite a lot of data in the literature suggesting that the ovaries function, indeed cycle normally, after hysterectomy if both ovaries have been retained. I should have thought that on present evidence it is really not valid to give implants to these women if they have retained ovaries.

Mr E. Cope (Gynaecologist, Oxford): Mr Campbell has done an intensive steroid study on eight anecdotal cases, and drawn the conclusion that there was no correlation between estrogen levels and flushes on the grounds that two women who did not flush had high levels but two further women who did not flush had levels which corresponded with the levels of the flushing patients. It seemed to me that the two that were at a low level were not peaking in the same way as the flushing patients were peaking. If a pellet is put in, and a steady state of estradiol is maintained at a high enough level, then there is no flushing. If, on the other hand, the patient's estrogen is at a constant low level, there is again no flushing. Each woman has a fairly wide band within which she flushes, and this might well be an end-organ effect.

I should like to ask Mr Campbell whether the particularly flat curve that those two patients had who were not flushing with a low level were not flushing because they were not peaking.

Mr S. Campbell (Gynaecologist, London): That is a very reasonable point of view. I should point out that the cases we studied were *not* anecdotal in that they were randomly selected. There did not seem to be a close relationship between these peaks and the occurrence of a hot flush, but I would like to do more frequent sampling before I could draw a firm conclusion on this point. I would agree that the two non-flushing patients, with low levels of estrogen, did not seem to peak as much as those who had flushes. This is especially true of estradiol values (Figure 1) where the percentage fluctuation about the mean RIA value is much higher in flushing patients. On present evidence we cannot get a rule for everybody, but with more frequent sampling we may further elucidate this matter. Mr Cope's observation however may well be valid.

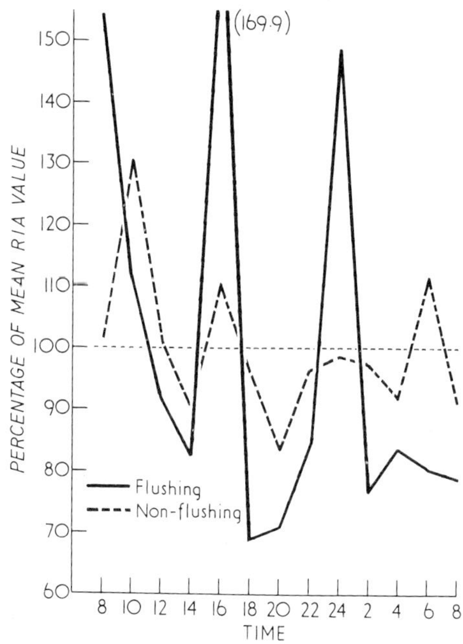

Figure 1 Diurnal variation of plasma estradiol in flushing and non-flushing patients

Professor I. D. Cooke: Perhaps we are being far too simplistic about the relationship between steroid levels and flushing. I wonder, in view of the central nervous system data on aromatization of androstenedione in the hypothalamus whether the observation of an androstenedione relationship to hot flushing may not be of some importance. We must begin to study central nervous system catecholamine levels in response to hormonal backgrounds before we can get a fuller understanding. We are looking at it very superficially at the moment.

Professor R. W. Beard: I should like to say something in support of Mr Campbell, and the suggestion that anecdotal cases have little significance. In the hormone world now we shall see individual patients in small groups, but studied in great depth, who will produce data of considerable significance.

Dr A. Jadresic (Hastings): I was very interested in Mr Campbell's academic exercise, and this would seem to correspond to other acute observations. Has he studied any correlation between LH suppression and remission of the climacteric syndrome with estrogens in long-running treatment? Conditions might be different to what he has observed in acute studies.

Mr S. Campbell: We are moving now to studying patients who are actually receiving therapy, and comparing the response to therapy with these 24-hour profiles. The only observation that I can make at the moment is that LH was a less sensitive index of estrogen status than FSH.

Professor I. D. Cooke: We have one or two anecdotal observations that LH is not necessarily suppressed to pre-menopausal levels. It can run along at moderately high levels even with complete remission of symptoms.

Dr P. A. van Keep (Gynaecologist, Geneva): We know that a number of women have post-menopausal estrogen production and that the peripheral conversion of androstenedione to estrone is related to factors such as age, body weight, liver disease, diabetes, etc. At the same time, we know that these factors are also known as risk factors with regard to endometrial carcinoma. It is therefore not too difficult to presume that the influence of estrone at the receptor level may play a role in the occurrence of endometrial carcinoma. If that is the case, a plea could be made for treatment with other estrogens than estrone, even in those women who have some post-menopausal estrogen production.

Professor I. D. Cooke: There is a very large 'if' in suggesting that the receptor level activity of estrone is important in carcinogenesis. If this can be shown, I should be much more inclined to pursue this line, but at present it is unproven. I would only accept circumstantial evidence in relation to clinical observation. Professor Lauritzen himself has said that there has been no reported increase in the incidence of endometrial carcinoma in patients who have had long-term estrogen therapy of varying sorts.

Professor R. W. Beard: Would Professor Cooke not agree that we should be thinking of the estrogens as separate compounds, rather than all under the same heading of estrogen?

Professor I. D. Cooke: Yes, of course, but we also have to think about intra-cellular metabolism. For example the Gurpide group have shown substantial conversion of estradiol to estrone within the endometrium itself (Gurpide, E. and Welch, M. (1969).

J. Biol. Chem., **244**, 5159.) Perhaps even the administration of different estrogens may end up as the same estrogen at the cellular level.

Dr K. J. Anderton (Gynaecologist, Sheffield): Mr Campbell has tried to demonstrate a relationship between hot flushes and the levels of individual hormones in these patients. Has he looked at the ratios of hormones, say estrone to estradiol, or estrogens to androgens, and the variation in these ratios in relationship to hot flushes?

Mr S. Campbell: That would be interesting to do. My data came quite recently and I have not done as full an analysis as I should like to do. In the two patients who had the highest levels of estrogen, estradiol levels were marginally greater than estrone, (E_1/E_2 ratio = 0·90) whereas in the non-flushing patients with low estrogen levels and in the 7 flushing patients the E_1/E_2 ratios were 1·60 and 1·73 respectively.

Dr Muriel Yates (General Practitioner, Liverpool): As a general practitioner who has only basic resources available, could I ask how practical it is to have estrogen estimations done, and what the costing to the National Health Service is likely to be. I have been following up menopausal women for a long time, and I should like to know how practical this would be out in the periphery.

Professor I. D. Cooke: Steroid assays would be an extraordinarily expensive way of doing this. Something simpler, such as a karyopyknotic index would give the basic information as to whether there is a reasonable amount of circulating estrogen. That would not show minor variations in estrogen levels but it might be useful as a primary objective. The epidemiological studies of de Waard *et al.* ((1972). *Acta Cytol.* (*Balt.*), 16, 273) from the Netherlands used urinary cytology, and others have used vaginal cytology as screening procedures.

Mr S. Campbell: I agree with Professor Cooke in that widespread steroid studies would be wasteful of resources. I believe that patients with menopausal symptoms but *without* flushes or those who have asked for HRT, because of something that they have read, should have an assessment of their estrogen status, preferably by blood or urine estrogen assay before contemplating treatment. Patients with vasomotor symptoms whom one meets much more commonly, do not require steroid assay studies.

Professor R. W. Beard: Dr Yates has raised an important philosophical question as the investigations are time-consuming and expensive, are they therefore worthwhile? I would put it another way. We should not be giving treatment in a blanket empirical fashion until we know what we are doing. Initially it may be expensive to do these investigations, but if they are worthwhile, then in the end they will prove cheaper and easier to do.

Professor I. D. Cooke: Perhaps one day we shall be interested in giving some of these patients with higher estrogen levels antiestrogens, and then determinations may be important.

Section B

ENDOCRINOLOGY

PART 2

Chairman: R. W. BEARD

7

Pharmacology of natural and synthetic estrogens

K. Fotherby

During the past two decades there has been much controversy regarding the relative potencies of the two synthetic estrogens, ethinylestradiol and its 3-methyl ether (mestranol), used as components of the oral contraceptives. It is only recently that some clarification of this problem has been achieved. In addition it has also been suggested that mestranol might have some biological activities different from those of ethinylestradiol. A similar controversy is taking place in regard to the estrogens used for treatment of post-menopausal women, with the added complication that the number of estrogens being used is larger. At least six different estrogens or their derivatives are used, ethinylestradiol, mestranol, estradiol valerate, estrone sulphate, estriol dihemi-succinate and stilbestrol. The matter is further complicated by the fact that the estrogens may be used in combination with a progestogen and that one of the preparations used, Premarin, is a mixture of compounds; although it contains estrone sulphate as the major component it also contains small amounts of other estrogen sulphates. Again the controversy concerns not only the relative potency of the various estrogens but also the possibility that there may be differences between the estrogens in the spectrum of effects that they produce and in the way that these effects are produced.

Biological potency of estrogens

In general terms, the potency of a compound will depend upon:
(1) the route of administration, whether oral or parenteral, and any changes undergone by the compound either during absorption from the gastro-intestinal tract or absorption from the site of injection.

(2) the way in which it is metabolized. The activity will be affected by the rate at which the administered compound is metabolized, whether it binds to the plasma proteins and the effect which it has upon the binding of endogenous hormones.
(3) its degree of interaction with the tissues; in many cases this will be determined by the extent to which it interacts with the tissue receptor proteins.
(4) the capability of the tissues to respond to the stimulus produced by the compound.

The relative potencies obtained will depend upon which particular end point is being measured (Table 7.1). There are obvious difficulties in determining relative potencies in humans. Even in animals where more 'standardized' preparations can be obtained, relative potency may show considerable variations. There are, for example, considerable species differences

Table 7.1 Comparative activity of various steroids in inhibiting nidation, ovulation and gonadotrophin in the rat

	Relative potency		
Steroid	*Anti-nidation*	*Anti-ovulation*	*Anti-gonadotrophin release*
Estradiol	100	100	100
Estrone	70	150	30
Estriol	12	15	10
Ethinylestradiol	70	170	300
Mestranol	20	85	100

From Desaulles and Krahenbuhl[36] and Kincl[37]

(Table 7.2) and this presents difficulties in finding a suitable animal model which can be used to predict potency in humans. Large variations occur in results even when the same test is used (Table 7.3), the relative potency of estradiol and estrone in the Allen–Doisy test varying ten-fold or more when different administration schedules are used[1]. The same variations are apparent if a biochemical end point, for example the effect on plasma lipid concentration, is used and the potency determined in this way does not correlate with estrogenic potency as determined by tests using the uterine weight or vaginal smear responses[2].

Many of the difficulties encountered in determining relative potency *in vivo* can be overcome by *in vitro* testing and this is the only way in which the relative interaction of the compounds with tissues can be determined.

However relative potency obtained in this way may not be directly relevant to the *in vivo* situation. Thus the interaction of ethinylestradiol and diethylstilbestrol with uterine cytosol preparations is about double that of estradiol[3]. Similarly ethinylestradiol binding to hypothalamus and pituitary tissue preparations is much greater than that obtained with mestranol[4]

Table 7.2 The relative parenteral potency of estrogens compared with their oral activity (unity)

Experimental animals	*Relation of parenteral to oral dose* Estradiol-17β	*Estriol*	*Estrone*
Mice	75	0·67	62
Rats	620	1·4	198
Guinea pigs	1·8	—	19
Monkeys	20	—	5·0

From Pedersen-Bjergaard[38]

Table 7.3 The ratio of potencies of estradiol and estrone found by different investigators using ovariectomized rats or mice in the Allen-Doisy Test

Animals	*Number and nature of injections*	*Estradiol: estrone ratio*
Rats	3 Oily	6
Rats	6 Aqueous	7
Mice	3 Oily	0·8
Mice	6 Aqueous	3
Rats	1 Oily	3
Mice	1 Oily	2
Mice	3 Oily	2
Mice	6 Aqueous	2
Mice	5 Oily	5–10
Rats	3 Oily	12

From Emmens[39]

Metabolism of estrogens

A study of the metabolism of the compounds will help in the elucidation of their biological potency. Until recently it was widely accepted[5] that ethinylestradiol was twice as potent as mestranol. In studying changes in the concentration of cortisol binding globulin produced by administration of the estrogens the mean figure for the relative potency of mestranol compared to ethinylestradiol was 64%[6] and was regarded as confirming the above findings. However, the confidence limits for this mean value varied from 39% to 86%. A recent careful study [7–9] showed that in contrast to previous studies these two estrogens were equipotent in terms of antiovulatory activity, effect on plasma gonadotrophins and endometrial response. It now seems likely that these variations can be explained in terms of the metabolism of mestranol. Most of the mestranol which is administered appears to be fairly rapidly converted to ethinylestradiol[10] and similar results have been found in a more detailed pharmokinetic study[11]. It seems very likely therefore that many of the estimates regarding the relative potency of mestranol and ethinylestradiol were merely reflecting the degree to which subjects receiving these estrogens were able to convert mestranol to ethinylestradiol.

Estradiol valerate is rapidly absorbed, the maximum concentration in blood being reached in about 30 minutes[12] and a similar pattern is seen after the oral administration of estradiol itself[13]. Estrone sulphate is also rapidly absorbed and under normal circumstances is the major estrogen circulating

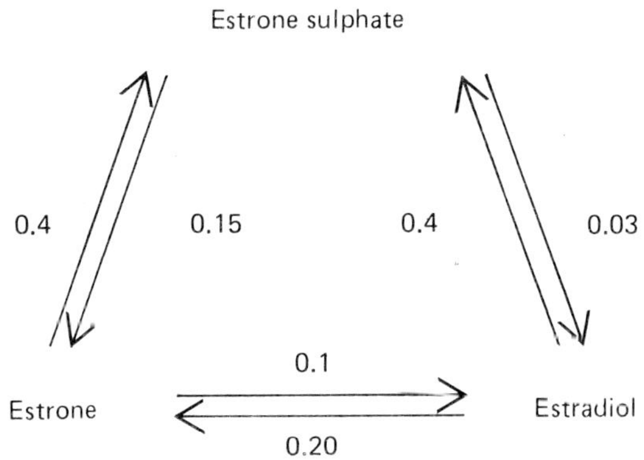

Figure 7.1 Interconversion of estradiol, estrone and its sulphate. (Values refer to transfer constants. From Longcope[15]).

the human. It reaches the peripheral circulation without undergoing significant metabolism by the liver. About 40% of the estrone and estradiol which is produced in the body is converted to estrone sulphate. The inter-relationships between estrone, estradiol and estrone sulphate are shown in Figure 7.1. The conversion of estrone to estradiol takes place to only a small extent but significant amounts of estradiol (about 20%) are converted to estrone[14–16]. From the equilibrium and transfer constants it has been calculated that a dose of estrone sulphate of 0·5 mg will give a plasma estrone production rate of 70 μg/day and an estradiol production rate of about 7 μg/day[14]. These values should be compared with the approximate production rates in post-menopausal women of about 40 μg/day for estrone and 5–7 μg/day for estradiol[17]. Estriol 16, 17-dihemisuccinate appears to be absorbed in the unchanged form[18], hydrolysis of the ester taking place rapidly in the liver.

Metabolic effects of estrogens

It has been suggested that synthetic estrogens may exert a greater effect on metabolic processes than 'natural' estrogens, interpreting this term to mean those compounds which after administration give rise in the circulation to estrogens which are similar to those produced endogenously.

Estrogens at high doses are known to lower serum cholesterol levels and to raise serum triglyceride levels; this effect may also occur with low doses, e.g. 20–40 μg mestranol[19]. Bolton *et al.*[20] found a rise in triglycerides when ethinylestradiol was administered in doses of 20–50 μg daily whereas administration of 0·625–1·25 mg/day Premarin had no effect. This latter finding was also noted by Notelovitz and Southwood[21]. However in a comparative study Robinson *et al.*[22] found that ethinylestradiol in a dose of 10 μg per day for one year had no effect upon cholesterol or phospholipid levels but changes were found with Premarin at doses of 0·625 mg and above daily.

Many reports, often conflicting, have been published regarding changes in glucose tolerance in women using oral contraceptives. Beck[23] concluded that the synthetic estrogens had no discernable effects on glucose tolerance or peripheral insulin metabolism in normal women at the doses used in the pill. Spellacy *et al.*[24] also found that ethinylestradiol, mestranol and Premarin did not change glucose tolerance although there was an increase in the fasting growth hormone levels except with Premarin. No change in glucose tolerance occurred when the dose of ethinylestradiol was increased 10 times to 0·5 mg/day. Notelovitz[25] also found no effect of Premarin on glucose tolerance. However in a dose of 1·25 mg daily this compound has been reported to decrease glucose tolerance[26]. Other workers have reported changes in glucose tolerance with quite small doses of mestranol, e.g.[27] and these reports suggest that mestranol may have a more pronounced effect than other estrogens. Most would agree that the changes produced by estrogens are more apparent in pre-diabetic subjects.

Similarly variations have been observed in the measurement of various coagulation factors. Elkeles *et al.*[28] in a comparison of ethinylestradiol, mestranol, Premarin and stilbestrol found that their administration had no significant effect on platelet adhesiveness but that platelet aggregation induced by ADP was increased by all estrogens tested. However, only the synthetic estrogens changed the electrophoretic mobility induced by ADP whereas Premarin and low doses of mestranol had no effect. In the study of Bolton *et al.*[20] a number of factors (plasma fibrinogen, platelet adhesiveness and partial thromboplastin time) remained unchanged by the administration of ethinylestradiol at doses of 20–50 μg daily or Premarin at doses of 0·625–1·25 mg/daily. Greig and Notelovitz[29] found that Premarin (1·25 mg daily) did not affect antithrombin III levels. Astedt and Jeppsson[30] found no change in the fibrinolytic activity of vein walls in women receiving estradiol at a dose of 10 mg daily for 10 days although it was decreased in similar studies using 250 μg ethinylestradiol daily for 10 days.

Other estimates of relative potency in humans

The concentration of certain proteins in plasma, particularly corticosteroid binding globulin and caeruloplasmin, is affected by estrogens and the response to estrogen appears to be dose related[31]. These workers carried out a comparison of changes following the administration of Premarin, stilbestrol and ethinylestradiol and found potency ratios of 1:14:200 respectively.

Rudel and Kincl[32] studied the antiovulatory activity of a number of estrogens in women who received the compound from day 5 to day 24 of the menstrual cycle. They found ethinylestradiol and mestranol to be about 100 times as active as estradiol and Premarin and stilbestrol were much less active. Earlier studies, with similar results, were performed by Howard *et al.*[33] and Tokuyama[34].

A few reports have appeared regarding the relative effectiveness of the various estrogens in the treatment of menopausal symptoms. All appear to be clinically effective. Kupperman *et al.*[35] devized a menopausal index, a numerical conversion factor of the severity of the eleven most common menopausal symptoms, to compare a number of estrogens and found the most effective to be ethinylestradiol 50 μg daily followed by estradiol 2 mg daily, Premarin 1·25 mg daily and stilbestrol 0·3 mg daily.

It is apparent from the above account that our knowledge of the relative potency and metabolic effects of the estrogens is still meagre. The increasing use of hormone replacement therapy makes it necessary to carry out properly designed and carefully controlled clinical trials which should include assessment of both short and long term changes in metabolic parameters.

References

1. Morgan, C. F. (1963). A comparison of topical and subcutaneous methods of administration of sixteen oestrogens. *J. Endocrinol.*,**26,** 317
2. Drill, V. A. and Riegel, B. (1958). Structural and hormonal activity of some new steroids. *Recent Progr. Horm. Res.*, **14,** 29
3. Korenman, S. G. (1969). Comparative binding affinity of estrogens and its relation to estrogenic potency. *Steroids*, **13,** 163
4. Eisenfeld, A. (1974). Oral contraceptives: ethinylestradiol binds with higher affinity than mestranol to macromolecules from the sites of anti-fertility action. *Endocrinology*, **94,** 803
5. Christie, G. A. (1970). Comparative potency of ethinyl oestradiol and mestranol. *Med. J. Austral.*, **2,** 202
6. Schwartz, U. and Hammerstein, J. (1974). The oestrogenic potency of various contraceptive steroids as determined by their effects on transcortin-binding capacity. *Acta Endocrinol.*, **76,** 159
7. Goldzieher, J. W., Maqueo, M., Chenault, C. B. and Woutersz, T. B. (1975). Comparative studies of the ethynyl estrogens used in oral contraceptives. I. Endometrial response *Am. J. Obstet. Gynecol.*, **122,** 615
8. Goldzieher, J. W., de la Pena, A., Chenault, C. B. and Cervantes, A. (1975). Comparative studies of the ethynyl estrogens used in oral contraceptives. III Effect on plasma gonadotropins. *Am. J. Obstet. Gynecol.*, **122,** 625
9. Goldzieher, J. W., de la Pena, A., Chenault, C. B. and Woutersz, T. B. (1975). Comparative studies of the ethynyl estrogens used in oral contraceptives. II Antiovulatory potency. *Am. J. Obstet. Gynecol.*, **122,** 619
10. Warren, R. J. and Fotherby, K. (1973). Plasma levels of ethynyloestradiol after administration of ethynyloestradiol or mestranol to human subjects. *J. Endocrinol.*, **59,** 369
11. Bolt, H. M. and Bolt, W. H. (1974). Pharmacokinetics of mestranol in man in relation to its oestrogenic activity. *Europ. J. Clin. Pharmacol.*, **7,** 295
12. Kolb, K. H. (1967). The metabolism of oestradiol valerate. Medizinische Mitteilungen, **28,** 16
13. Fishman, J., Goldberg, S., Rosenfeld, R. S., Zumoff, B., Hellman, L. and Gallagher, T. F. (1969). Intermediates in the transformation of oral estradiol. *J. Clin. Endocrinol.*, **29,** 41
14. Ruder, H. J., Loriaux, L. and Lipsett, M. B. (1972). Estrone sulfate: production rate and metabolism in man. *J. Clin. Invest.*, **51,** 1020
15. Longcope, C. (1972). The metabolism of estrone sulfate in normal males. *J. Clin. Endocrinol.*, **34,** 113
16. Longcope, C. and Williams, K. I. H. (1974). The metabolism of estrogens in normal women after pulse injections of ^{3}H-estradiol and ^{3}H-estrone. *J. Clin. Endocrinol.*, **38,** 602
17. Longcope, C. (1971). Metabolic clearance and blood production rates of estrogens in postmenopausal women. *Am. J. Obstet. Gynecol.*, **111,** 778

18. van der Vies, J. (1965). Fate of oestriol-16,17 dihemisuccinate after oral administration to rats. *Acta Endocrinol.*, **48,** 630
19. Aitken, J. M., Lorimer, A. R., Hart, D. M., Lawrie, T. D. V. and Smith, D. A. (1971). The effects of oophorectomy and long-term mestranol therapy on the serum lipids of middle-aged women. *Clin. Sci.*, **41,** 597
20. Bolton, C. H., Ellwood, M., Hartog, M., Martin, R., Rowe, A. S. and Wensley, R. T. (1975). Comparison of the effects of ethynyloestradiol and conjugated equine oestrogens in oophorectomized women. *Clin. Endocrinol.*, **4,** 131
21. Notelovitz, M. and Southwood, B. (1974). Metabolic effect of conjugated oestrogens on lipids and lipoproteins. *South African Med. J.*, **48,** 2552
22. Robinson, R. W., Higano, N. and Cohen, W. D. (1960). Effect of long-term administration of estrogens on serum lipids of postmenopausal women. *N. Engl. J. Med.*, **263,** 828
23. Beck, P. (1973). Contraceptive steroids: modifications of carbohydrate and lipid metabolism. *Metabolism*, **22,** 841
24. Spellacy, W. N., Buhi, W. C. and Birk, S. A. (1972). The effect of estrogens on carbohydrate metabolism: glucose, insulin and growth hormone studies on one hundred and seventy-one women ingesting Premarin, mestranol and ethinyl oestradiol for six months. *Am. J. Obstet. Gynecol.*, **114,** 378
25. Notelovitz, M. (1974). Metabolic effect of conjugated oestrogens on glucose tolerance. *South African Med. J.*, **48,** 2599
26. Goldman, J. A. and Ovadia, J. L. (1969). The effect of estrogen on intravenous glucose tolerance in women. *Am. J. Obstet. Gynecol.*, **103,** 172
27. Gow, S. and MacGillivray, I. (1971). Metabolic, hormonal and vascular changes after synthetic oestrogen therapy in oophorectomized women. *Br. Med. J.*, **2,** 73
28. Elkeles, R. S., Hampton, J. R. and Mitchell, J. R. A. (1968). Effect of oestrogens on human platelet behaviour. *Lancet*, **ii,** 315
29. Greig, H. B. W. and Notelowitz, M. (1975). Natural oestrogens and antithrombin III levels. *Lancet*, **i,** 412
30. Astedt, B. and Jeppsson, S. (1974). Oestradiol and the fibrinolytic activity of vein walls. *J. Obstet. Gynaecol. Br. Commonwlth*, **81,** 719
31. Musa, B. U., Seal, U. S. and Doe, R. P. (1965). Elevation of certain plasma proteins in man following estrogen administration: a dose–response relationship. *J. Clin. Endocrinol.*, **25,** 1163
32. Rudel, H. W. and Kincl, F. A. (1966). The biology of antifertility steroids. *Acta Endocrinol, Suppl.* 105, **51,** 7
33. Howard, R. P., Keaty, E. C. and Reifenstein, E. C. (1956). *J. Clin. Endocrinol.*, **14,** 509
34. Tokuyama, T., Leach, R. B., Sheinfield, S. and Maddock, W. C. (1954). *J. Clin. Endocrinol.*, **14,** 509
35. Kupperman, H. S., Blatt, M. H. G., Wiesbader, H. and Filler, W. (1953). Comparative clinical evaluation of estrogenic preparations by the menopausal and amenorrheal indices. *J. Clin. Endocrinol.* **13,** 688
36. Desaulles, P. A. and Krahenbuhl, C. (1964). Comparison of the antifertility and sex hormonal activities of sex hormones and their derivatives. *Acta Endocrinol.*, **47,** 444
37. Kincl, F. A. (1972). Oestrogens as antifertility agents. International Encyclopaedia of Pharmacology and Therapeutics. Section 48, Vol. II (M. Tausk, ed.) pp 347–384 (Oxford: Pergamon Press)

38. Pedersen-Bjergaard, K. (1939). *Comparative Studies Concerning the Strengths of Estrogenic Substances* (London and New York: Oxford University Press)
39. Emmens, C. W. (1939). Report on biological standards. V. Variables affecting the estimation of androgenic and oestrogenic activity. Medical Research Council (Brit) Special Report Series No. 234, 1939

8

Estrogen target organs and receptor

R. W. Taylor

α-Estrogen has widespread effects on the mammalian body and psyche. It interferes extensively with the plasma binding and thus with the activities of other hormones. Most dramatically of all it produces well defined and easily demonstrable changes in what are generally called the 'target tissues' (Figure 8.1)[1, 2]

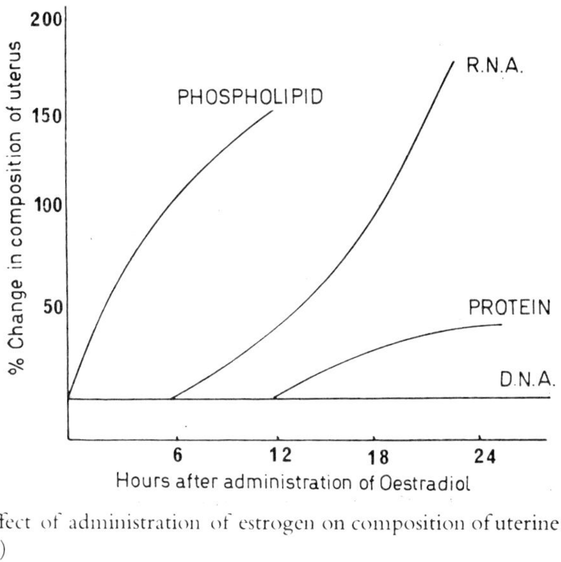

Figure 8.1 Effect of administration of estrogen on composition of uterine tissue. (After Meuller, 1965)

The characteristic of target tissues is the presence of highly specific protein receptor molecules within the cells which fasten firmly to estradiol. By this definition the target tissues are those derived from the Müllerian duct, the breast, the hypothalamus and the anterior pituitary gland[3].

The nature of the cell response to estrogen stimulus depends upon the character of the cell nucleus and will therefore vary from one tissue to another. Thus the glandular cells of the endometrium proliferate under the influence of estrogen while the cells of the endosalpinx secrete a fluid which is very important in determining normal fertility. However the interaction of the steroid molecule with the receptor proteins of the cytoplasm and its subsequent movement into the nucleus appears to be similar in all target tissues. Because human endometrium is comparatively easy to obtain and to work with we elected to study the mode of estrogen action in this tissue and the outline of the process is based upon these studies.

The movement of estrogen within the target cell

The events which follow the entry of the estradiol molecule into the cell are a matter of some conjecture but the best interpretation at present is illustrated in Figure 8.2[4]. The estradiol becomes fixed to the receptor protein and the whole complex moves towards the nuclear membrane. The original receptor

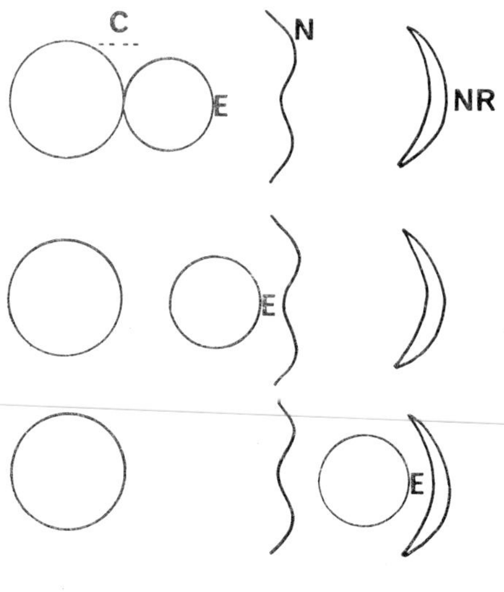

Figure 8.2 Hypothetical model for estrogen transport into target tissue nuclei. (From Jungblutt[4], courtesy of Pergamon Press)

splits and the smaller fraction to which the estradiol has become attached moves into the nucleus. There it becomes fixed to a separate nuclear receptor.

The specificity of the estrogen–receptor reaction

The specificity of the receptor molecule is high. The estradiol when it gains entry into a target cell remains unaltered. This is in sharp contrast to the events which occur in organs such as the liver where the steroid is metabolized and many new compounds produced[5].

Experiments using the 17α isomer of estradiol show that retention within the uterus is poor, suggesting that the 17β configuration is important[6]. However 17-methyl estradiol, 17α ethinylestradiol, hexestrol, diethyl stilbestrol and dienestrol are all retained within the target cell in a way similar to that of 17β estradiol[5]. The presence of an unsaturated steroid ring with an attached hydroxyl group may be the significant feature common to these compounds. Estriol is retained to a lesser extent within the target cell

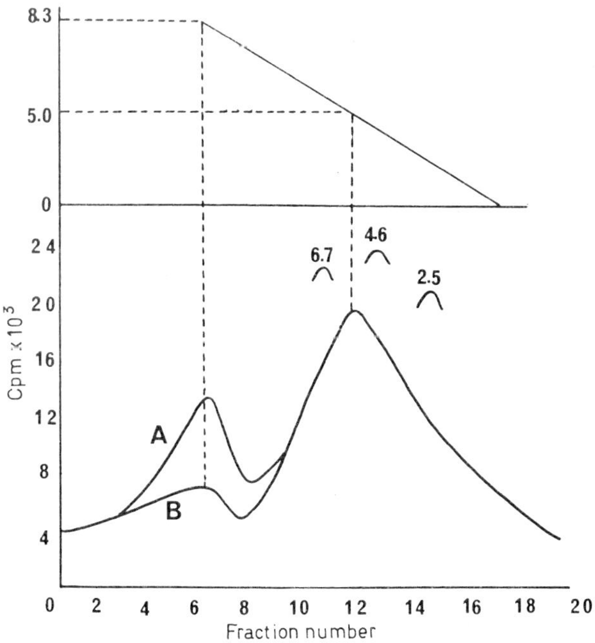

Figure 8.3 Sucrose gradient profile ³H-labelled-estradiol cytoplasmic receptor. Shows binding of labelled hormone at 8S and 4-5S (A) and elimination of specific 8S binding by pre-treatment with excess, unlabelled estradiol (B)

and estrone is retained only after it has first been altered to 17-estradiol[5]. Testosterone, cortisone and progesterone are not retained by estrogen receptors[7].

The nature of the receptor molecule

The cytoplasmic receptor is an acidic protein having a molecular weight of about 236 000[8]. It separates in the 8–10S range a sucrose gradient (Figure 8.3). The estradiol binding is acid labile, destroyed by trypsin but unaffected by RNAase or DNAase[9].

The nuclear receptor is a smaller molecule than is the cytoplasmic receptor. It separates as a 4–5S protein in a sucrose gradient. The estradiol binding is also acid labile, the attachment being to a non-histone component of the nuclear chromatin[10]. This binding is destroyed by trypsin but unaffected by DNAase or RNAase.

The quality of the estradiol–receptor binding

In a series of *in vitro* experiments, employing tritium labelled estradiol and separating firmly bound from free estradiol by precipitation with dextran/

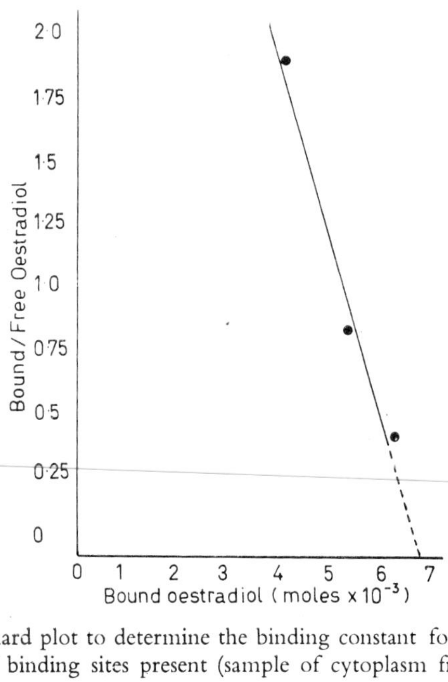

Figure 8.4 A Scatchard plot to determine the binding constant for estradiol receptors and the number of binding sites present (sample of cytoplasm from follicular phase endometrium)

charcoal a series of Scatchard plots were constructed[11]. One such plot is illustrated (Figure 8.4). The slope of the line gives the dissociation constant and the intersect on the abcissa indicates the number of such binding sites available[12]. The number of cytoplasmic binding sites in edometrium and endosalpinx varies from 4 to 6000, with the probability that the number is higher in the endometrium. The dissociation constant varies from 2 to 4×10^{-10} M[13]. By the nature of the experimental techniques this may be somewhat overestimated but it nevertheless indicates a remarkably high affinity of the receptor for estradiol. It is calculated that circulating estrogens are bound to serum proteins with dissociation constants of the order of 10^{-3}–10^{-6} M[13]. The affinity of target tissues for estrogen may thus be from 1 to 10 million times greater than is the affinity of the serum proteins. For this reason, estrogen-dependent tissues may obtain their necessary stimulus from minute levels of circulating hormone, an extremely economical system.

The influence of endogenous hormones on estrogen binding

Brush *et al.*[14] first suggested that the uptake of estrogen and its intracellular distribution might be different in the two phases of the normal menstrual cycle. This was confirmed and the role of progesterone, progestational agents and anti-estrogens suggested[11]. The number of cytoplasmic binding sites appears to increase with estrogen stimulation over a considerable period of time but there is no obvious increase during the short time of the average menstrual cycle. This may perhaps explain the refractory period often noted between the application of local estrogen cream and the relief of atrophic vaginitis. However, as the estrogen stimulus of the first part of the menstrual cycle proceeds, progesterone receptors appear, reaching their maximum number at about the time of ovulation. This would explain the fact that progesterone does not have a noticeable effect upon the endometrium unless it has previously been primed by estrogen[15]. The proportion of intracellular estrogen that gains access to the cell nucleus falls from a mean 80% in the follicular phase to 19% in the luteal phase. This is a progestational effect, not an effect of long continued estrogen stimulation. It is not seen in conditions of cystic hyperplasia or endometrial carcinoma but it can be induced by progesterone or progestational agents[11].

Advancing age sees a diminution in the number of estrogen receptors but they never disappear and their number increases to that found in the normal reproductive years when an estrogen stimulus is applied.

Anti-estrogens

The term anti-estrogens is variously used. To some, an anti-estrogen is a substance which blocks the fixation of estradiol by the cytoplasmic receptor.

Compounds such as stilbestrol come into this category. However, because the cells treat some compounds like this as estrogens, the clinical effect may be indistinguishable from the natural steroid. To the clinician, an anti-estrogen is a compound which prevents some of the effects of estrogen on tissues. This implies that they prevent the steroid molecule reaching the target cell nucleus. Using a technique employing the human endosalpinx[11] a number of compounds have been tested for their effectiveness in reducing the proportion of administered labelled estradiol which gains access to the cell nucleus. Clomiphene citrate and 'Tamoxiphen' (ICI) reduce the proportion of estradiol bound to the nuclear fraction of the target cells by 70–80%. They are thus comparable to progesterone in this respect.

References

1. Meuller, G. C. (1965). In: *Mechanisms of Hormone Action*, p. 228. (New York: Academic Press)
2. Jeffcoate, T. N. A. (1975). In: *Principles of Gynaecology*, 4th, ed. p. 73. (London: Butterworth)
3. Littge, W. G. and Whalen, R. E. (1970). *Steroids*, **15,** 605
4. Jungblutt, P. W. (1968). *Advances in Biosciences*, Vol. 2, pp. 157 (G. Raspe, ed.). (Braunschweig: Pergamon Press)
5. Jensen, E. V. and Jacobsen, M. (1962). *Rec. Prog. Horm. Res.*, **18,** 387
6. Terenius, L. (1968). *Cancer Research*, **28,** 328
7. Toft, D., Shyamala, G. and Gorski, J. (1967). *Proc. Nat. Acad. Sci. U.S.A.*, **57,** 1740
8. Puca, G. A., Nola, V. and Bresciani, F. (1971). *Advances in Biosciences*, **7** (In prep. New York: Pergamon Press)
9. Gorski, J., Toft, D., Shyamala, G., Smith, D. and Notides, A. (1968). *Recent Progress in Hormone Research*, **24,** 45. (New York: Academic Press)
10. King, R. J. B. (1967). *Arch. Anat. microse, Morph. exp.*, **56,** 570
11. Taylor, R. W. (1974). The mechanism of action of oestrogen in the human female. *J. Obstet. Gynaec. Brit. Cwlth.*, **81,** 856
12. Scatchard, G. (1949). *N.Y. Acad. Sci., Annals*, **51,** 660
13. Westphal, U. (1961). In: *Mechanisms of Action of Steroid Hormones*, pp 33. (New York: Pergamon Press)
14. Brush, M. G., Taylor, R. W. and Maxwell, R. (1966). *J. Obstet. Gynaec. Brit. Cwlth.*, **73,** 954
15. Crocker, S. and King, R. J. B. (1974). Personal Communication

Discussion on Section B:

Endocrinology (Part 2)

Chairman: *Professor R. W. Beard*

Professor R. W. Beard: We have heard some of the modes of action of estrogens, and ways of assessing their modes of action, and also their sites of action.

Dr N. G. Mussalli (Obstetrician, Welwyn Garden City): The speakers have told us of the anabolic effects of estrogens. Could they tell us something about the effect on adipose tissue, and especially the effect on cyclase and lipase?

Dr K. Fotherby (Biochemist, London): Lipase is the principal enzyme on which the estrogens are supposed to act but a number of other factors are also involved, which is probably why the overall picture that one sees varies considerably. I did not have the time to go into it fully but I wanted to show that the different reports on changes in the various plasma lipids in people treated with estrogens show a considerable variation in the responses which have been obtained.

Professor V. Wynn (Human metabolism, London): I believe what the questioner had in mind was the mode of action of estrogens on lipid metabolism as such, and this is very complex. The most fundamental action of an estrogen is probably to induce certain hepatic enzymes, particularly fatty acid synthetase, and acetyl-coA-carboxylase Both these enzymes are important in terms of fatty acid triglyceride synthesis. The other site of action of an estrogen that one could pick out—I am only mentioning the controlling sites of estrogen activity—would be phosphorenyl-pyruvate-carboxy-kinase, which is very important in terms of gluconeogenesis.

If I may, while we are talking about the metabolic effects of estrogens, pick up a point made by Dr Fotherby concerning estrogen effects on carbohydrate metabolism. It is perfectly true that estrogens, given alone, in moderate doses, have little discernable effect on glucose tolerance. They do, however, have quite a distinct effect on fasting glucose levels causing hypoglycaemia, the mode of action being interference with glucagon secretion and a change in the portal blood insulin to glucagon ratio. That is why there can be a hypoglycaemic effect in pregnancy.

Dr Fotherby mentioned metabolic changes in connection with the Pill, but there have been remarkably few studies of carbohydrate or any other metabolic parameter in post-menopausal women. We have to remember however that the pill in its usual form is a combined steroid preparation, and if the estrogen is combined with a 19-nortestosterone—that is to say a progestogen derived from a 19-nor steroid—then quite distinct changes in carbohydrate metabolism occur, which do not occur, to any extent, when estrogen is used alone, or when estrogen is combined with an acetoxy-progesterone derived progestogen.

Mr B. Eton (Gynaecologist, Hastings): Professor Taylor has pointed out that estrogens increase the number of receptors in certain gynaecological cancers. Could he describe the effects of high-dosage progestogens in that context, bearing in mind their therapeutic use?

Professor R. W. Taylor (Gynaecologist, London): They have exactly the same effect as they have in normal cells. The response to be got from a tumour can be calculated, providing it is a piece of actively growing tumour, by counting the number of estrogen receptors. One can work backwards from there to work out how many progesterone receptors there are, and so tell which patients will respond to progestational therapy. The effect of the progestogen is to prevent the estrogen from getting into the cell nucleus.

Mr E. S. Saunders (Gynaecologist, London): Are what are called 'natural' estrogens any different from the so-called synthetic estrogens? I have the feeling that the pharmaceutical firms take advantage insofar as they say that the hormones which are called natural hormones are all made from natural ingredients, namely the urine of pregnant mares. In fact they used to be made that way, but nowadays they are made synthetically, because the biochemists know their chemical structure. The public is being misled. Patients often ask if an estrogen is a nautral estrogen but these tablets are not a natural estrogen. Could Dr Fotherby clear up the question? Is there really such a difference in the value of the treatment between the so-called 'natural' hormones and the others?

Dr K. Fotherby: I wanted to retain the term 'natural estrogens' for those compounds which are used therapeutically, and which after administration produce *in vivo* compounds of the same structure as those which are produced endogenously. In this case one could call Progynova (estradiol valerate) a natural estrogen to the extent that after administration it increases the blood concentration of estradiol, a naturally occurring hormone. The same thing could be said for Premarin, or estrone sulphate. I do not like the term 'natural estrogen' because one has to define fairly closely what it means. Also, although these compounds may give rise *in vivo* to estrogens similar to those produced by the ovary or the adrenal, the way in which they are produced and the pattern of concentration in the circulation is different. Obviously endogenously produced steroids are secreted at a reasonably constant rate throughout the period of the day, taking into account diurnal variations and so forth, whereas oral treatment with compounds of the type like Progynova, or estrone sulphate provides pulse administration, intermittently increasing quite markedly the blood concentrations of estradiol, estrone or estrone sulphate. This pattern of concentration is different from that to be seen under *in vivo* situations. That may have quite a marked bearing on the biological effects that they produce.

Professor R. W. Taylor: It depends which effect one is looking at, too. The administration of pulsed estrogen makes no great difference if one is looking at its effect on, say, the vaginal epithelium, or the endometrium. Pulses can be given once in 24, or even once in 48 hours, and the same effect can still be produced. The other metabolic effects are more likely to be influenced by the type of estrogen given.

Dr K. Fotherby: That will depend on the time course for the particular biological activity which is being considered. In the case of vaginal smears, this will extend over a long period of time which is why the pulse effect and continuous administration produce roughly similar results. There may well be differences in metabolic effects.

Professor R. W. Beard: We should like to know whether we should be giving a compound like Harmogen (piperazine estrone sulphate), or whether we can give stilbestrol to women for long term therapy. Can we answer that question?

Dr K. Fotherby: We cannot answer that, because it depends on so many variables, as regards dose, and for how long, and the way in which the dose will be given, and so on.

Professor R. W. Beard: Let me be more specific. If we give Harmogen, for example we shall be giving one tablet for many many weeks, possibly years. Is this a safer compound, as opposed to say stilbestrol?

Dr K. Fotherby: I do not think that we are in any situation to answer this question. We need some very rigorously controlled, properly designed clinical trials, and I have seen no reports of any such so far in the literature.

Dr H. S. Jacobs (Gynaecological endocrinologist, London): Were the figures given by Dr Fotherby for the transfer constants of estrone, estrone sulphate and estradiol obtained in post-menopausal women, or in pre-menopausal women? They might differ.

Dr K. Fotherby: The figures were for pre-menopausal women, and there may well be some variations in the post-menopausal, although I do not think that they will be vastly different from the figures that I produced. At least two groups of investigators have measured the transfer constants, and both sets of results agree reasonably well.

Dr D. G. May (General Practitioner, Surbiton): Professor Taylor touched on the capacity of estrogen to combine with carcinoma cells. Obviously in the post-menopausal woman, it would be inadvisable to give hormones to a woman who has had a hormone-dependent tumour removed. Would it also be inadvisable to give them to somebody who has had another carcinoma, say an adeno-carcinoma of the colon, removed?

Professor R. W. Taylor: From the point of view of the individual tumour cell, there would be no particular problem. There are no estrogen receptors in carcinoma from the colon. We have looked at the gut and at a number of other tumours as well. There might be a positive benefit if one was looking in terms of general metabolic effect, because one of the effects of estrogens is to stimulate the immunological defence mechanism. Estrogen therapy certainly does no harm, and might do some good.

Mr C. H. Naylor (Gynaecologist, London): Do estrogens have any effect on the immune response?

Professor R. W. Taylor: It is not my field but from my recall of the literature I think that they enhance the immune response.

Section C

PSYCHOLOGICAL ASPECTS

Chairman: C. H. NAYLOR

9

Emotional response to the menopause

Margaret Christie Brown

The menopause is a time of change, both physical and psychological. I shall be concentrating on the psychological aspects, although the interaction of emotion on hormone and hormone on emotion makes any division rather false.

Although the incidence of major psychological illness, particularly severe depression, is sometimes said to be increased at the menopause, I shall leave this point for others to comment on. I shall discuss the frequently occurring complaints of anxiety, misery and minor depression that occur at this time.

The menopause coincides with middle age, and these two factors and the implications of them, can impinge on one another and greatly confuse the effects and way of coping with either. It is this combination of factors which causes difficulty in understanding the problems and I want to discuss some of the factors involved.

First of all, let us look at the various phases of life we pass through, of which middle age is one. It is a phase of life common to us all, men and women. The way we deal with such phases, whether puberty, adolescence, marriage or parenthood, depends on again, a number of factors: Our general situation and degree of contentment, our genetic make up and, probably the most important of all, the expectations we have about the new stage we are to go through. Our expectations are based on past experience and the experience of the people around us so that a mother who always had very painful periods will produce a different environment and expectations for her daughter, to one who had no trouble at all. Similarly obviously, a child brought up in a family where mother and father showed each other love and affection has a different expectation of marriage to the child brought up in a warlike or divided family. So that life continuously demands that we adjust to new phases.

What is different for women, is the way these phases of development have an accompanying drama, so that at puberty there is the sudden rather miraculous regular appearance of blood, heralding the reproductive era, at parturition there is the appearance of a baby and at the menopause, the end of this reproductive era, the loss of periods. With these demonstrations of fact, it is less easy for the woman to deny their implications, than it is for the man, so that quite apart from hormonal imbalance at these times, causing extra difficulty, there is considerable emotional and philosophical readjustment to make, in the case of the menopause to the recognition of the passage of time, the loss of youth and potential and the approach of death.

Let us consider further the implications of these facts of life. These are all to do with frightening ideas of loss, change and end.

At puberty one faces the loss of childhood, of protection and of parents. Some never tolerate these losses and remain largely dependent people. Sometimes they transfer the dependence to a spouse, sometimes they retain parents as the major security figure.

At parturition comes the loss of freedom, both physically and emotionally—again some never tolerate this; extramarital relationships may develop or the woman may bring her mother into the home to do the entire mothering while she continues her career as if no change had occurred.

At the menopause many changes occur—parents die, children leave home, etc. The ability to cope with new phases in life depends on the appropriate maturity of the individual. The more emotionally mature a person is, the more she is capable of adjustment to change and loss. There are many ways of defining maturity but perhaps a simple one in this context is that the mature person does not feel herself to be entirely dependent on another person and is flexible enough to change aims and goals as this becomes appropriate and necessary.

The achievement of maturity and the satisfaction of the period of life which is to come, is related to the ability to let go of the preceding phase. This ability may depend on the degree of satisfaction achieved within it.

We should examine factors which make it difficult to let go of the preceding phase of life. Firstly, it may have been too satisfying and protected, and parents may have encouraged dependence and fear of the world because of their own inability to let go. Secondly, paradoxically, it may not have been satisfactory enough so that the individual continues to seek what was missing as a child when she is an adult and it is no longer appropriate or achievable. So that the ability to let go of the preceding phase may depend on the degree of satisfaction achieved within it. The passage of time is easier to tolerate if well spent. The middle aged person in the greatest distress, is the one who feels she missed opportunities or failed to have what she most needed.

I should now like to consider some of the early factors of development which may lead to difficulty in maturing, a sense of failure and an inability to adjust.

A large part of female psychology is involved with implications drawn from the perception of the anatomical differences between the sexes. With the discovery at a very young age that the boy has advantageous parts which she does not, comes a period of envy and a sense of inferiority which may lead to the need to find compensations and which may also lead to a permanent resentment towards the male and a permanent devaluing of the female aspects of her. One child may find compensation for these uncomfortable resentments by totally involving herself in identifying with mother and denying her envy by overvaluing her female function—her whole sense of self esteem lying in her domestic reproductive role. The loss of this role may seem to be the loss of all that is valuable in her and even her reason for living.

Another child may have compensated for her lack of penis by proving she is as good a man as the rest and by becoming a tomboy. Tomboys tend to despise feminine things and idealize masculine ones. They are frequently very successful in life because proving success is so very important to them—their self esteem rests in achievement. This kind of woman is often very resentful when she realizes that in sexual matters she is vulnerable in a way that the man is not. For her, from the moment she has intercourse she risks pregnancy or risks side effects from the prevention of pregnancy. Because of this fact, we can see pregnancy, parturition, lactation and care of the child form a natural logical part of female sexuality. Often it is a resented part and today the trend is to deny this link between sex and reproduction but it is there, even if only seen in the extremely energetic efforts made to produce a perfect method of contraception in order better to separate the two. Particularly today, sex and reproduction are almost the only fields which are totally representative of femaleness or maleness.

The female who was strongly a tomboy often has difficulty in accepting her reproductive role but may manage to displace her need for achievement on to the production of children—take this away from her and she feels again the loss of self esteem and a great sense of regret over lost career opportunities—in other words she sees herself as no longer having the opportunity for achievement. She often blames husband and children for this and may try to continue to achieve through her children—putting extra pressure on them for success. The marriage of a child, likely around this time, takes this compensation away since the child is no longer under her control and depression may set in.

On the other hand the woman who has not come to terms with her reproductive capacity may find it difficult to let go of a phase that she has never yet fulfilled, yet still partly hoping to fulfil it. There are several women seen each year at Chelsea who panic after 40 when they have not had a child—they could not take up the challenge when it was there—they cannot bear to pass the challenge when the time comes. Particularly relevant here were a couple married 15 years who had never consummated the marriage and who waited until the wife was 44 before trying to deal with their infertility.

Therefore, where overvaluing, undervaluing or imposing of other attributes on the function of reproduction has occurred, difficulty is to be expected with the menopause. Many women say that they thought they would be pleased at no longer having to worry about pregnancy after the menopause but are surprised to find that it seems to take away the whole purpose of life and sex. This feeling is particularly strong in those bought up as Roman Catholics in whom there is the added complication of the teaching that the purpose of copulation is conception.

One of the difficulties of the menopause which Kinsey has pointed out is the fact that many women, conditioned by upbringing against sexual pleasure, slowly, within the security of love and marriage, reach a state of disinhibition and satisfaction, just as the man, often with much of his sexual drive quenched by early rejection, begins to lose interest and potency. At around 50 he is likely to be very involved in his work, perhaps threatened by younger men; possibly facing his own feelings of failure to realize his ambitions and trying to deny his failing sexual interest. Perhaps he is trying to prove his potency with a younger woman, more attractive and exciting and therefore more likely to arouse his flagging sexual interest. His loss of interest in his wife will certainly be experienced by her as a loss of love and arouse fears of being rejected, left alone and unloved. This loss of interest in sex by her husband may also be experienced by the wife as a deliberate aggressive withholding, with the arousal of her anger and resentment which then has to be coped with.

Many mild psychological symptoms and physical symptoms experienced at these crisis points of change in our lives may then be psychosomatic. This means that painful feelings of anxiety, anger or fear may be displaced unconsciously into distressing but less emotionally disturbing symptoms, which the patient hopes may be coped with by medical means, since they may seem impossible to deal with by any other means. Thus, symptoms arise which make for an acceptable complaint that can be looked at and cared for by husband and doctor without embarrassment. For example, a feeling of bitter resentment towards the husband is not an acceptable patient response, and the husband or doctor who would then feel there was nothing he could do about it, but sleeplessness, headaches, backache and depression are well known acceptable symptoms to have at this time of life. This displacement is, of course, unconscious and is in no way a sort of malingering. However, the patient will, also unconsciously, often try to hide from the doctor the real cause of her distress and will resist talking about it, as her way of dealing with it is to deny and displace it.

To give an example of some of these points. In the more immature woman, the loss of parents, likely around the menopause, may be experienced as more than just sadness. The loss may produce a feeling of panic and a fear of inability to cope. An example of this was a woman complaining of various symptoms of anxiety and loss of libido which were attributed by her doctor and herself as due to the menopause. On careful questioning however, the symptoms coincided with her mother remarrying and going to live in America, leaving her to look after her own teenage son, husband and house for the first time in her married life. Her mother had had a flat downstairs and looked after them all. The patient had become pregnant by accident and had continued to deny her adult state to the point at which her child had become severely disturbed and she had attended a child guidance clinic with him for 4 years. Faced with the loss of security and need to take responsibility she panicked. It was difficult for her to face the reality of the situation and needless to say she disliked my interpretations and produced a particularly dramatic response to taking estrogen—as she herself said, she couldn't face looking into her relationship with her mother all over again as she had had to do at the child guidance clinic with her son.

Where the marriage is an unsuccessful one, a woman may have used her children as an emotional replacement of husband and invested all her good loving feelings in the child. The loss of the child by its marriage may arouse intense feelings of loss, rage and envy towards the new member of the family who she is expected to love. This may place a burden of having to control emotions with which the woman cannot cope, on top of the hormonal upheaval she may also be coping with.

The woman who has a hysterectomy has to deal with all her feelings more acutely with no time for adaptation. Where no discussion has been possible before an operation the anxieties are often denied and suppressed and then rather like delayed mourning, may cause trouble for years. I saw recently a patient who had experienced this. She remembered feeling rather shocked when told she should have a hysterectomy but apparently went through the operation with no feelings of anxiety. Since then however, she has suffered with 'nerves' and loss of libido—has been on diazepam, has been charged with shop lifting and has felt frightened and agoraphobic ever since—despite estrogen replacement.

Surveys have shown that the group of women least likely to have menopausal symptoms are single women who have not suffered from dysmenorrhea. The reasons for this must be multifactorial but one important factor is that these women have come to terms gradually over a number of years with non-fulfilment of a female role. It may have been a deliberate way to avoid the vulnerability of being female or it may have been by force of circumstances, in either case she is likely to have faced many of these issues many times and learned to tolerate them over a number of years. So that, rather like living with a seriously ill member of the family, the mourning is done while the patient is alive and often death welcomed as a relief.

I have tried to stress the fact that the presentation of symptoms at the menopause is a complicated process with many emotional ramifications and I have mentioned that hormonal changes may be one important factor in this process. We have just come to the end of a double blind trial with estrogen replacement therapy in which we have made a number of detailed assessments of psychological symptoms and attempted to assess the post-menopausal adjustment of patients by questionnaire combined, in some cases, with interviews. Unfortunately many of these results are not yet available but a preliminary result based on clinical impression may be of interest. 22 patients were interviewed on three occasions, before trial, half way through and at the end. The interviews on the last two occasions were of a global assessment nature and the point of interest was that out of 22 patients, 15 gave a clear unequivocal account of general improvement in a sense of well being during the half of the trial at which they were later found to have taken the estrogen rather than the placebo. Four of 22 gave a mixed reaction throughout the 12 months and three out of 22 seem to have found life more difficult when taking the estrogen. I stress this is merely a clinical impression and not entirely double blind since it was not always possible to stop the patient reporting on hot flushes which, of course, gave an obvious indication of when the estrogen was being taken. However, it was remarkable how so many patients said the same thing which was 'I felt I could cope better'.

I should finally like to make the point that the menopause is a time of loss and I believe women should not fall into the trap of feeling guilty about their sadness or of putting doctors in the position of feeling that they must produce some universal panacea so that no distress is felt at all. With any loss of any value there is mourning. Indeed we see the importance of mourning and psychiatrists frequently have to deal with troubles following the inability to mourn. It may, therefore, be important for women to experience some distress as they re-appraise their position at this time of life and perhaps we can only enjoy the next stage by a process of gradual letting go which is one of the purposes of mourning.

10

Psychiatric aspects of the menopause

C. Barbara Ballinger

Introduction

There has been considerable difference of opinion about the significance of emotional symptoms occurring at the time of the menopause and their relationship, if any, to hormonal changes at this time.

Jeffcoate[1] argued that symptoms of emotional disturbance at this time of life were in no way related to the hormonal changes of the menopause and should not be treated with estrogen preparations. In contrast, Malleson[2] and Wilson and Wilson[3] considered that symptoms of depression, emotional lability and irritability occurring at the time of the menopause were due to estrogen lack and should be treated accordingly with estrogen replacement.

Considering the treatment of emotional symptoms at the time of the menopause, a similar variation of opinion is found. Claims have been made for the use of hormone preparations[4] and antidepressant drugs[5] in the treatment of menopausal symptoms. Another study[6] showed little difference between the effects of stilbestrol and an antidepressant drug in the relief of menopausal symptoms but both preparations were more effective than placebo.

More recent surveys[7, 8] of menopausal complaints indicate that vasomotor symptoms increase suddenly at the time of cessation of menstrual periods when circulating estrogen levels fall. Symptoms such as depression, irritability and insomnia were frequently reported in these surveys but did not show such a clear relationship to the cessation of menstrual periods.

The aim of the present study was to screen a group of women from the general population between the ages of 40 and 55 years for psychiatric symptoms and relate changes in psychiatric morbidity to chronological age, menopausal status and vasomotor symptoms.

Method

As previously described[9] all women between the ages of 40 and 55 years on the lists of six General Practitioners working from the same premises in the City of Dundee were approached by letter and asked if they would take part in this survey.

The 60-item General Health Questionnaire (GHQ) as described by Goldberg[10] was used to screen the subjects for psychiatric morbidity. The GHQ is a self-administered questionnaire which has been developed for the detection of non-psychotic psychiatric illness and gives a measure of current emotional disturbance. The GHQ was scored as recommended by Goldberg[10] and all women scoring 12 or more were identified as psychiatric 'cases'.

The GHQ was also used for the assessment of vasomotor symptoms. The term 'hot flush' was avoided in view of Donovan's criticism[11] that this term was used at the time of the menopause for symptoms which had been present before that time and the answers to Question 9 of the GHQ 'Have you recently been having hot or cold spells' and Question 10 'Have you recently been perspiring (sweating) a lot' were noted instead.

Information concerning menstrual periods and social factors was also requested using a brief questionnaire.

Results

Of the 760 women approached 539 (71%) returned completed questionnaires and 155 (28·8%) of the women who responded scored 12 or more on the GHQ and were identified as psychiatric 'cases'.

Menopausal status

37 women were excluded from this classification either because they had had a hysterectomy or they did not give the relevant information.

228 women reported regular menstrual periods and were considered pre-menopausal. 81 women reported that they had missed between 3 and 12 menstrual periods just prior to completing the questionnaire and were considered menopausal. The post-menopausal group included 109 women up to and including 5 years post-menopausal and 84 women 6 or more years post-menopausal. The proportion of psychiatric 'cases' in each group is

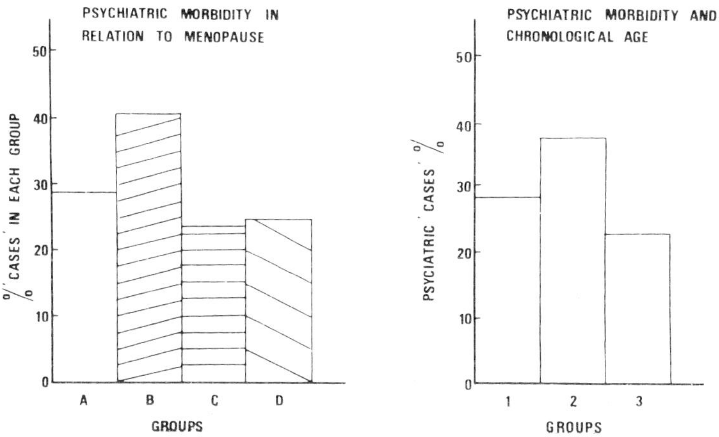

Figure 10.1 Variation in psychiatric morbidity with menopausal status (A–D) and chronological age (1–3). A—pre-menopausal; B—menopausal; C—up to 5 years post-menopausal; D—6 or more years post-menopausal; 1—age 40 to 44 years; 2—age 45 to 49 years; 3—age 50 to 54 years. (Reproduced with kind permission of the Editor of *British Medical Journal*)

shown in Figure 10.1. The difference between the menopausal group and the rest reaches statistical significance ($\chi^2 = 8{\cdot}02$, 3 d.f. $p < 0{\cdot}05$).

Chronological age

The subjects were grouped according to their age on 1st January, 1974. 159 women were 40 to 44 years of age inclusive, 167 women were 45 to 49 years of age inclusive, and 213 women were 50 to 54 years of age inclusive. The proportion of psychiatric 'cases' in each group is shown in Figure 10.1. The difference in psychiatric morbidity between the women of 45 to 49 years of age and the rest reaches statistical significance ($\chi^2 = 9{\cdot}78$, 2 d.f. $p < 0.01$).

Menopausal status and chronological age

The distribution of psychiatric morbidity according to both chronological age and menopausal status is shown in Figure 10.2.

The women of 40 to 44 years of age were predominantly pre-menopausal (83·5%) and the women of 50 to 54 years of age were predominantly post-menopausal (73%).

23·6% of the pre-menopausal women age 40 to 44 years were identified as psychiatric 'cases' compared with 39% of pre-menopausal women age

45 to 49 years. This difference reaches statistical significance ($\chi^2 = 4{\cdot}98$, 1 d.f. $p < 0{\cdot}05$). The difference in psychiatric morbidity between the pre-menopausal women of 45 to 49 years of age and those of 50 to 54 years of age does not reach statistical significance. There is no significant variation in the level of psychiatric morbidity with chronological age within the menopausal and post-menopausal groups. There is no significant variation in psychiatric morbidity with menopausal status within any of the three groups according to chronological age.

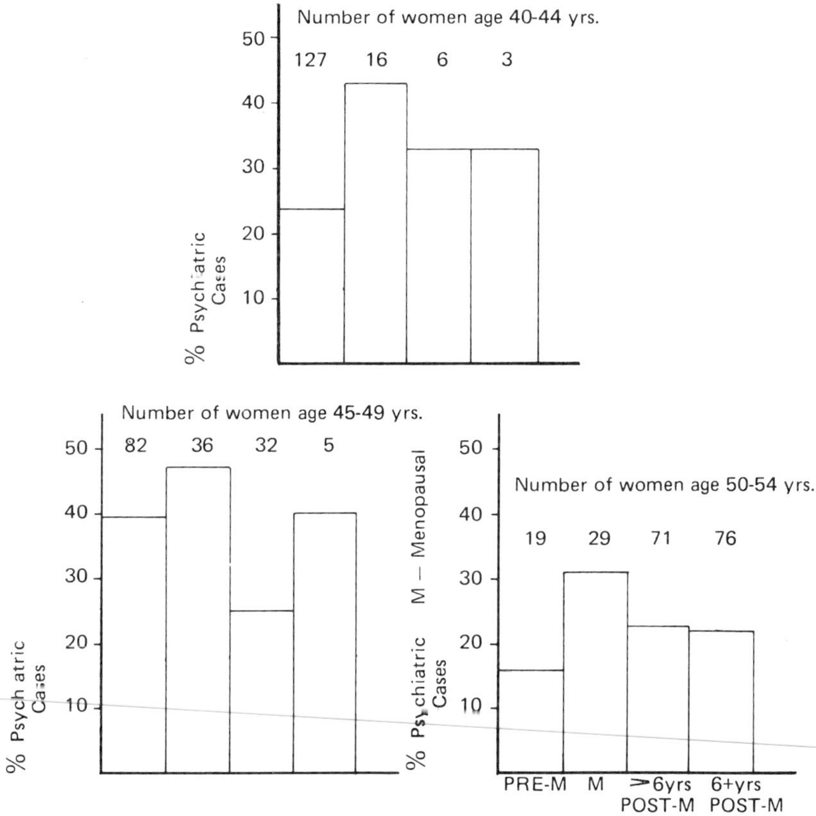

Figure 10.2 Variation in psychiatric morbidity with menopausal status in three age groups

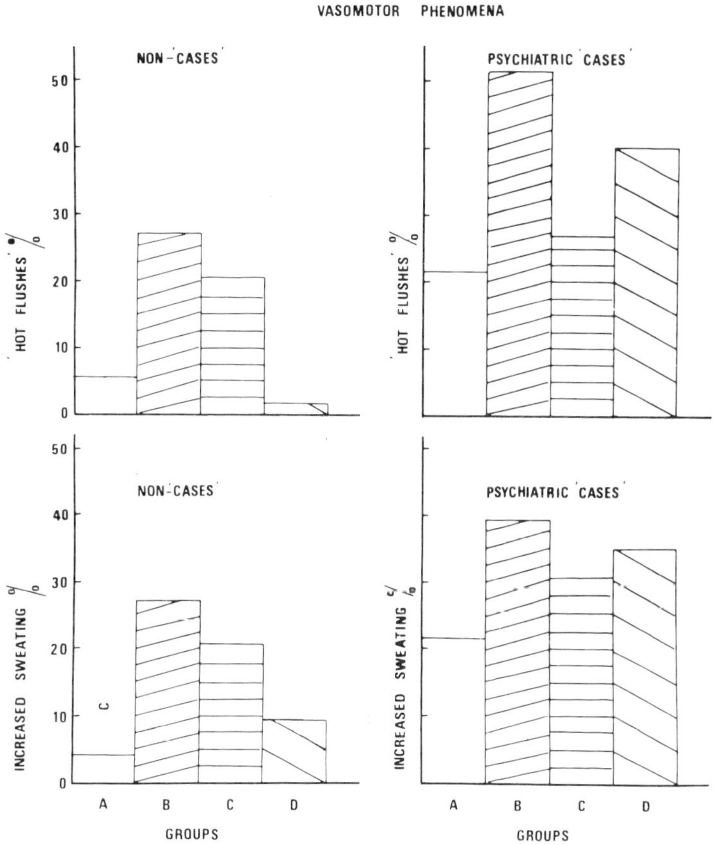

Figure 10.3 Proportion of subjects reporting increase in vasomotor symptoms in relation to menopausal stautus (A–D). A—pre-menopausal; B—menopausal; C—up to 5 years post-menopausal; D—6 or more years post-menopausal. (Reproduced with kind permission of Editor of *British Medical Journal*)

Vasomotor phenomena

Figure 10.3 shows the variation in the proportion of women who reported vasomotor symptoms occurring more or much more than usual in relation to menopausal status. The 'cases' and 'non-cases' are shown separately. The 'non-cases' show a significant increase in these complaints in the menopausal group and this increase is maintained in those women up to 5 years post-menopausal. The pattern of change in the psychiatric 'cases' is less clearly defined.

Table 10.1 shows the proportion of women in each group according to

Table 10.1 Vasomotor symptoms in psychiatric 'cases' and 'non-cases' in relation to menopausal status

Hot or cold spells	*Pre-M.*		*M.*		*Up to 5 yrs. post-m.*		*6+ years post-m.*	
	Psych. N–65	*Non-Psych. N–163*	*Psych. N–33*	*Non-Psych. N–48*	*Psych. N–26*	*Non-Psych. N–83*	*Psych. N–20*	*Non-Psych. N–64*
Absent	51%	76%	27%	50%	19%	36%	35%	48%
Present—no change	28%	18%	21%	23%	54%	43%	25%	50%
Present—increased	21%	6%	52%	27%	27%	21%	40%	2%

N—number of subjects in each group

menopausal status who reported hot and cold feelings absent, present but no more than usual and present more or much more than usual. Considering the pre-menopausal women the difference between the psychiatric 'cases' and the 'non-cases' reaches statistical significance for both absence of hot and cold feelings ($\chi^2 = 12{\cdot}7$, 1 d.f. $p < 0{\cdot}001$) and the presence of these symptoms more or much more than usual ($\chi^2 = 11{\cdot}24$, 1 d.f. $p < 0{\cdot}001$).

Considering the menopausal women there is no significant difference between the psychiatric 'cases' and the rest regarding absence of hot and cold feelings but the difference between the psychiatric 'cases' and the rest for reported increase in these feelings reaches statistical significance ($\chi^2 = 4{\cdot}06$, 1 d.f. $p < 0{\cdot}05$).

Considering those women up to 5 years post-menopausal, the difference between the psychiatric 'cases' and the rest does not reach statistical significance for either absence or increase in hot or cold feelings.

Considering those women 6 or more years post-menopausal there is no significant difference between the psychiatric 'cases' and the rest for absence of hot or cold feelings but a highly significant difference between the psychiatric 'cases' and the rest for reported increase in these feelings ($\chi^2 = 20{\cdot}25$, 1 d.f. $p < 0{\cdot}001$).

Discussion

The results of this survey indicate a significant variation in psychiatric morbidity with both menopausal status and chronological age. It is difficult to separate these two factors and, to some extent spurious, as the menopause may be considered as a well-defined episode in the ageing process in women.

When psychiatric morbidity is looked at in relation to both chronological age and menopausal status (Figure 10.2) a significant increase in psychiatric morbidity is seen first in the pre-menopausal women of 45 to 49 years of age. This increase is maintained over the year of the menopause and is followed by a significant reduction in psychiatric morbidity immediately following the menopause. The majority of pre-menopausal women of 45 to 49 years of age are within 5 years of the menopause as very few women of 50 to 54 years of age are still pre-menopausal.

The pre-menopausal increase in psychiatric morbidity is not accounted for by an excess of those family and social problems which have been found to be related to psychiatric morbidity at this time of life[9]. It may be related to culturally determined expectations of considerable discomfort at the time of the menopause and the fall immediately after the menopause may occur because these expectations are not fulfilled.

It is also possible that the pre-menopausal increase in psychiatric morbidity is related to biochemical or endocrine changes occurring just prior to the menopause. It has been postulated[12] that there are changes in the sensitivity of the feedback mechanism in relation to estrogen and LH prior to the menopause.

There is little evidence in this survey to support the view that emotional disturbance at the time of the menopause is related to reduction in estrogen levels. The timing of the change in psychiatric morbidity is different from that of the change in frequency of vasomotor symptoms which are considered to be most clearly related to the change in estrogen levels[13].

The association between reported vasomotor symptoms and psychiatric morbidity varies with menopausal status. As seen in Table 10.1, complaints of hot or cold feelings were least common in the pre-menopausal women and were much more likely to be made by those women identified as psychiatric 'cases' than by the others. In the menopausal and post-menopausal groups women with evidence of psychiatric disturbance were no more likely to report the presence of hot or cold feelings than those without evidence of psychiatric disturbance. However, considering those women who were 6 or more years post-menopausal, the psychiatric 'cases' were significantly more likely to report that these symptoms were occurring more or much more than usual. This suggests that those menopausal women with evidence of current emotional disturbance are less tolerant of vasomotor symptoms and are perhaps more likely to present for treatment than those women who do not have evidence of current emotional disturbance. A similar conclusion was reported by Foldes[5] in a study of the use of an antidepressant drug in the treatment of climacteric symptoms.

Summary

539 women from the general population were screened for psychiatric illness using the General Health Questionnaire. The level of psychiatric morbidity increased just prior to the menopause; this increase was maintained over the year of the menopause and immediately following the menopause the level of psychiatric morbidity decreased. In contrast vasomotor symptoms did not increase until the year of the menopause and this increase was maintained until 5 years after the menopause.

Menopausal and post-menopausal women with evidence of psychiatric disturbance were no more likely than those without evidence of psychiatric disturbance to report the presence of vasomotor symptoms but appeared to be less tolerant of these symptoms.

It seems unlikely from the timing of the changes in psychiatric morbidity and vasomotor symptoms that changes in estrogen levels underlie the variation in psychiatric morbidity at the time of the menopause but it may be of value to look further at those biochemical endocrine changes which occur just prior to the menopause.

Acknowledgments

I thank Drs Jean Ferguson, John Ferguson, E. D. B. Denovan, J. B. Malcolm, W. H. Gossip and Carol Henderson for permission to approach their patients; and Professor I. R. C. Batchelor and Professor James Walker for their advice and help in the preparation of this paper.

I thank the Editor of the *British Medical Journal* for kind permission to reproduce Figures 1 and 3 from the *British Medical Journal* of 9th August 1975 p. 344 and p. 345.

References

1. Jeffcoate, T. N. A. (1960). Drugs for menopausal symptoms. *Brit. Med. J.*, **1**, 340
2. Malleson, J. (1953). An endocrine factor in certain affective disorders. *Lancet*, **ii**, 158
3. Wilson, R. A. and Wilson, T. A. (1963). The fate of the non-treated post-menopausal woman: A plea for the maintenance of adequate oestrogen from puberty to the grave. *J. Amer. Geriat. Soc.*, **11**, 347
4. Comninos, A. C. (1972). Hormonal and nonhormonal treatment of menopause. *Psychosomatic Medicine in Obstetrics and Gynaecology. 3rd Int. Congr., London 1971*, p. 622 (Basel: Karger)
5. Foldes, J. J. (1972). Psychosomatic approach to the menopausal syndrome. Treatment with opipramol (Insidon). *Psychosomatic Medicine in Obstetrics and Gynaecology. 3rd Int. Congr., London 1971*, p. 617 (Basel: Karger)
6. Wheatley, D. (1972). The use of psychotropic drugs in the female climacteric. *Psychosomatic Medicine in Obstetrics and Gynaecology. 3rd Int. Congr., London 1971*, p. 612 (Basel: Karger)

7. Jaszmann, L., van Lith, N. D. and Zaat, J. L. A. (1969). The perimenopausal symptoms: The statistical analysis of a survey. *Med. Gynaecol. Sociol.*, **4,** 268
8. McKinlay, S. M. and Jeffreys, M. (1974). The menopausal syndrome. *Brit. J. Prev. Soc. Med.*, **28,** 108
9. Ballinger, C. B. (1975). Psychiatric morbidity and the menopause; screening of a general population sample. *Brit. Med. J.*, **3,** 344
10. Goldberg, D. P. (1972). *The Detection of Psychiatric Illness by Questionnaire.* 1st Ed. (London: Oxford University Press)
11. Donovan, J. C. (1951). The menopausal syndrome: A study of case histories. *Amer. J. Obstet. Gynaecol.*, **62,** 1281
12. Adamopoulos, D. A., Loraine, J. A. and Dove, G. A. (1971). Endocrinological studies in women approaching the menopause. *J. Obstet. Gynaec. Brit. Cwlth*, **78,** 62
13. Daw, E. (1974). Lutinising hormone (L.H.). Changes in women undergoing artificial menopause. *Current Med. Res. and Opinion*, **2,** 256

11

Psychological changes following hormonal therapy

M. Dorothea Kerr

There is much controversy regarding the presence or absence of psychological and psychiatric symptoms in the climacteric, let alone controversy whether gonadal hormonal therapy ameliorates these symptoms.

I have been a practising psychiatrist in the United States for 20 years and became interested in the effect of hormones on psychiatric symptoms about 1968. Adhering to the concept that the patient you are most interested in is yourself, I noted that gonadal hormones, first as an oral contraceptive then cyclic estrogen–progestin treatment improved my own pre-menstrual depression, irritability and headaches as well as menstrual dysmenorrhea.

Questioning my office menopausal and post-menopausal patients then in psychotherapy, several told of relief of emotional symptoms such as headaches, mood depression and insomnia by estrogens prescribed by their gynaecologists. The majority gave similar statements—that the relief was definite, began within a time period of 1–3 months, and that symptoms returned in varying degrees in the estrogen withdrawal periods of their induced cycle. Their subjective improvement certainly was as good as I had observed many times with pharmacotherapy. I wondered if estrogens were a naturally occurring tranquillizer and antidepressant.

I began investigating women age 40+ referred to me with psychological difficulties for menopausal symptoms including the vasomotor, psychological and psychosomatic subtypes. I found that the psychological changes of anxiety, depression, tension and irritability apparently begin long before the actual termination of periods and correlate fairly well with estrogen levels as determined by vaginal smear stained by the Shorr method.

Central to the patient's psychological symptoms is an insidious awareness of a sense of internal frustration or lack—an inability to feel gratified—and an inability to feel and to function as she has usually done. This is a deep feeling at first vaguely felt and extremely disturbing to a woman as she becomes aware of it. This profound sense of internal inadequacy is expressed as the symptom of intermittent, often cyclic, depression or 'blues'. The patient complains of sudden, involuntary, easily precipitated crying spells, or a sensitivity to rejection especially by those close to her or an intolerance of loneliness or perhaps all three. She speaks of a need for babying, of being cared for. The depression may be expressed outwardly as irritability so that she quarrels with and alienates her family and associates. Concomitant with the depression, there is often increased fears (anxiety) and tensions.

I have the clinical impression that women who have psychological and psychosomatic changes to altering hormone levels at other times in their adult life such as premenses, menses, pregnancy, postpartum and when using oral contraceptives have similar responses to hormonal change in their climateric period.

Benedek and Rubenstein in 1942[1] by daily psychodynamic interviews and vaginal smears found very similar symptoms to those I describe in the menopause during the pre-menstrual phase; anger, excitability, fatigue, crankiness, crying spells and fear of mutilation. They described frustrations as seeming unbearable, gratification of needs imperative, and all emotions less controlled than at any other time in the cycle. This regression to more infantile ways of responding and coping and the increased irritability of the sympathetic nervous system were seen by the authors as resulting from the low estrogen levels of the pre-menstrual phase.

In 1965 Neugarten and Kraines[2] did an interesting study of 480 women comparing symptoms reported by menopausal women with symptoms reported by women at other age periods. The two highest symptom groups were the adolescent (13–18) and the menopausal (45–54). The women in the 45–54 group who reported themselves as non-menopausal had lower symptom scores than those who reported themselves menopausal. Adolescents most frequently reported emotional or psychological symptoms while the menopausal women tended to report somatic symptoms. The authors felt the change in sex hormones during adolescence and menopause primarily responsible for producing an increase in sensitivity to and frequency of symptoms.

Ivey and Bardwick in 1968[3] studied 26 normal female college students over two menstrual cycles and found pre-menstrual anxiety scores significantly higher than those at ovulation. There were consistent themes of hostility and depression as well as themes of non-coping. Bardwick states in her 1971 book

Psychology of Women[4] that 'human behaviour is clearly very variable, and this variability originates in the reaction of the hypothalamus and central nervous system to internal and environmental stimuli. When we look at specific behaviour, women seem very different from other female primates and mammals, whose sexual arousability, for example, is stimulated solely by high estrogen levels. But if we take a closer look at *general mood shifts, feelings of self-esteem* and *self-depreciation, depression and well-being*, we begin to discern the physiologically linked affect cycle which underlies the specific behaviour.'

During the 1930s in the United States it was generally agreed that the menopausal vasomotor symptoms and mild depression were relieved by estrogenic hormones[5, 6]. There was considerable disagreement as to results in severe depressive illnesses. An influential study in 1940 by Ripley, Shorr and Papanicolaou[7] on hospital inpatients reported an improvement in the patient's feeling of well-being but no specific influence on the depressive illness itself, especially the true involutional melancholia with feelings of unreality, suspiciousness, hypochondriacal and nihilistic delusions. The use of estrogen as a therapy for depression sharply declined thereafter.

About the time that estrogens were discovered in the 1930s, the psychogenetic theories of emotional and somatic symptoms were coming into vogue. Psychiatry in the United States beginning in the 1940s was primarily interested in psychoanalytical, behavioural and cultural theories of aetiology. The generally accepted view as given by McCandless in 1964[8] is that 'while the climacteric in women is frequently signalled by the physiologic manifestations of ovarian involution, these symptoms tend to focus on, rather than cause the psychological problems of the climacteric. Emotional difficulties, when they occur, derive from discontinuity in the transition of the sociobiologic role, before and after cessation of menses'—a rather elaborate way of describing what many call 'the empty nest syndrome'. In accordance with aetiology, the treatment of choice has been psychotherapy[9]. In the last few years tranquillizers and antidepressants have become popular therapy in the climacteric. Again, most of the American literature refers to them as adjuncts to psychotherapy or substitutes for the patient resistant to psychotherapy since psychotherapy is still our cardinal psychiatric method[10, 11].

During this time there have been several reports of successful treatment of mild to moderate menopausal and post-menopausal psychological and psychosomatic symptoms by gynaecologists and internists[12-14].

Many of the reported studies tend to lack good experimental control and tend to overlook the power of suggestion or the influence of a sympathetic physician. Estrogen therapy for psychological difficulties was adversely affected in the United States in 1973 by the influential Medical Letter[15], a therapy compendium written by faculty members from several medical schools. They stated unequivocally that estrogens have no demonstrable effect on anxiety, depression or any other type of emotional symptoms.

Hopefully, the biochemists will soon clarify the climacteric events so that we can proceed clinically on surer grounds. One such use of a biochemical indicator, the plasma enzyme monoamine oxidase, in estrogen therapy of severe depression is currently in progress in the United States. Central catecholamine insufficiency has been postulated by Schildkraut[16] to be the basis of mental depression based primarily on pharmacological studies involving reserpine, amphetamine, imipramine and MAO inhibitors. The catecholamine theory of depression involves mainly norepinephrine[17-19] and monoamine oxidase is one of the enzymes responsible for catabolism of norepinephrine. Nies[20] in 1971 found platelet and plasma MAO to be elevated with age (higher at each decade), sex (higher in women), and depression (elevated in depressive *vs.* normals).

In 1972 Klaiber *et al.*[21] found that the daily administration of 5 mg of conjugated oral estrogens significantly reduced the elevated plasma monoamine oxidase activity of a group of moderately depressed out-patients. At the same time, estrogen suppressed an EEG index ('driving' responses to photic stimulation) found elevated in depressed patients compared to non-depressed controls. That study, however, did not systematically investigate the effects of estrogen administration on the symptoms of depression.

Currently, Klaiber and his group are continuing a double-blind study of high dose (up to 30 mg daily) conjugated estrogen therapy for severe, chronically depressed, therapy-resistant, inpatient women from age 20–55 (40% being menopausal and post-menopausal)[22] Of the 40 treated patients up to the present time about 60% showed significant improvement in their depression rating scales after at least 3 months of therapy as compared to the placebo patients[23]. As in his previous study, estrogen therapy significantly lowered the elevated plasma MAO activity of the depressed patients but it took 3 months to achieve significant results.

In Klaiber's experience, the doses of estrogen that produces estrogenic response in vaginal tissues are considerably lower than those required to affect plasma MAO activity, particularly in depressed women. His results indicate an estrogen resistance in severely depressed women, for example, the severely depressed inpatients on 5–20 mg conjugated estrogens dosage daily had less MAO suppression after 3 months than non-depressed women on 5 mg daily after 1 month. Incidentally, side effects were few in these patients on large doses of estrogen. In summary, Klaiber and his group feel their results indicate that oral conjugated estrogens are an effective therapy for severe endogenous depression and that endogenously depressed women have elevated plasma MAO activity which is reduced toward normal levels concomitant with the estrogen therapy.

In my outpatient clinical psychiatric experience, I have found estrogen in the menopausal age patient to produce a feeling of normal well-being and to improve the entire emotional state of the patient. In proper dosage, they ameliorate psychosomatic target symptoms such as headaches, epigastric pain, insomnia, paraesthesias, palpitations, arthralgias and myalgias;—generalized symptoms as weakness and fatigue; and emotional components as anxiety, tension, mood depression and irritability. The pure vasomotor symptoms of hot flushes and sweats are relieved within a few days; the other symptoms are gradually relieved over a 1–3 month period[24]. The majority of menopausal symptoms come on gradually and are quickly or gradually relieved depending on dosage. The longer a depression is permitted to deepen, the more difficult it is to treat as seems true with other therapies of depression[25].

Some patients may require ten times or more the average dosage of estrogen before there is symptomatic improvement. The vaginal smear stained by the Shorr stain and method can be an invaluable aid in the regulation of dosage. If symptoms persist, with a smear showing full estrus (85–90% of cornified cells), one can be sure that the symptoms are not menopausal and probably of psychogenic origin. To obtain full estrus in the smear usually requires 5·0–7·5 mg mixed equine estrogens (Premarin), 0·3–0·4 mg ethinyl estradiol (Estinyl) or 3–4 mgm diethylstilbestrol. In some women a much higher, and in others a much lower dosage is necessary to obtain an estrus smear[25].

The more common side effects have been mastalgia, bloating and weight gain. The most important side effect and the most difficult to handle is breakthrough bleeding despite my use of cyclic sequential estrogen and progestin. It usually can be stopped by increasing the estrogen in the early phase of the cycle, or by increasing the dose of progestin in the later cycle stage. I must admit that breakthrough bleeding has been the most troublesome and disquieting symptom to my patients on long-term, moderate to high dose estrogen therapy. Patients whose emotional symptoms have responded well to estrogen yet have persistent breakthough bleeding have preferred hysterectomy to discontinuing estrogen therapy.

To conclude, I hold that any patient whose psychiatric illness arises in the menopause, or is aggravated in the menopause, or is aggravated at phases in the menstrual cycle should be given a therapeutic trial of hormone therapy in conjunction with psychiatric management[24, 25]. Depression is an ubiquitous phenomenon and the earlier the treatment, the better the response. One can have a high index of suspicion for the lady who may have menopausal depression through her previous hormonal history—her response to hormonal depths and heights throughout her life. Early hormonal treatment to this patient may prevent a prolonged, painful even disabling illness.

Regardless of whether one accepts a beneficial influence of estrogens on psychological symptoms in the menopause, remember that the presence of psychoneurosis or psychosis is not a contraindication to the use of hormones. The menopause presents additional difficulty for the woman already attempting to adjust to the myriad dysfunctions of an emotional illness. Alleviating the menopausal element often restores her to her premorbid adjustment with which she has learned to live quite comfortably.

References

1. Benedek, T. and Rubinstein, B. (1942). The sexual cycle in women: The relation between ovarian function and psychodynamic processes. *Psychosom. Med. Monogr.* (Washington, D.C.: National Research Council)
2. Neugarten, B. L. and Kraines, R. J. (1965). 'Menopausal symptoms' in women of various ages. *Psychosomat. Med.*, **27,** 266
3. Ivey, M. and Bardwick, J. M. (1968). Patterns of affective fluctuations in the menstrual cycle. *Psychosomat. Med.*, **30,** 336
4. Bardwick, J. M. (1971). *Psychology of Women: A Study of Bio-cultural Conflicts.* (New York: Harper & Row)
5. Hawkinson, L. F. (1938). The menopausal syndrome. *J. Amer. Med. Ass.*, **iii**, 390, July
6. Wiesbader, H. and Kurzok, R. (1938). The menopause. A Consideration of symptoms, etiology and treatment by means of estrogens. *Endocrinology*, **23,** 32
7. Ripley, H. S., Shorr, E. and Papanicolaou, G. N. (1940). The effect of treatment of depression in the menopause with estrogenic hormones. *Amer. J. Psychiat.*, **96**, 905
8. McCandless, F. D. (1964). Emotional problems of the climacteric. *Clin. Obstet. Gynecol.*, **7,** 489
9. Detre, T. (1968). Severe emotional reactions precipitated by the climacterium. *Psychosomatics*, **9** (supp.): 31
10. Douglas, H. S. (1969). Role of psychotropic therapy in estrogen-deficient menopausal patients. *Medical Annals of D.C.*, **38,** 437
11. Litkewitsch, H. (1963). Antidepressant-tranquilizer regimen in menopausal patients. *J.A.M.W.A.*, 819
12. Cameron, W. J. (1966) Endocrine therapy in the menopause. *Gen. Pract.*, **33,** 2, 110
13. Greenblatt, R. G. (1952). Newer concepts in the management of the menopause. *Geriatrics*, **7,** 263
14. Kantor, H. L., Michael, C. M., Bowles, S. H., Shore, H. and Ludvigson, H. W. (1966). The administration of estrogens to older women, a psychometric evaluation. Proceedings of the *Seventh International Congress of Gerontology*, Vienna
15. *Medical Letter* (1973), January
16. Schildkraut, J. J. (1965). The catecholamine hypothesis of affective disorders: a review of supporting evidence. *Amer. J. Psychiat.*, **122,** 509
17. Kety, S. S., Javoy, F., Thierry, A., Julou, L. and Glowinski, J. (1967). A sustained

effect of electroconvulsive shock on the turnover of norepinephrine in the central nervous system of the rat. *Proc. Natl. Acad. Sci. USA*, **58,** 1246

18. Maas, J. W., Fawcett, J. and Dekirmenjian, H. (1968). 3-methoxy-4-hydroxy phenylglycol (MHPG) excretion in depressive states. *Arch. Gen. Psychiat.*, **19,** 129
19. Post, R. M., Gordon, E. K., Goodwin, F. K. and Bunney, W. E. Jr. (1973). Central norepinephrine metabolism in affective illness: MHPG in the cerebrospinal fluid. *Science*, **179,** 1002
20. Nies, A., Robinson, A. S., Ravaris, C. L. and Davis, J. M. (1971). Amines and monoamine oxidase in relation to aging and depression in man. *Psychosomat. Med.*, **33,** 470
21. Klaiber, E. L., Braverman, D. M., Vogel, W., Kobayashi, Y. and Moriarty, D. (1972). Effects of estrogen therapy on plasma monoamine oxidase activity and EEG driving responses in depressed women. *Amer. J. Psychiat.*, **128,** 1492
22. Klaiber, E. L., Braverman, D. M., Vogel, W. and Kobayashi, Y. (1974). The use of steroid hormones in depression. *First World Congress Biol. Psychiat.*, Argentina
23. Klaiber, E. L. (1975). Personal communication
24. Kerr, M. D. (1968). Psychohormonal approach to the menopause. *Modern Treatment*, **5,** 587
25. Cohen, E. J. and Sonkin, L. S. (1968). Treatment of the menopause. *Modern Treatment*, **5,** 545

12

Estrogens, plasma tryptophan levels in perimenopausal patients

M. Aylward

Introduction

General considerations

At the present time there is an apparent wealth of detailed information on the physico-chemical properties and biological roles of estrogens. This plethora of undoubtedly valuable knowledge not only provides a greater understanding of the effects of these hormones on metabolic processes and biochemical events at tissue, cellular, and sub-cellular levels but also clarifies the sensitive biological control systems which regulate gonadal hormones in the female. Yet, it is readily apparent that the relative lack of information and data on the climacteric as a total process in the human female is the cause of much concern. The present limited knowledge of the menopause and post-menopausally related events taken with the urgent need to clarify certain issues regarding the advisability of therapeutic intervention with estrogenic compounds indicate that detailed investigations on the menopause and its sequelae are still amongst the most needed in biomedical research. Perhaps the aspect most neglected in our increasing awareness of the mechanisms underlying climacteric complaints is that which relates to psychological impairment in general and to any specific psychological effects of estrogens in particular.

Considering the many and complex factors which may contribute to psychological disturbance during the climacteric, it is not surprising that little research has been undertaken to evaluate the consequences of declining ovarian function on the pattern of psychological disorders encountered. It has been suggested[1, 2] that the only symptoms directly associated with endogenous estrogen withdrawal and specifically relieved by estrogen replacement therapy are the autonomic vasomotor disturbances and those associated with atrophic vaginitis. However studies undertaken in South Wales, which form the basis of the present communication, lend considerable support to the observations of others[3–5] that estrogens not only benefit physical symptoms, but also improve the emotional state in the climacteric.

Plasma-(L) tryptophan and depression

There is increasing evidence[6–8] of abnormal indoleamine metabolism in depressive patients, manifesting as reduced levels of 5-hydroxytryptamine (5-HT) and 5-hydroxyindoleacetic acid (5-HIAA) in the brains, and decreased levels of 5-HIAA in the lumbar cerebrospinal fluid (CSF) of such patients. Indirect evidence indicates[9] that the rate-limiting step in the synthesis of brain 5-HT is the concentration of L-tryptophan in brain, and not a deficiency of the enzyme, tryptophan-5-hydroxylase: the concentration of L-tryptophan in the normal mammalian brain is significantly lower than the Michaelis constant (K_m) of this enzyme for its substrate[10]. Furthermore, it has been demonstrated[11] that drugs which accelerate 5-HT synthesis also increase brain tryptophan concentration. It would appear that the rate of 5-HT synthesis is controlled largely by brain tryptophan concentrations. Thus, increasing the availability of tryptophan to the brain may conceivably influence brain function. Yet most of the plasma-tryptophan is not readily available since it is bound to plasma albumin[12]. Recently, however, it has been shown[13] that increasing the amount of unbound plasma tryptophan, i.e. '*free*' species, also increases brain tryptophan.

Tryptophan is displaced from its binding sites to plasma albumin both *in vitro* and *in vivo* by clinically effective anti-inflammatory drugs[14–16] and by natural estrogens[15, 17]. Thus the natural estrogens which depress the proportion of protein-bound plasma-tryptophan might contribute to a beneficial effect on mental depression: the corollary to this proposal implies that endogenous estrogen deficiency is likely to be associated with abnormally low concentrations of *free* plasma-tryptophan and hence a predisposition to features of mental depression.

Mental depression at the climacteric

Psychological disturbance in perimenopausal patients

The alterations in affective state which, at present, are given the rather nebulous and ill-defined term *Mental Depression* include a number of different disease entities. Whereas changes in mood and drive are commonly encountered and well recognized responses evoked by environmental events, it is the exaggerated quality of such responses which identifies depressive illness. The variability both in therapeutic response and in the evolution of the disorder in depressive syndromes, which may even manifest similar clinical features, suggests that different metabolic lesions operate as aetiological factors. The period immediately preceding the menopause and the post-menopausal years are often accompanied by disturbing psychological alterations[5] which are exhibited, to a varying degree, by approximately half of all women during their climacteric. In a study still in progress in South Wales[20] 56% of a randomly selected population of 596 post-menopausal women, in whom the period of climacteric amenorrhea ranged between 6 and 28 months, exhibited features of mental depression. In this group the most common symptoms were: inability to make decisions (79%), apathy or inner unrest (65%), irritability and aggressiveness (51%), depressive thought content (47%), sleep disturbances (46%), psychomotor retardation (38%), loss of libido (37%), and loss of emotional reaction (18%). Whilst the provocation of these features of mental depression cannot be divorced from complex environmental, psychological, and genetic factors, consideration of these factors alone can lead to an underestimation of alterations in body biochemistry which may play a major role in perimenopausal depressive states. A basic ignorance of the primary mechanisms involved in the depressive process has precipitated a high incidence of speculative hypotheses, yet several theories promoted in the last decade relating to disturbances of electrolytes, endocrine systems, adenylate cyclase activity, and biogenic amines, merit serious consideration. It is the aim of this paper to report the concepts, and the associated experimental work, which has been confined to investigation of the role of indoleamines in perimenopausal depression in studies undertaken in South Wales.

Plasma tryptophan levels in perimenopausal patients

Total plasma-tryptophan levels have been found normal in depressive patients. However, the concentrations of *free* plasma-tryptophan in female depressive patients are significantly lower than in corresponding female control subjects[18, 19]. In a preliminary attempt[17] to establish whether the levels of *free* plasma-tryptophan in post-menopausal women were in any way associated with the occurrence of features of mental depression, fasting levels of *free* and *total* plasma-tryptophan levels were measured[16] in 18 women who had undergone abdominal hysterectomy and bilateral oophorectomy within 2 years of the investigation, and in a randomly selected group of female osteoarthritic patients of similar age and socio-economic status as the control group. The Hamilton Depression Scale[21] (HRS) was used to score the severity of individual symptoms of mental depression. Table 12.1 shows that both the concentration and percentage of fasting *free* plasma-tryptophan are significantly lower ($P < 0.001$) in the post-menopausal group than in controls. However there is no significant difference in *total* plasma-tryptophan concentrations between the two groups ($P > 0{\cdot}5$).

Table 12.1 Fasting levels of free and total plasma-tryptophan in surgically castrated post-menopausal patients and corresponding female controls

Patients	*Age (yrs.)*		*Plasma-tryptophan levels*					
			Total (μg/ml)		*Free* (μg/ml)		*Free* (%)	
	Mean	*SE*	*Mean*	*SE*	*Mean*	*SE*	*Mean*	*SE*
Post-menopausal group (n = 18)	44·6	1·6	12·42	0·81	0·82*	0·11	6·6*	0·59
Control group (n = 12)	44·5	1·4	12·16	0·79	1·36	0·05	11·2	0·53

* Post-menopausal group *vs.* Control group $P < 0{\cdot}001$

The individual HRS scores in patients of both groups were ranked and the ranks summed. Kruskal and Wallis' test was used to detect differences in HRS ranks at different *free* plasma-tryptophan concentrations. These data are given in Table 12.2 and indicate that severity of depression is greatest in patients with *free*-tryptophan concentrations 0·48–0·79 μg/ml ($K = 5{\cdot}213$, $P < 0{\cdot}001$). All 14 of the patients with *free*-tryptophan levels in the range 0·48–0·79 μg/ml were from the post-menopausal group: the remaining four post-menopausal patients had *free*-tryptophan levels in the range 0·81–1·20 μg/ml (Table 12.2).

In the same study[17] the post-menopausal patients were allocated at random to treatment with either estrone–piperazine sulphate (3·0 mg/d) or placebo for three 21-day courses with a break of 7 days between each course. The trial was carried out under double-blind conditions. Assessments at monthly intervals included standard objective and subjective measures of clinical response, vaginal cytology, and HRS scores, together with measurement of

Table 12.2 Analysis by Kruskal and Wallis' Test of Hamilton Depression Scale Scores in post-menopausal patients and corresponding female controls related to fasting free plasma-tryptophan levels

Number of patients	*Range of freeplasma-tryptophan* (μg/ml)	*K*	*P*
14	0·48–0·79	5·213	$< 0·001$
7	0·81–1·20	2·72	$= 0·05$
9	1·31–1·54	1·16	$> 0·10$

fasting plasma-tryptophan levels. After 3 months treatment with estrone-piperazine sulphate the group (10 patients) mean *free*-tryptophan concentrations was 1·30 μg/ml (SE = 0·09) compared with a mean value of 0·75 μg/ml (SE = 0·06) which represents a highly significant increase ($P < 0·001$). In contrast the group in receipt of placebo (eight patients) showed no significant change in mean levels of *free* plasma-tryptophan throughout the 3-month period and at the final assessment the group mean *free*-tryptophan concentration of 0·81 μg/ml (SE = 0·06) remained significantly lower than corresponding controls ($P < 0·001$). With regard to symptoms of mental depression, the individual changes at each examination (differences between baseline and 4-week, 4-week and 8-week, 8-week and 12-week HRS scores were ranked and the ranks summed. The mean ranks for different *free* plasma-tryptophan concentrations are shown in Table 12.3. Amelioration in depression scores is greatest in the group of patients with levels of *free* tryptophan greater than 1·30 μg/ml ($F = 2·8$, $0·01 > P > 0·001$). There was a highly significant direct correlation between improvement in HRS scores and *free* plasma-tryptophan concentrations (Spearmans Correlation Test: $D^2+1 = 44$; $n = 18$; $P < 0·001$).

These observations in a small population of women exhibiting features of endogenous estrogen withdrawal and mental depression following hysterectomy and bilateral oophorectomy revealed not only a definite relationship between severity of mental depression and *free* plasma-tryptophan levels but also a significant amelioration in both physical and mental symptoms with an orally administered 'natural' estrogen.

These results prompted a further more comprehensive evaluation[20] of the postulated correlation between *free* plasma-tryptophan levels and mental depression in a large population of perimenopausal patients in South Wales. At the present time 642 patients have been admitted to the study. For the purposes of the present article reference is only made to the data obtained

Table 12.3 Analysis by ranking procedure of the results of Hamilton Scale Scores in post-menopausal patients related to fasting free plasma–tryptophan concentrations

Number of patients	*Mean free tryptophan concentrations in plasma after 3 months* (μg/ml)	*Mean rank for different plasma levels*
8	0·46–0·75 'Low'	2·2
4	0·81–1·21 'Intermediate'	6·72
14	1·32–1·56 'High'	12·96

thus far which lends support to the existence of perimenopausal depression as a distinct entity associated with abnormal indoleamine metabolism and specifically relieved by estrogen replacement therapy.

CORRELATION BETWEEN FREE PLASMA–TRYPTOPHAN AND PERIMENOPAUSAL DEPRESSION

In almost every case admitted to the South Wales study the first sign of approach of the menopause was the occurrence of irregularities in the menstrual cycle. The menstrual pattern was taken as the basis for further analysis of complaints, which were assessed by employing the Kupperman Menopausal Index Score[22] and the Hamilton Rating Scale[21], thus allowing complaints or symptoms to be studied in relation to the biological age[23]. The relation between the values for fasting *free* plasma–tryptophan and Mean Symptom Score (HRS) in the first 79 patients on the first occasion they were seen is shown in Figure 12.1. The inverse correlation is statistically highly significant ($r = -0{\cdot}8016$; $P < 0{\cdot}001$). This correlation has proved significant, to a varying degree, in a further 292 patients subsequently studied. During periods of exacerbation of psychological symptomatology, as judged by marked increases in both the total Hamilton Rating scores for depression, and also in the sub-scores relating to depressed mood, there were significant decreases in *free* tryptophan levels. Similarly during phases of remission of symptoms of mental depression free levels of the amino acid rose significantly.

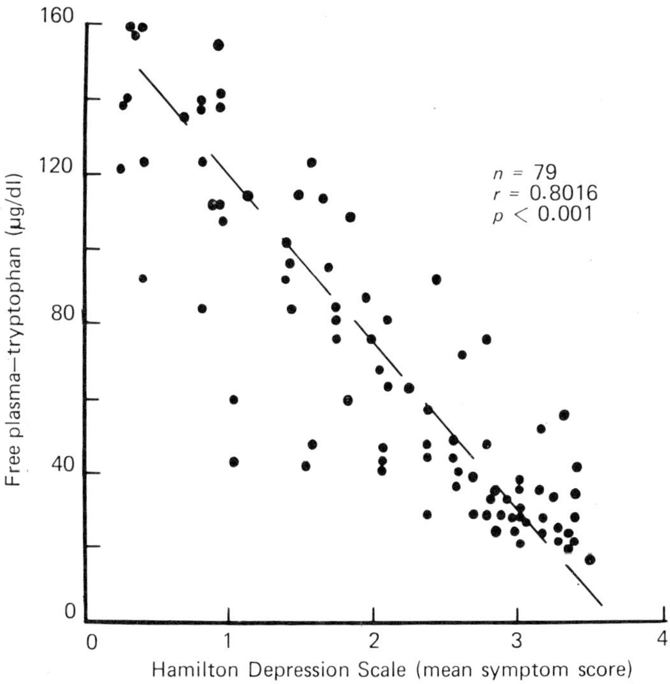

Figure 12.1 Relationship between 'fasting' *free* plasma–tryptophan levels and HRS depression scores in 79 perimenopausal patients at first attendance

ENDOGENOUS PLASMA–ESTROGEN AND FREE PLASMA–TRYPTOPHAN

In the same 79 patients described above fasting levels of estrone, estradiol, and total estrogens in plasma were measured employing radioimmunoassay techniques[24, 25] and the relationship between these measurements and fasting *free*-plasma–tryptophan concentrations are plotted in Figure 12.2. The correlations are statistically significant: for free-tryptophan *vs.* plasma 17β-estradiol, $r = 0{\cdot}8301$, $P < 0{\cdot}001$; for free-tryptophan *vs.* estrone, $r = 0{\cdot}8119$, $P < 0{\cdot}001$. The relationship of these measurements over longer periods of time have been investigated in 95 patients followed up for at least 3 years. From data obtained in this group it would appear that there exists a direct correlation between free-plasma–tryptophan levels and total endogenous estrogen concentrations in the range of plasma estrogen concentrations from 0·5 to 1100 μg/ml.

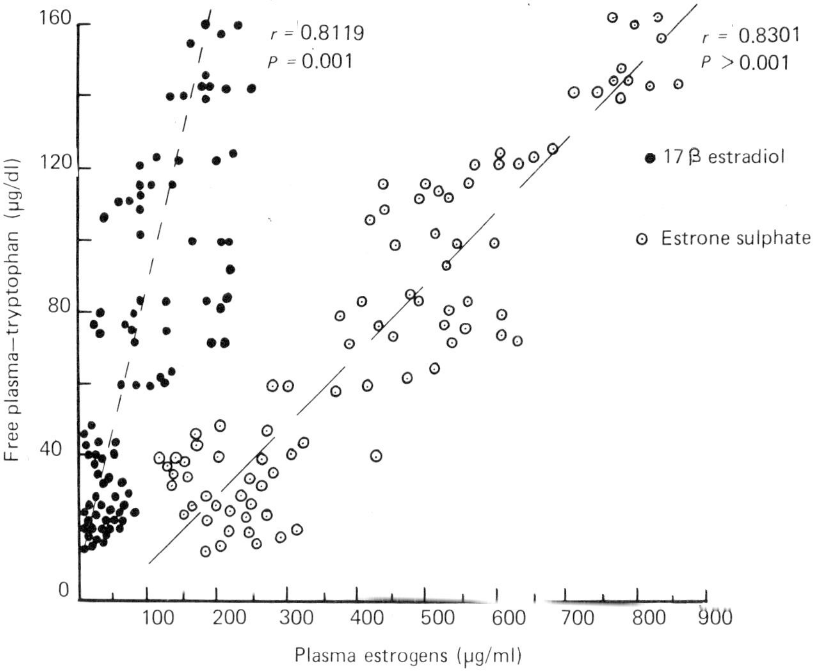

Figure 12.2 Relationships between 'fasting' levels of *free* plasma–tryptophan and plasma estrone and estradiol in 79 perimenopausal patients at first attendance

Estrogen replacement therapy and climacteric depression

Controlled clinical trials

In a report[26] of one of several controlled clinical trials undertaken on patients in the South Wales study population, two treatments were compared in a double-blind between-patient trial: estrone–piperazine sulphate (3·0 mg/d) and placebo (lactose) respectively, administered throughout a 21 day course. Prior to admission to the trial proper patients received placebo only under single-blind conditions for a 21-day period. 'Placebo-responsive' patients were withdrawn and the remainder (65 patients) were randomly allocated to the two treatments but were stratified according to age, duration of menopausal symptoms, 'menopausal index' score[22], and whether menopause had been spontaneous or followed surgical castration. 33 patients received the active treatment and 32, the placebo. In Figure 12.3 are plotted the differences between pre-treatment values for plasma levels of estrone,

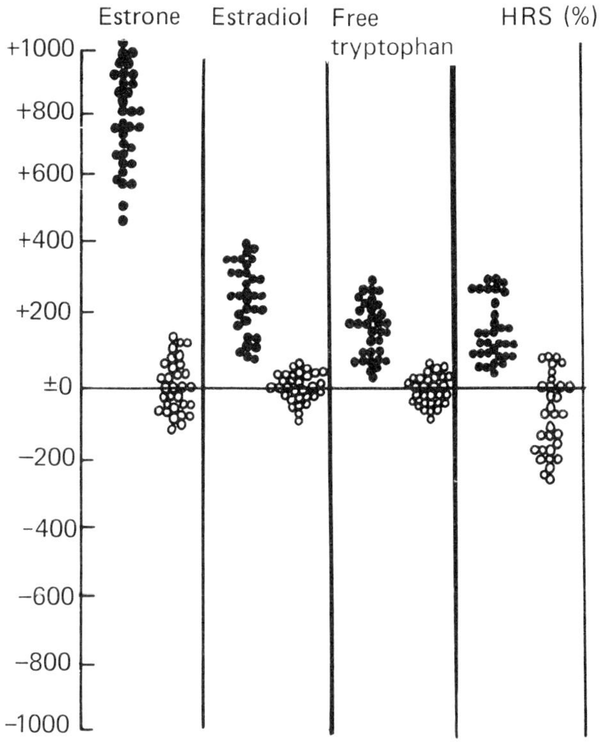

Figure 12.3 The difference between the values for the plasma estrone, estradiol, free tryptophan and the HRS depression score (% change) before and after 21 days treatment with estrone–piperazine sulphate (●) and placebo (○) in 65 perimenopausal patients

estradiol, and *free*-tryptophan together with percentage change in HRS depression scores, and each subsequent value at one month. The results in the 33 patients who received estrone–piperazine sulphate indicate that in almost all these patients, there was a marked increase in the plasma estrone, estradiol, and *free*-tryptophan and an amelioration of mental depression scores (Figure 12.3). The results in the 32 patients who received placebo indicate that the levels rose and fell in almost equal numbers of the patients whilst the HRS depression scores revealed a deterioration in the majority of the patients. In the placebo group as a whole there was no significant change in any of the measurements of plasma estrogens and *free*-tryptophan. (Figure 12.3).

Whilst it is admitted that the placebo effect is so great in any studies of therapy at the menopause, necessitating great care when interpreting results; the results of this study weigh heavily in favour of there being a definite beneficial effect of 'natural' estrogens in perimenopausal depression which does not reflect a placebo response. Furthermore, the objective changes in *free* plasma–tryptophan observed only in the estrogen-treated patients provides indirect evidence that a metabolic lesion underlies psychological disturbances in many perimenopausal patients and is likely to be related to endogenous estrogen withdrawal.

In the South Wales Study[20] using clinical criteria only it has been possible to distinguish several patients with severe mental depression which responded dramatically to treatment with estrone–piperazine sulphate. Figure 12.4 shows an example. This patient assessed under double-blind conditions

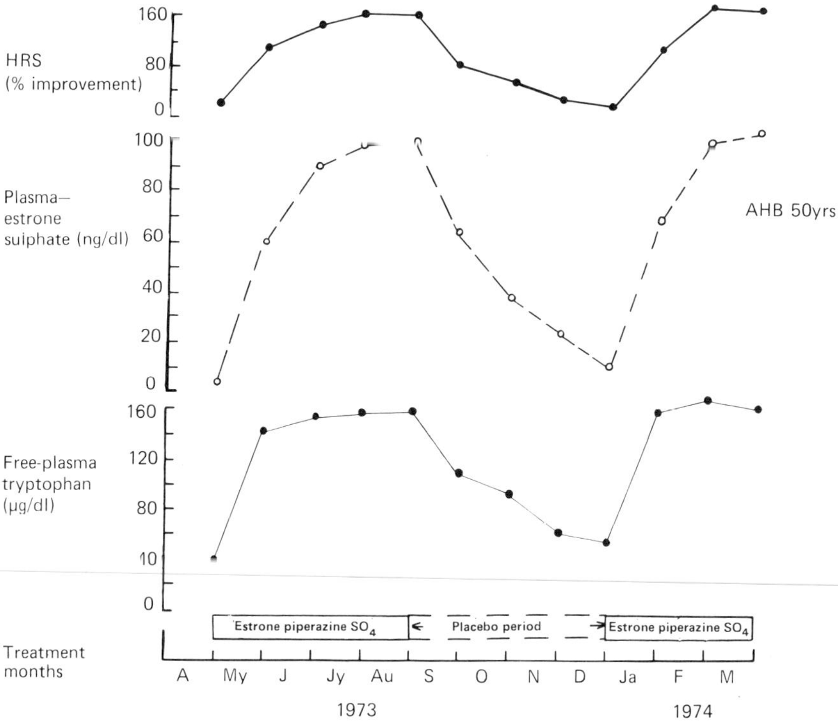

Figure 12.4 The *free* plasma–tryptophan, plasma–estrone sulphate and percentage improvement in Hamilton Depression Scale Score in a patient during treatment with estrone–piperazine sulphate (3 mg/d) and with placebo

exhibited marked improvement in HRS depression score accompanied by significant increases in both *total* plasma-estrogen and plasma *free*-tryptophan levels when in receipt of estrone–piperazine sulphate. When the active treatment was substituted by placebo there was a profound deterioration in mental depression and significant decreases in *free*-tryptophan and estrogen levels. However, restoration of active treatment was accompanied by marked improvement in all indices (Figure 12.4).

Estrogens, unesterified fatty acids and tryptophan levels

When plasma unesterified fatty acid (UFA) concentration increases, the *free* fraction of tryptophan also increases as UFA displaces the amino acid from its binding sites to plasma albumin[12]. Increased plasma UFA concentrations in rats is associated with significant increase in *free* plasma–tryptophan[27], and increased plasma UFA within minutes of exposure to stress occurs in human subjects[28]. These observations indicate that often disregarded environmental disturbances may be relevant to the design and interpretation of experiments on tryptophan. At present the effects of estrogen replacement therapy on changes in UFA levels in perimenopausal women are being evaluated[29]. Results to date indicate no significant changes in plasma levels of cholesterol, triglycerides or UFA in patients in receipt of either estrone–piperazine sulphate or estradiol valerate for periods ranging from 3 months to 2 years. Fluctuations in UFA levels in plasma are thus unlikely to be responsible for the increased *free* plasma–tryptophan levels found in perimenopausal patients treated with 'natural' estrogens.

Conclusions

The climacteric heralds the insidious approach of a large number of clinical problems which are thought to be associated with the decline in endogenous estrogen production and function that follows the menopause. A great variety of disturbing psychological alterations which, in fact, appear well in advance, in the pre-menopausal period, correlate fairly well with diminishing levels of endogenous estrogen.

Unfortunately, the evidence in favour of estrogens' beneficial effects on climacteric depression has, in the past, been based on uncontrolled studies. In the present article an attempt has been made to describe controlled clinical trials in which treatment of the perimenopausal patient with 'natural' estrogens is associated with a definite improvement in mental depression. It is proposed that the data reviewed provides sufficient evidence to support a relationship between declining estrogen levels and the psychological changes associated with the ageing woman. The recognition of perimenopausal depression is advocated as a distinct entity specifically related to endogenous estrogen deficiency, and disturbed indoleamine metabolism. Evidence is presented which implies that perimenopausal depression associated with endogenous withdrawal and abnormally low levels of *free* plasma–tryptophan should be specifically treated with appropriate 'natural' estrogen preparations without recourse to the ever proliferating tranquillizers and antidepressants which have but a limited place in the treatment of this syndrome.

Acknowledgments

I wish to thank my colleague Jeffrey Maddock for his technical advice and co-operation in providing some of the data for this article, my Secretary Sandra Thomas for her untiring and efficient assistance in the preparation of the manuscript, and my wife for her help in the management of the patients.

References

1. Utian, W. H. (1973). Comparative trial of P1496, a new non-steroidal oestrogen analogue. *Brit. Med. J.*, **1,** 409
2. Jones, W. H., Cohen, E. J. and Wilson, R. B. (1973). Clinical aspects of the menopause. In: K. J. Ryan and D. C. Gibson (eds:). *Menopause and Aging*, pp. 2–4. (D.H.E.W. Publication, N.I.H. No. 73–319, Bethesda Public Health Service)
3. Dapunt, O. (1967). Das klimakterische Syndrom. *Zbl. Gynäk.*, **89,** 300
4. Winter, G. F. (1967). Natürliche konjugierte Oestrogene im Klimakterium. *Zbl. Gynäk.*, **89,** 296
5. Kopera, H. (1973). Estrogens and psychic-functions. In P. A. van Keep and C. Lauritzen (eds.). *Frontiers of Hormone Research: Ageing and Estrogens*, **vol. 2.** pp. 118–33 (Basel: Karger)
6. Coppen, A., Prange, A. J., Whybrow, P. C. and Noguera, R. (1972). Abnormalities of indoleamines in affective disorders. *Arch. Gen. Psychiatr.*, **26,** 474
7. Ashcroft, G. W., Crawford, T. B. B., Cundall, R. L., Davidson, D. L., Dobson, J., Dow, R. C., Eccleston, D., Loose, R. W. and Pullar, I. A. (1973). 5-Hydroxytryptamine metabolism in affective illnesses: the effect of tryptophan administration. *Psychol. Med.*, **3,** 326
8. Ridges, A. P. (1975). Biochemistry of depression: a review. *J. Int. Med. Res.*, **3,** (Suppl.) (2), 42
9. Jequier, E., Robinson, D. S., Levenberg, W. and Sjoerdsma, A. (1969). Tryptophan-5-hydroxlase activity and brain tryptophan metabolism. *Biochem. Pharmac.*, **18,** 1071
10. Eccleston, D., Ashcroft, G. W. and Crawford, T. B. B. (1965). 5-Hydroxyindole metabolism in rat brain. A study of intermediate metabolism using the technique of tryptophan loading. II. Applications and drug studies. *J. Neurochem.*, **12,** 493

11. Tagliamonte, A., Biggio, G., Vargiu, L. and Gessa, G. L. (1973). Increase of brain tryptophan and stimulation of serotonin synthesis by salicylate. *J. Neurochem.*, **20**, 909
12. McMenamy, R. H. and Oncley, J. L. (1958). Specific binding of L-tryptophan to serum albumin. *J. Biol. Chem.*, **233**, 1436
13. Knott, P. J. and Curzon, G. (1972). Free tryptophan in plasma and brain tryptophan metabolism. *Nature, London*, **239**, 452
14. McArthur, J. N., Dawkins, P. D. and Smith, M. J. H. (1971). The displacement of L-tryptophan and dipeptides from bovine serum albumin *in vitro* and from human plasma *in vivo* by anti-inflammatory drugs. *J. Pharm. Pharmacol.*, **23**, 393
15. Aylward, M. and Maddock, J. (1973). Total and free plasma tryptophan concentrations in rheumatoid disease. *J. Pharm. Pharmacol.*, **25**, 570
16. Aylward, M. and Maddock, J. (1974). Plasma L-tryptophan concentrations in chronic rheumatic diseases and the effects of some antirheumatic drugs on the binding of the amino acid to plasma proteins *in vitro* and *in vivo*. *Rheumatol. Rehabil.*, **13**, 62
17. Aylward, M. (1973). Plasma tryptophan levels and mental depression in postmenopausal subjects: Effects of oral piperazine–oestrone sulphate. *I.R.C.S. Med. Sci.*, **1**, 30
18. Coppen, A., Eccleston, E. G. and Peet, M. (1972). Total and free tryptophan concentration in the plasma of depressive patients. *Lancet*, **ii**, 1415
19. Maddock, J., Jackson, D., Rees, P., Thomson, J. and Aylward, M. (1976). Plasma tryptophan levels and sleep in depressed female patients. (In preparation)
20. Aylward, M., Maddock, J., Parker, R. J., Holly, F., Murray, R., Jackson, D. and English, H. (1976). Epidemiology of perimenopausal complaints in an urban population. (In preparation)
21. Hamilton, M. (1960). A rating scale for depression. *J. Neurol. Neurosurg. Psychiat.*, **23**, 56
22. Kupperman, H. S., Blatt, M. G. H., Wiesbader, H. and Filler, W. (1953). Vasomotor disturbances and the menopause. *J. Clin. Endocrinol. Metab.*, **13**, 688
23. Jaszmann, L. (1973). Epidemiology of climacteric and post-climacteric complaints. In: P. A. van Keep and C. Lauritzen (eds.). *Ageing and Estrogens: Front. Hormone Res.*, **2**, pp. 22–34 (Basel: Karger)
24. Kirkham, K. E. and Hunter, W. M. (1971). *Radioimmunoassay Methods*, (Edinburgh and London: Churchill Livingstone)
25. Abraham, G. E. (1974). Radioimmunoassay of steroids in biological fluids. *Acta Endocrinol.*, 183 (Suppl.)
26. Aylward, M., Holly, F. and Parker, R. J. (1974). An evaluation of clinical response to piperazine–oestrone sulphate ('Harmogen') in menopausal patients. *Curr. Med. Res. Opin.*, **2**, 417
27. Curzon, G. and Knott, P. J. (1975). Rapid effects of environmental disturbance on rat plasma unesterified fatty acid and tryptophan concentrations and their prevention by antilipolytic drugs. *Br. J. Pharmacol.*, **54**, 389
28. Taggart, P. and Carruthers, M. (1971). Endogenous hyperlipidaemia induced by emotional stress of racing driving. *Lancet*, **i**, 363
29. Aylward, M., Maddock, J. and Rees, P. (1976). Natural oestrogen replacement therapy and blood clotting. *Brit. Med. J.*, **1**, 220

13

Double blind psychometric studies on the effects of natural estrogens on post-menopausal women

S. Campbell

Claims as to the beneficial effects of estrogen therapy on symptomatic and psychological changes of the menopause vary enormously. On the one hand there are the rather exaggerated claims of Wilson and Wilson[1] who believe estrogen to be a panacea for all post-menopausal ills and the media who are at present promoting HRT as the 'happy pill', while on the other hand there are workers like Utian[2, 3] who believe that the only effects of estrogen therapy are to control vasomotor symptoms and atrophic vaginitis. Utian, in one of the few well documented placebo controlled trials found that estrogen had no effect on insomnia, irritability, depression, palpitations, backache or libido although he did observe a 'mental tonic' effect with oral estrogen.

Because of the dearth of good placebo studies published to date on the effect of estrogens on post-menopausal symptomatology and psychological changes, we carried out two randomized double-blind placebo trials. The first (lasting 4 months) contained patients with severe menopausal symptoms and data from 64 patients were obtained; the second (lasting 1 year) was designed for patients with less acute symptomatology and contained 56 patients.

Patients and methods

All patients in the trials were post-menopausal or had infrequent periods with at least 3 months between menses. The patients were informed that the tablets given to them would be of different strengths and the patient's

General Practitioner was informed in every case that a placebo trial was being conducted.

In the first study each patient was monitored for 4 months. For 2 of these months they took Premarin 1·25 mg daily in 3 weekly courses, with one treatment-free week between each course, and for 2 months they ingested a placebo tablet also for 3 weeks in every 4. The patients in the 4-month study had severe post-menopausal symptoms which did not justify a prolonged placebo trial. In particular, 44 of the 64 patients in the short study had severe vasomotor symptoms. However, 20 patients had negligible vasomotor symptoms and differences in the response to treatment of these patients when compared with the flushing patients will be discussed.

The second study was similar to the first except that each patient was monitored for 12 months, 6 months of which they took Premarin 1·25 mg for 3 weeks in every 4, and 6 months of which they ingested placebo on an identical schedule. Most of these patients had vasomotor symptoms but they were of a less intense nature than those of the short trial patients and the majority presented with a different complaint.

Patients filled in questionnaires on admission to the study (control values) and at each 2-monthly attendance; 24 patients were lost from the 2-month trial initially, because of insufficient instruction on how to complete the form but this deficiency was corrected when we obtained the services of our Research Assistant, Jane Minardi. It should be stressed, however, that neither she nor the attending doctors were aware of which particular tablets the patient was ingesting. Eleven patients (9%) left the trials before completion, seven while taking placebo and four while taking Premarin. Six of these patients left for incidental reasons, such as moving from the district, but five left the trial because of side effects attributed to the therapy; four of these patients were taking placebo and one was taking Premarin. The patient taking Premarin complained of chest pain, tension, swelling and aching of the legs, but also complained of these symptoms while on placebo. Two of the patients on placebo left the trial with a similar list of symptoms while two further placebo patients left because vasomotor symptoms had returned and they were unwilling to continue.

Symptometric and psychometric evaluation was carried out by the following tests:

1. Graphic Rating Scales (GRS)

Graphic rating scales[4, 5] are a widely accepted, sensitive method of measuring emotional change. A line of fixed length is provided for every symptom and emotional state to be studied and a description of the extremes of the symptom or emotional state is stated at each end of the line. The subject makes a self rating of his or her present state by making a mark on the line, usually at some intermediate point. The scales are filled in at regular intervals by the patient and the distance from one end of the line measured at each visit to give a quantitative assessment of change. A sample of a graphic rating scale assessment is shown in Figure 13.1.

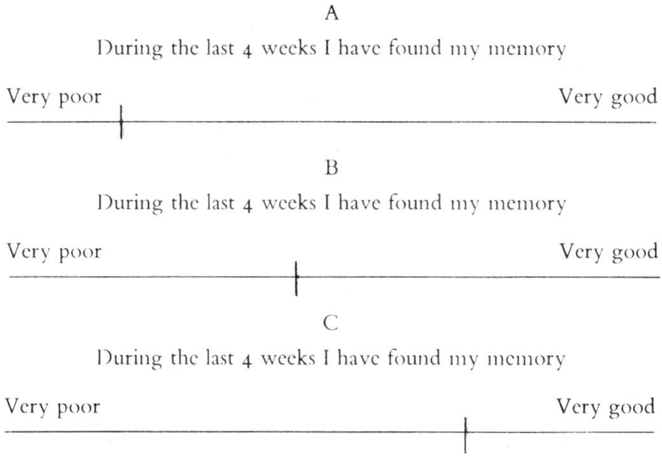

Figure 13.1 Typical graphic rating scale recording for memory scores A. for control; B. after placebo tablet for 6 months; C. after Premarin tablet for 6 months

2. Beck Self-Rating Questionnaire (Beck Score)

This is a self-rating questionnaire which measures changes in levels of depression and was devised by Beck *et al.*[6] in America. It is a measure of quite severe depression and is not as sensitive as the graphic rating scales. It was used in this trial principally to establish any relationship between depression and the incidence of menopausal symptoms. However, it was also used to monitor changes on drug or placebo and only these aspects will be discussed in this paper.

3. Eysenck Personality Inventory (EPI)

This is a widely used personality test which provides scores on neuroticism and extroversion and it was used to provide a measure of possible predisposition to menopausal symptoms. More recently it has been shown that there is a slight fall in neuroticism and rise in extroversion scores on recovery from depression and therefore changes in the score on drug and placebo were also examined.

4. General Health Questionnaire (GHQ)

This questionnaire was devised for epidemiological studies as a way of detecting potential cases of psychiatric disorder by Goldberg[7]. The higher the score the more likely it is that the individual has a psychiatric problem. It does not provide a diagnosis and it was used in an attempt to correlate

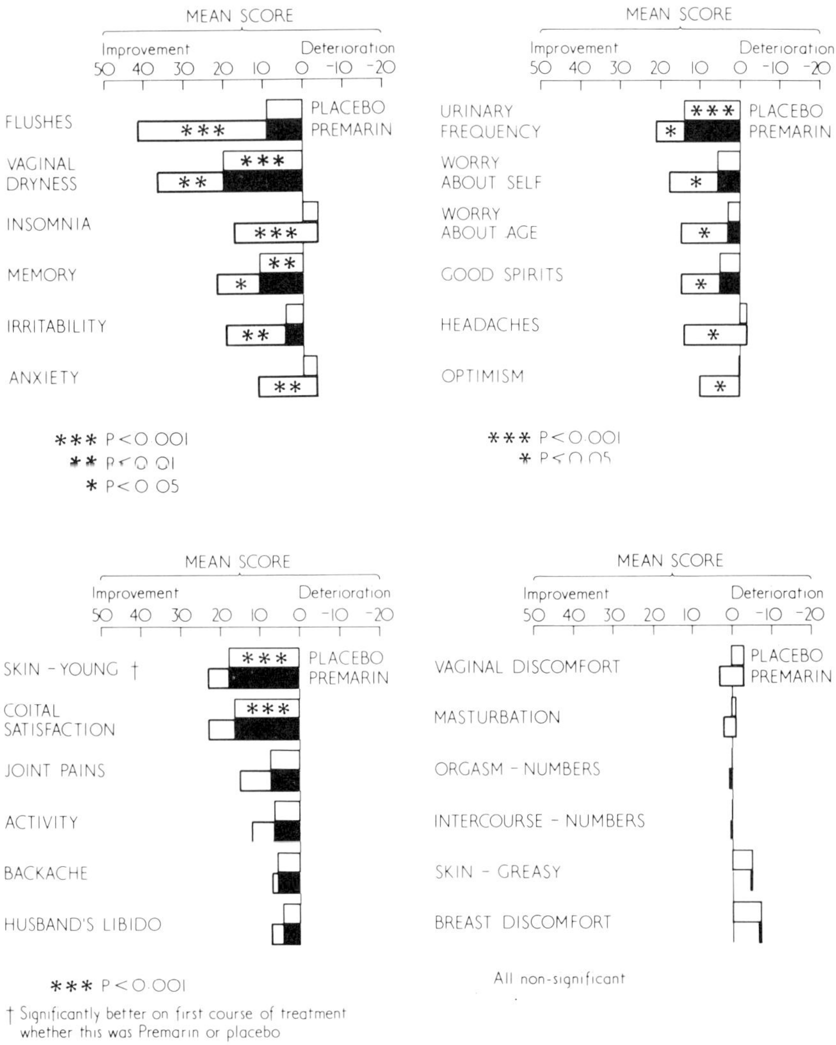

Figure 13.2 Differences in graphic rating scale scores for Premarin and placebo therapy in the four-month study

severity of symptoms with psychiatric illness. However, as with the Beck and EPI scores we also used this test to monitor changes between drug and placebo.

Results and Discussion

Four-month study

A statistical comparison was made between the graphic rating scale assessments after both courses of treatment. There was no statistical difference between the first and second courses of treatment no matter which tablet was taken, suggesting that the placebo effect was similar whether it was ingested before or after the Premarin. Changes in the mean GRS score on placebo relative to control and Premarin relative to placebo were analysed statistically using Student's '*t*' test and are presented in Figure 13.2.

The importance of the placebo effect in any study such as this is illustrated by finding highly significant placebo effects on vaginal dryness, urinary frequency and coital satisfaction which are inexplicable except as part of a general psychological uplift which all patients experience in going to a clinic and receiving sympathy and medical attention for their menopausal ailments. The significant placebo effect on 'youthful skin' is more understandable in view of the beauty parlour publicity and explains the continuing success of these institutions.

Beneficial effects of Premarin over placebo were expected for vasomotor symptoms and vaginal dryness and these are clearly demonstrated in this study. However, benefits of estrogen therapy over placebo were also observed for many other symptoms including significant reductions in insomnia, irritability, headaches, anxiety, urinary frequency and significant improvements in memory, good spirits and optimism. The improvement in such a large number of symptoms is to some extent a domino effect, i.e. a reduction in vasomotor symptoms will create a favourable response in a large number of other associated symptoms. This can be demonstrated by studying the 20 women who had severe 'menopausal' symptoms but who had no flushes; in this group significant improvements on estrogen therapy were observed only for vaginal dryness, memory and anxiety (including worry about self and worry about age). The improvement in insomnia which was highly significant in the flushing patients was not apparent in this group indicating that insomnia is clearly related to vasomotor symptoms. However, the improvement in memory and anxiety scores in this sub-group does suggest that the 'mental tonic' effect described by Utian[3] is an entity and is independent of vasomotor symptoms.

Twelve-month study

For this analysis, a mean score for the whole 6-month treatment period was determined for each patient. Again there was no statistical difference between the first and second courses of treatment, no matter which tablet was taken.

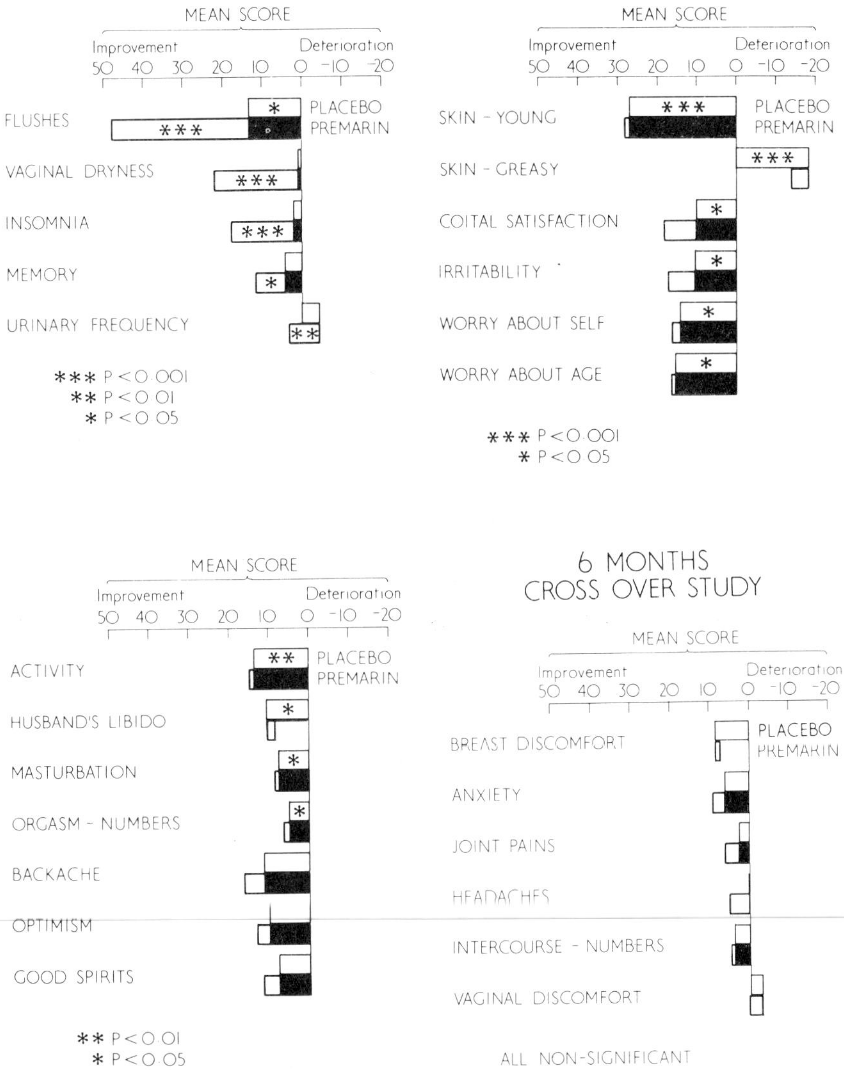

Figure 13.3 Differences in the graphic rating scores for Premarin and placebo therapy in the twelve-month study

Changes in the mean GRS score on Premarin and placebo were analysed as before and the results are presented in Figure 13.3. As expected the longer placebo trial showed alterations in the placebo effect. For example, the highly significant placebo effect on vaginal dryness and urinary frequency demonstrated in the short trial now disappeared. Conversely, the longer treatment period with Premarin resulted in an enhanced improvement in these symptoms. With 'youthful skin' however, the positive placebo effect was maintained and in addition there was now a significant increase in skin greasiness with the placebo tablet (this is recorded in Figure 13.3 as a deterioration, although in patients with dry skin this effect would probably be regarded as beneficial). It is thus clear that patient judgements on skin texture and appearance is highly subjective and is of no reliance when judging the value of estrogen therapy.

The beneficial effects of estrogen on vasomotor symptoms, vaginal dryness, insomnia, memory and urinary frequency observed in the short study were maintained and in some instances enhanced by the prolonged therapy. The other symptoms previously reported as showing significant improvement in the 4-month study did not reach significance which is explained by the fact that as vasomotor symptoms were less severe in this group, the domino effect was also less marked. Nevertheless, there was a small shift towards improvement in 15 of the 19 remaining symptoms (Figure 13.3) and it is likely that this reflects an overall increase in morale due to the elimination of flushes and atrophic vaginitis and also the 'mental tonic' effect again shown by an increased memory score. Certainly there is no evidence of a direct estrogen effect on symptoms such as back ache, joint pains or libido. It is interesting that the effect of estrogen on libido as reflected by masturbation, orgasm, frequency of coitus and coital satisfaction showed no significant enhancement despite the marked improvement in vaginal dryness, indicating that the ability to have sexual intercourse and the desire to have sexual intercourse are not necessarily related. Husbands libido also did not appear to change with the patient's altered estrogen status.

The difficulty in assessing the effect of estrogen therapy by the standard personality and depression scoring systems is highlighted by the results presented in Figure 13.4. The Beck score, the GHQ and the neuroticism score as assessed by the EPI all showed highly significant improvement on both placebo and Premarin over control values, but although the effect of Premarin was slightly greater, the difference was non-significant. This suggests that these tests are not sufficiently sensitive when monitoring changes in women who for the most part do not have psychiatric problems. These results also re-emphasize that in menopausal women strong placebo effects can persist for as long as 6 months.

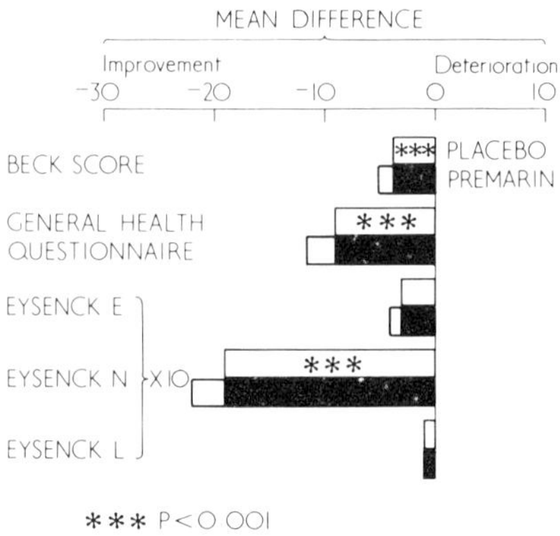

Figure 13.4 Differences in the Beck score, GHQ and Eysenck personality scores for Premarin and placebo therapy in the twelve-month study

Summary

A 4-month double-blind placebo trial with Premarin (conjugated equine estrogens) was performed on 64 patients with severe menopausal symptoms. Using the graphic rating scale system of assessment, a statistically significant improvement was observed with Premarin in 12 psychological and symptomatic scores (Table 13.1). From a study of 20 patients without vasomotor symptoms it appears that many of these symptomatic improvements resulted from the abolition of flushes and the treatment of vaginal atrophy and dryness (i.e. a domino effect). Nevertheless, there did appear to be 'mental tonic' effect with estrogens as shown by an improvement in the memory and a reduction in the anxiety scores.

A second 12-month double-blind placebo trial was also performed on 56 patients with less severe menopausal symptoms and a statistically significant improvement in five psychological and symptomatic scores was observed with Premarin as assessed by the graphic rating scales (Table 13.1). Despite the lessening of the domino effect, there was a small improvement in 15 of the remaining 19 symptoms and it is likely that the cumulative effect of these small improvements indicates an overall enhancement of well-being. The strength of the placebo effect was particularly well observed in the three standard psychiatric scoring systems, the Beck score (for depression), the General Health Questionnaire and the Eysenck Personality Index (for

Table 13.1 Symptoms significantly improved by estrogen therapy when compared with placebo

2-month cross over study (64 patients)	*6-month cross over study (56 patients)*
1. Hot flushes	1. Hot flushes
2. Insomnia	2. Vaginal dryness
3. Vaginal dryness	3. Insomnia
4. Irritability	4. Urinary frequency
5. Poor memory*	5. Poor memory
6. Anxiety*	
7. Worry about age*	
8. Headaches	
9. Worry about self*	
10. Urinary frequency	
11. Optimism	
12. Good spirits	

* Significant improvement in 20 patients without flushes

neuroticism). All three showed highly significant placebo effects extending for 6 months with a small but non-significant improvement with Premarin over placebo. It is suggested that these tests are not sufficiently sensitive to assess psychologic or symptomatic changes in menopausal women and that this is best achieved by the graphic rating scales.

Acknowledgement

This chapter, presented by S. Campbell, was written jointly by Campbell, S., Beard, R. J., McQueen, J., Christie Brown, Margaret E. and Minardi, Jane.

References

1. Wilson, R. A. and Wilson, Thelma, A. (1963). The fate of the nontreated post-menopausal woman: a plea for the maintenance of adequate estrogen from puberty to the grave. *J. Am. Geriatr. Soc.*, Vol. XI, No. 4, 347
2. Utian, W. H. (1972). The true clinical features of post-menopause and oophorectomy and their response to oestrogen therapy. *South Afr. Med. J.*, **46,** 732
3. Utian, W. H. (1975). Definitive symptoms of post-menopause incorporating use of vaginal parabasal cell index. In: P. A. van Keep and C. Lauritzen (eds). *Frontiers in Hormone Research: Estrogens in the Post-Menopause*, pp. 74–93. (Basel: S. Karger)
4. Guilford, S. (1936). *Psychometric Methods*, New York

5. Lader, M. H. and Wing, L. (1966). Physiological measures, sedative drugs and morbid anxiety. *Institute of Psychiatry Maudsley Monographs* (Oxford: Oxford University Press)
6. Beck, A. T., Ward, C. H., Mendelson, M., Mock, J. and Erbaugh, J. (1961). An inventory for measuring depression. *Arch. Gen. Psychiatr.*, **4**, 561
7. Goldberg, D. P. (1972). The detection of psychiatric illness by questionnaire. *Institute of Psychiatry Maudsley Monographs* (Oxford: Oxford University Press)

14

Double blind cross-over study of estrogen replacement therapy

Jean Coope

Estrogens relieve hot flushes at the menopause and they have been used successfully in this country in small doses for many years.

The present argument is about whether other symptoms such as depression, weakness and dizziness respond to estrogen. If they do, are we justified in giving replacement therapy for the rest of our patients' lives? Are estrogens effective and are they safe?

We set up a double-blind cross-over study of 30 menopausal women in general practice[1]. We used conjugated equine estrogens because the manufacturers claimed that there were no adverse effects on blood clotting with this therapy. The trial took place in a mixed industrial and rural group practice of 6500 patients on the edge of the Pennine hills. 35 women aged 40–61 years presenting at the surgery with one or more menopausal symptoms included in the Kupperman Menopausal Index were given a code number and randomly allocated to two groups on a double-blind basis. They were told that they would be given during the following six months two preparations, one of which was estrogen and the other a harmless inert tablet. Neither they nor the doctor would be informed which preparation they received first.

Table 14.1 shows the number of women presenting with symptoms and how severely they were affected.

The patients were assessed clinically by the Menopausal Index described by Kupperman and Blatt in 1953[2]. Also the symptoms were recorded separately. Hot flushes were counted in the week before assessment Assessments took place before therapy and each month for 6 months.

Clotting studies were carried out by Dr Leon Poller at Withington Hospital and are reported separately (Chapter 27).

Vaginal cytology was carried out and the Karyopyknotic Index calculated, at the beginning, cross-over and end of the trial. Weight and blood pressure were recorded and patients were asked to report side effects, particularly pain or swelling in the legs.

Table 14.1 Number of patients presenting with symptoms and their severity

Symptom	*No. moderately or severely affected*	*No. mildly affected*	*No. completely relieved on placebo*	*No. completely relieved on estrogen*	*P value estrogen v. placebo (mean scores)*
Hot flushes	19	8	4	10	0·78 (proportional reduction = 0·04)
Paraesthesiae	6	14	4	6	0·14
Insomnia	2	17	6	7	0·25
Nervousness	14	8	4	10	0·12
Depression	12	5	4	5	0·93
Vertigo	4	6	4	3	0·90
Weakness	9	12	5	9	0·11
Arthralgia	8	9	3	5	0·26
Headaches	6	9	5	5	0·16
Palpitations	5	11	3	9	0·21
Formication		8	2	4	0·30
Menopausal index score	21	9	2	3	0·07

Group I were given Premarin (conjugated equine estrogens) 1·25 mg daily during three 21-day courses with a 7-day gap between each. Group II were given lactose tablets identical in taste and appearance with Premarin. After three months Group I received placebo and Group II Premarin for three months.

Five patients left before completion of the study. One woman moved and was lost to the trial, and two on estrogen failed to attend for clinical assessment at three months. Two patients with long psychiatric histories developed severe headaches and depression, the code was broken and they were found to be on estrogen and they were subsequently withdrawn from the trial.

Results

Both groups showed a striking improvement in the first 3 months. Although the estrogen group produced lower mean scores the response of all symptoms to placebo was so marked that no significant difference was found on statistical analysis using the Mann–Witney U test. After the cross-over, patients who were withdrawn from estrogen showed a sudden deterioration and returned to their initial level of symptoms. Patients who progressed from placebo to estrogen showed a further improvement which did not reach the 0·05 level of significance (see Figure 14.1).

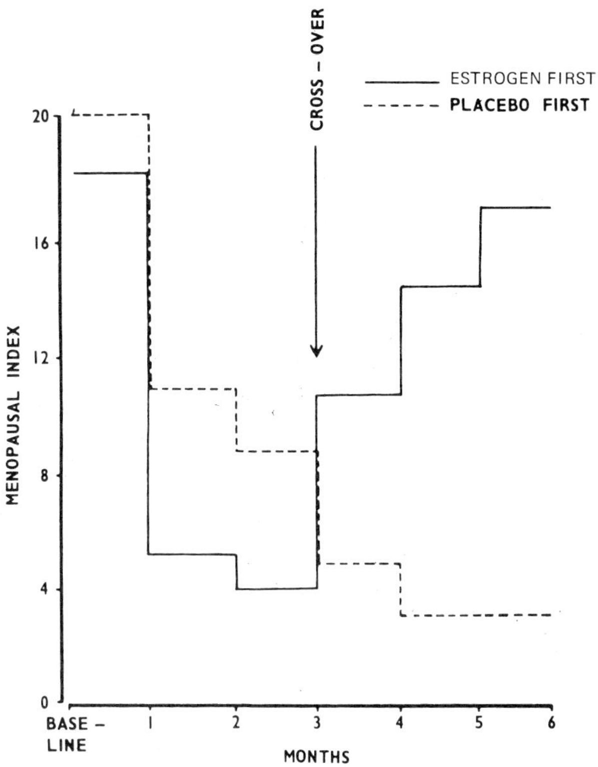

Figure 14.1 Kupperman Menopausal Index during the 6-month trial

When we looked at individual symptoms such as insomnia, arthralgia, vertigo, depression and palpitations, a similar picture emerged: (Figures 14.2–7). Individual patients showed striking response to estrogen, but

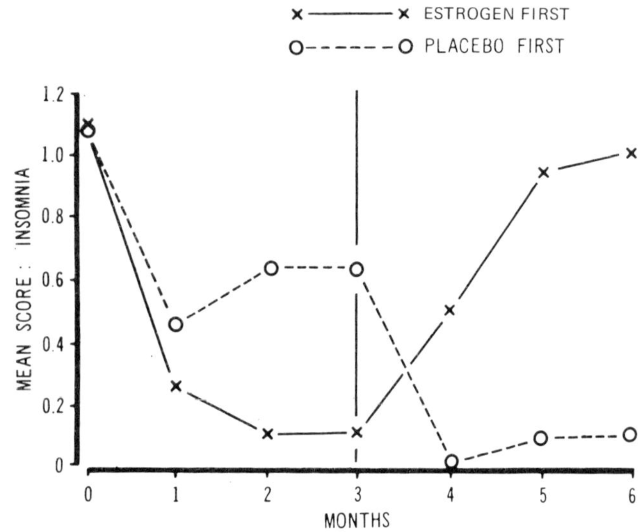

Figure 14.2 Assessment of insomnia during the 6-month trial

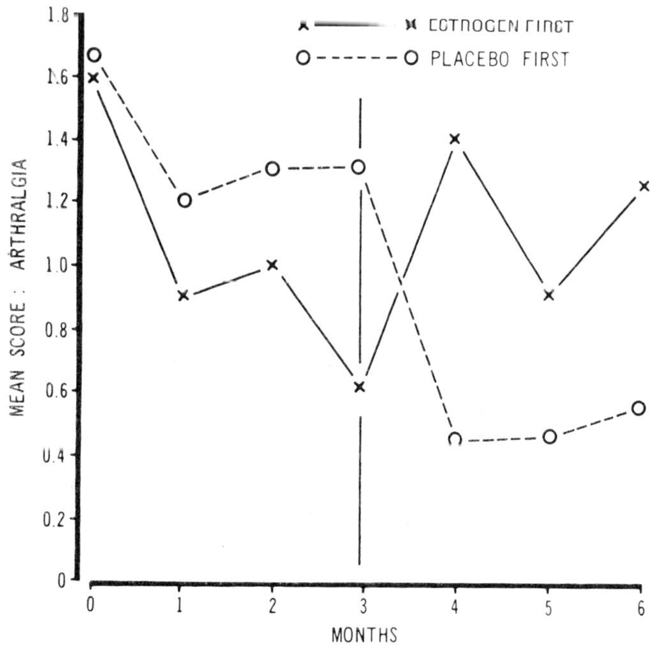

Figure 14.3 Assessment of arthralgia during the 6-month trial

analysis of the mean scores of the group showed a high placebo response which was not significantly different from the response to estrogen. Headaches (Figure 14.7) showed approximately equal scores, and many patients seemed to develop headache when taking estrogen; there would seem to be insufficient grounds for regarding headache as a menopausal symptom.

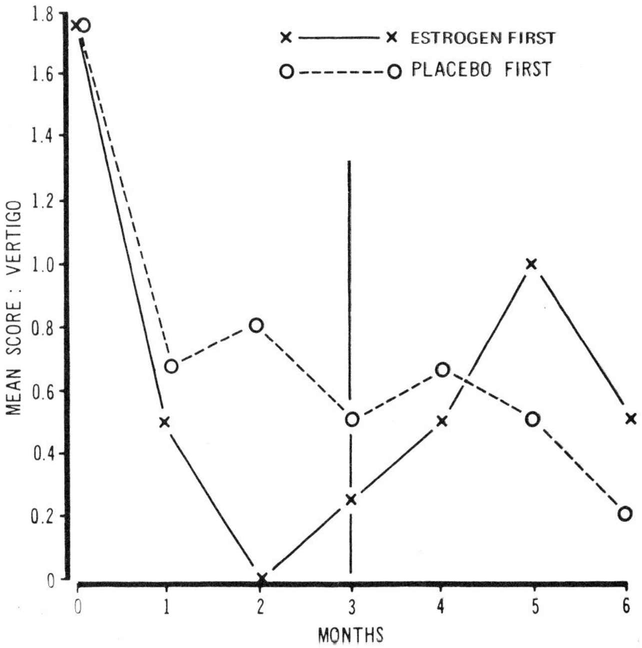

Figure 14.4 Assessment of vertigo during the 6-month trial

However, when we looked at hot flushes separately using the hot flush count (Figure 14.8) we found a significant proportional reduction on estrogen compared with placebo. Even here there is a high placebo response. This is reflected in the clinical observation that patients often complain that their hot flushes are worse when they are under stress. Relief of stress often improves their symptoms. The significant proportional difference between estrogen and placebo would imply that hot flushes are the most sensitive clinical indicator of the need for estrogen. Although placebo produced an improvement in flushes in most patients, it was usually necessary to give estrogen to abolish flushes completely.

The menopausal index, which combines estrogen-responsive symptoms such as flushes, with other less responsive symptoms such as headaches, is not as useful as the hot flush count in assessing the need for estrogen.

Weight and blood pressure showed no change on estrogen or placebo.

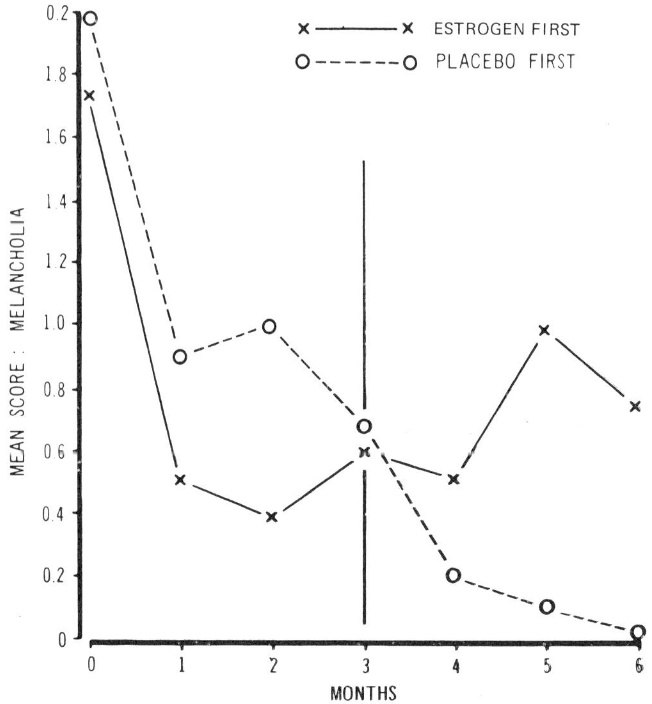

Figure 14.5 Assessment of melancholia during the 6-month trial

Vaginal cytology showed no correlation between Karyopyknotic Index and level of symptoms, as measured by the hot flush count or the Menopausal Index. These findings are similar to those reported by Wachtel and Gordon[2] in their study of 140 women in the London area.

Although the Karyopyknotic Index (Figure 14.9) showed a significant rise ($P<0{\cdot}05$) on estrogen compared with placebo, there was no significant correlation between improvement in symptoms and changes in the karyopyknotic index. The karyopyknotic index was not found to be a useful indicator of the initial need for estrogen, or a useful guide to therapy in this age group.

Side-effects were minimal (Table 14.2). It is interesting that nausea and breast discomfort occurred on placebo more commonly than on estrogen.

These were the side-effects which patients expected would occur on estrogen.

Clotting studies showed a significant increase in coagulation factors on natural estrogens and have been reported in detail by Dr Poller. His paper

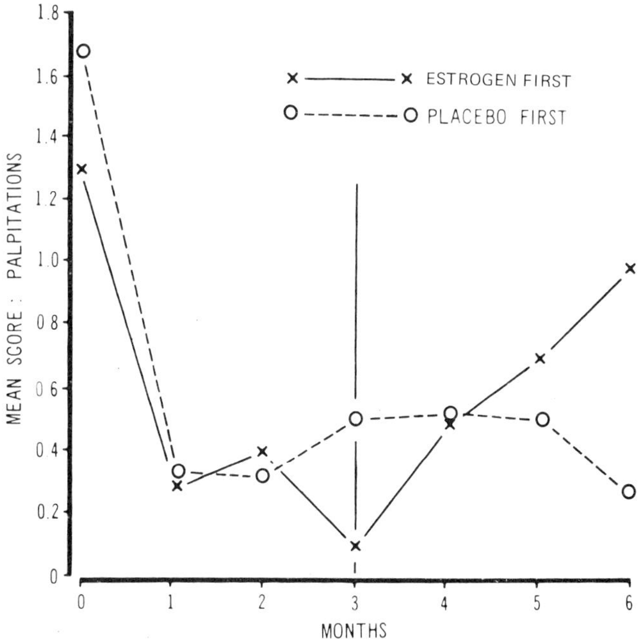

Figure 14.6 Assessment of palpitations during the 6-month trial

includes clinical details of the four patients who developed superficial venous thromboses during the trial. About one-third of patients showed no improvement on any therapy. These were mostly suffering from weakness, depression or headaches, and hot flushes were not predominant. 22 out of 30 women showed some improvement if only marginal, and embarked on long-term replacement therapy.

The loss of the placebo response in the second 3 months is interesting. It is probably related to the information we gave our patients. They knew they would receive *either* hormone *or* inert tablets and when hot flushes returned they knew that they were taking an inert preparation. The assessment might have been more objective if patients were told they would receive two hormones and that hot flushes might return, but it was considered more ethical to be completely frank with the patients, particularly in the clinical situation of general practice.

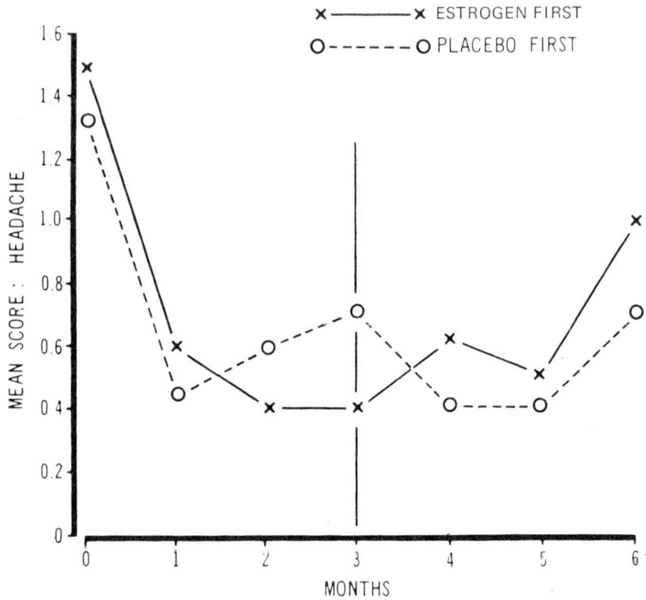

Figure 14.7 Assessment of headache during the 6-month trial

Table 14.2 Number of patients with side-effects

Symptom	*Placebo*	*Estrogen*
Nausea	2	0
Breast discomfort	2	1
Interval headache	0	1
Urinary infection	0	2
Nasal stuffiness	0	1
Rise in diastolic blood pressure> 90 mmHg	0	2
Rise in systolic blood pressure > 160 mmHg	0	3
Weight gain > 3 kg	2	2

The placebo response might conceivably have been even higher if patients had expected to receive estrogen throughout. Our women knew that there was a 50% chance of their receiving placebo.

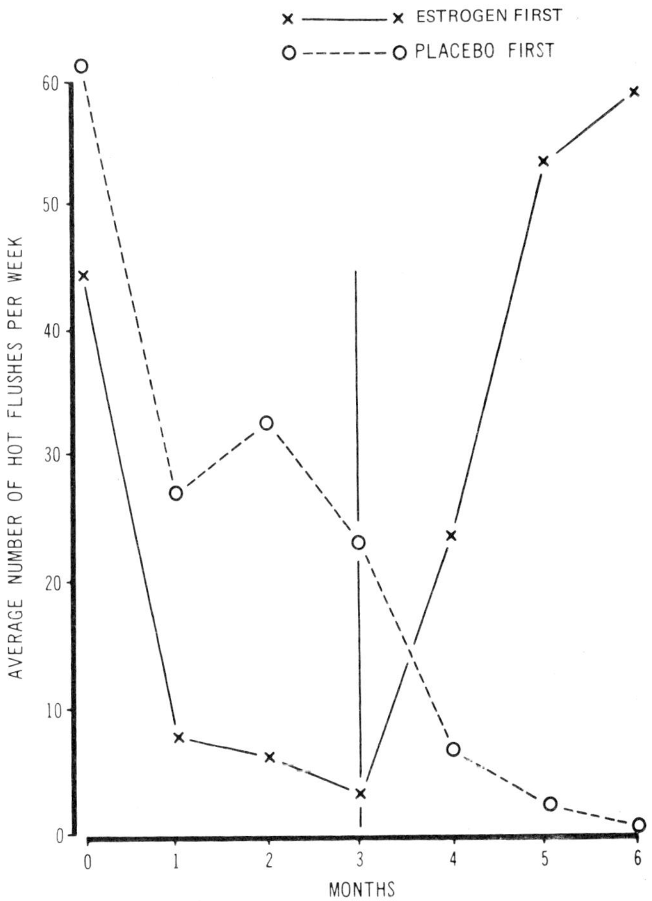

Figure 14.8 Hot flush count during the 6-month trial

The method of patient information is vitally important in a trial of this nature. If our patients had been told that they would receive a *non*-hormonal preparation I think the placebo effect would have been lower. The enormous publicity given to hormone replacement therapy in the lay press is reflected in the placebo response obtained. Possibly a longer trial would have shown a greater difference between estrogen and placebo. Our patients on long-term therapy are being followed up; however, any benefit must be set against the long-term risk of clotting problems, and findings reported by Dr Poller leave room for misgivings on this score.

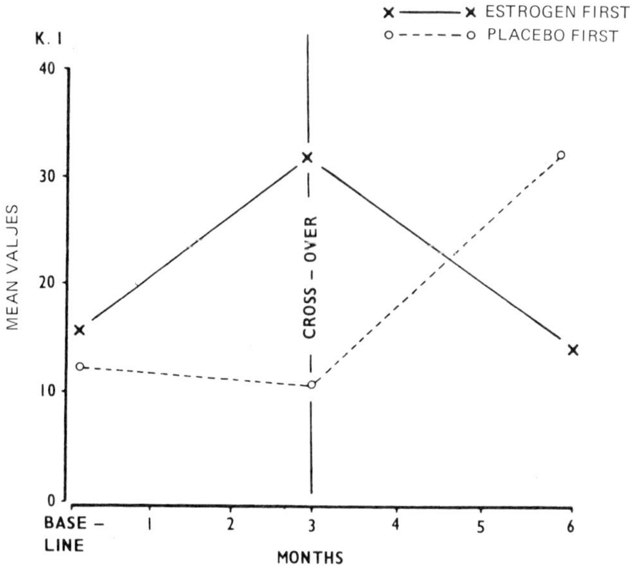

Figure 14.9 Karyopyknotic Index during the 6-month trial

Acknowledgement

Thanks are due to Ayerst Laboratories, Ltd., for their help and support throughout the trial.

References

1. Coope, J., Thomson, J. and Poller, L. (1975). *Br. Med. J.*, **4**, 139–143
2. Kuppermann, H. S., Blatt, M. U. G. and Wiesbaden, U. (1953). *J. Clin. Endocrinol.*, **13**, 88

Discussion on Section C:

Psychological Aspects

Chairman: *Mr. C. H. Naylor*

Mr C. H. Naylor (Chairman): We have heard in the various studies presented this afternoon that much use has been made of placebos. However, I should like to direct the first question to Dr Kerr. What part should or does the husband play in determining the emotional resources that the patient can draw upon, and should we have a scoring on the psychometric charts, indicating the husband's attitude?

Dr M. Dorothea Kerr (Psychiatrist, New York): I would certainly agree as a general principle that the husband should be included in any assessment. However, it is difficult enough to measure the woman's emotional responses without getting involved in those of the male.

Dr H. Minhas (Gynaecologist, Leeds): Hormone replacement therapy improves the texture of the skin, the texture of the hair, and halts osteoporosis. In other words, it halts the process of degeneration. Will it also improve a woman's life expectancy? We already have statistics to show that women live longer than men. Are we merely going to add to the number of years that women have to live alone?

Mr S. Campbell (Gynaecologist, London): We have no evidence that HRT will improve the life expectancy of women and indeed tomorrow's session may well show that we are putting our patients at some risk of thromboembolism. A more real problem is that by improving the woman's feeling of wellbeing, she will make sexual demands on her husband which he cannot possibly meet.

However, from our graphic rating scale assessments, libido was not significantly improved, so that it appears that the male will be spared undue stresses in his sexually declining years.

Dr P. A. Van Keep (Gynaecologist, Geneva): I could call myself a menopausologist. I was most interested in the first three papers, but I was slightly disappointed that nothing was said about the social aspects of the menopausal syndrome. We can safely say that the menopause is a completely different event for women in the higher social classes than it is for women in the lower social classes. This is of great relevance to our practical attitudes towards women who come and ask for help. The woman in a high social class can find her way to treatment, but the poorer woman, in a lower social class will be disappointed. She does not know what to say, what her complaints are, or what causes her complaints. She is more anxious than the more affluent woman. There is a further point, which Dr Jaszmann has already referred to and that is the role of the woman's job or occupation. Dr Jaszmann's sample included only a few women who worked but we were able to check on this factor using a much larger sample. We found that having a job, for women in a higher social class, has a strong protective effect against all unpleasant effects of the menopause, whereas in the lower social classes, it has exactly the opposite effect and it is these poorer women who need our help.

Dr C. Barbara Ballinger (Psychiatrist, Dundee): In our study there was no statistical difference in social class as far as I could classify it on husband's occupation. That was why I gave no figures. Social factors certainly play a large part. The sort of factors which did correlate with increased psychiatric morbidity were such things as children marrying or leaving home within the last year, and numbers of children. Women who had more than two children were more likely to have symptoms at this time. But this did not account for any change in psychiatric morbidity with the menopause and did not account for the hump in psychiatric morbidity in the pre-menopausal groups.

Mr C. H. Naylor: We are lucky to have a general practitioner with us. Dr Coope looks after patients in an industrial area and in the countryside. Did she notice any difference between the two sorts of ladies?

Dr Jean Coope (General Practitioner, Bollington): The number of patients was very small, but they ranged through all social groups, apart from class 5. We had several managing directors' wives, teachers, nurses, factory workers, home helps and cleaners. The women who were most in need of help were the poorer women, who were often under great stress. I would agree about the difficulties of running a job in a factory and running a home. Very often these women are saddled with grandchildren, they are going through tremendous family crises, and they have a lot of hard work. The better-off women seemed to want the estrogens for slightly different reasons. They wanted estrogens because of the publicity in the lay press, and the social class 1 women often wanted estrogens so that they could be glamorous hostesses. Of course we know that estrogens do not really increase libido, or at least in our study they did not, but some patients believed that they would. The poorer women were very often physically ill and were rather a different group. When we consider the numbers of patients in our practice, we must have several hundred women who are at risk from menopausal symptoms, of whom only thirty came for help during a period of about 9 or 10 months. The other women managed without it.

Dr M. Aylward (Clinical Research Consultant, Merthyr Tydfil): The pattern of severity of symptoms within the social classes has changed in our studies during the past year or 18 months. Prior to 18 months ago the patients that suffered the most were those in the lower social classes. Following the publicity that estrogen replacement has received, people in the upper social classes have been the most disturbed at their not receiving estrogen, and most patients now come from social classes 1, 2 and 3A.

Dr R. C. Greenberg (Community Psychiatrist, London): We know that in New York during the Great Depression the upper classes were the people throwing themselves out of windows. Is it not possible that what we have just been told is related to the changed economic climate, and therefore the greater depression of the so-called upper classes?

Mr C. H. Naylor: We ought to leave out any question concerning politics!

Dr R. C. Greenberg: It is not politics. It is a matter of real psychiatry. We know that true depressive illness increases in certain upper socio-economic classes during economic crises, whereas the lower socio-economic classes improve because the differential alters. To come to my two questions. First, to bring forward a point to which I have been trying to get an answer with reference to something Mr Campbell said this morning. Every time that I looked at his charts, two o'clock in the morning stared me in the face, and something that looked like diurnal variation. I should like to hear what the psychiatrists have to say about that. Early morning waking and diurnal variation are characteristics of endogenous depression.

I would also like to draw attention to the studies of Dr and Mrs Vasilou, the psychiatrists who run the Institute of Anthropos in Athens. They are studying psychiatric changes in the family in a society that is changing from a rural to an industrial society pretty rapidly. The attitudes that they have noticed are that people—women in particular—are changing from the traditional attitudes of the family, sacrifices for the children and planning for the future, to those of our kind of society where people are more interested in the here and now.

Mr C. H. Naylor: What, if anything, does Mr Campbell feel is the significance of the readings, and does he see a diurnal variation?

Mr S. Campbell: Of course there is a diurnal variation in androstenedione and testosterone, but that is the adrenal diurnal variation and not related to depression, or even to wakefulness. The spike at two o'clock in prolactin and in growth hormone is well known, and is related to deep sleep. This is well described in the literature. We certainly cannot relate this to the wakefulness of endogenous depression.

Mr C. H. Naylor: In answer to the second part of Dr. Greenberg's question, this afternoon we had very clearly defined for us a clinical syndrome, namely the psychiatric effects of the menopause. We have been asked whether that is changing in relation to other movements in our society. We cannot really answer that question this afternoon. It would require another symposium.

Dr E. J. Salter (Psychiatrist, Nottingham): As I understand it, a double-blind trial is one where the patient does not know what she is receiving and cannot know what she is receiving. I would question whether it is possible to do a double-blind trial with a drug that is so effective in treating a symptom such as hot flushes. I would submit that it is not possible to do a double-blind trial on depression in a patient whose hot flushes are being treated so effectively. I accept that hot flushes make people very unhappy, and that they can be made happy again following treatment. What I find difficult to accept is that seriously depressed people can be treated with estrogens. I do not think that most of those who spoke really believe that but I am not quite sure about Dr Kerr from the States. What kind of patients with depression would Dr Kerr treat with estrogens, bearing in mind that many of the severely depressed patients on this side of the Atlantic might be considered to be schizophrenic in the States, and that many of the patients in this country, to whom we give psychotherapy, would not be considered severely depressed?

Mr C. H. Naylor: That is a complicated question. First, the criticism of a double-blind trial. The questioner has asked whether the patients who derive benefit from it do not twig that they are on the estrogen, and not the placebo. Would that be correct.

Mr S. Campbell: I think that the questioner is wrong. The patients did not realise whether they were on estrogen or on placebo, hence the powerful placebo effects on the most unlikely symptoms such as vaginal dryness. Even in the six-months' cross-over trial prolonged placebo effects were demonstrated. These patients did not know, and neither did we.

Mr C. H. Naylor: I am not sure whether the second point was relevant—the ability of psychiatrists in this country to make a diagnosis of schizophrenia, and those in the States. Can I put it to Dr Kerr that we should like to know how she reaches a diagnosis of depression, and how she would treat it using estrogens?

Dr E. J. Salter: I am really anxious about gynaecologists treating serious depression.

Dr M. Dorothea Kerr: The patients were evaluated by many scales; psychiatric examination, Hamilton depression and anxiety scales as well. As for gynaecologists treating severely depressed patients, I would share the questioner's anxiety but in the dosages of estrogen used, I doubt that the gynaecologist would find it very effective.

Mr C. H. Naylor: We have come to the end of a very busy and successful first day, and that must be a good omen for Tuesday and Wednesday.

Section D

LIPID METABOLISM

Chairman: T. M. COLTART

15

The menopause and coronary heart disease

M. F. Oliver

Introduction

It is surprising that the influence of the menopause on coronary heart disease (CHD) has not received more attention in recent years. The subject seems to have been ignored by gynaecologists, endocrinologists and cardiologists—each presumably believing that the other is a repository of important information. But when one comes to assemble what is known about the interrelationship between the menopause and CHD, many gaps appear and it is clear that more studies are needed.

Epidemiology

It has been said on many occasions that the myocardial infarct rate in women lags 10–15 years behind that of men and there is no reason to alter this statement now. The male excess is still clearly evident in 1973 (Table 15.1). This sex difference is virtually absent in the Japanese, Bantus and U.S. negroes[1] for reasons which are not clear, although they may be partly nutritional since atherosclerosis is relatively uncommon in these races.

There has been a striking change in the coronary death rate in young and middle-aged women during the last 12–15 years (Figure 15.1). Between the years 1958 and 1972, there was a 50% increase in deaths from coronary heart disease in women aged 35–44 years and a 36% increase in women aged 45–54 years, but there was a negligible increase in women aged 55–64 years. This increase in the younger age groups was not evident before 1958. One can only speculate about the reasons for this abrupt and striking change. Greater cigarette smoking is likely to have contributed to the increased incidence

Table 15.1 Mortality from myocardial infarction by age and sex (RG, England and Wales, 1972)

Decades	*Males*	*Females*	*M : F Ratio*
35–44	546	80	6·8 : 1
45–54	2391	408	5·9 : 1
55–64	6022	1627	3·7 : 1
65–74	13110	5279	2·5 : 1

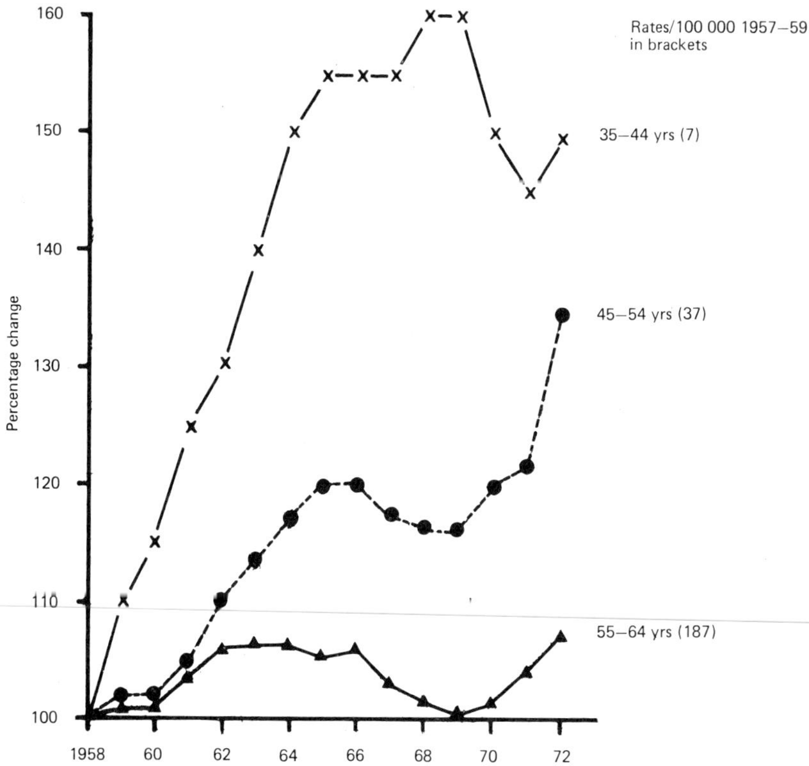

Figure 15.1 Percentage change in death rates from CHD, females. England and Wales (three-year moving averages with 1957–59 = 100)

in the 35–44 age group and there have been equally striking alterations in cigarette smoking habits in young women over approximately the same period of time. The Tobacco Research Council[2] has shown a 60% increase in cigarette smokers in women aged 20–29 over the last 15 years, and they are heavy cigarette smokers.

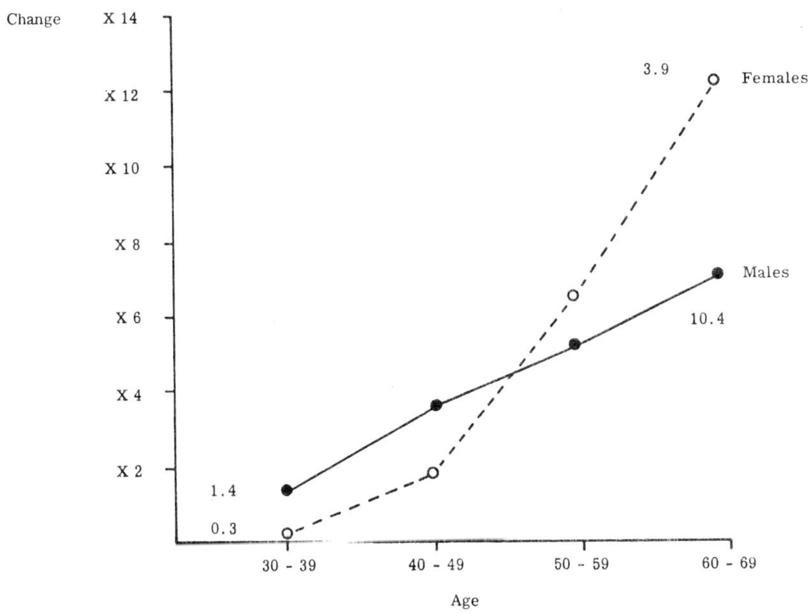

Figure 15.2 Acute heart attacks: incidence rates/1000 and change by age and sex (Edinburgh Community Study, 1972)

A community survey conducted in Edinburgh in 1972 reported the incidence of heart attacks in the city as a whole[3]. While acute heart attacks were, of course, more common in men at all ages up to 69 (the maximum age of the study), the rate of change was appreciably greater in women (Figure 15.2). While it can be argued that the relatively less marked increase in incidence in men is due to the fact that there were fewer men left to die from coronary disease in the 60–69 age group or proportionately more dying from other conditions, it can also be argued that the more rapid rate of increase in women relates to the menopause.

Premature menopause

The surgical removal of both ovaries from pre-menopausal women is followed by the premature development of clinical features of CHD[4] but the surgical removal of one ovary from women of comparable age does not influence the incidence of CHD 20 years later. After bilateral ovariectomy, the serum lipid levels are higher than after unilateral ovariectomy.

Again, there is a significant increase in the incidence rate of CHD in women followed for 10–20 years after menstruation had stopped spontaneously before the age of 40[5]. The serum cholesterol and triglycerides of these women are significantly higher than in women who continued to menstruate until a normal menopause. The serum lipids increase with the length of time since the menopause.

There have been a number of supporting studies suggesting that a premature menopause is associated with the premature onset of coronary heart disease but there is one which is in conflict[6]. In this study the incidence of CHD was the same in women who had a bilateral oophorectomy as in women who had a hysterectomy alone and there was no significant difference in serum cholesterol or beta-lipoprotein values between the two groups. The striking feature of this study is the high incidence of CHD in the control (hysterectomy) group and this is similar to the expected experience observed for normal women in the Framingham Study. It is possible that hysterectomy alone was associated in a considerable number of these women with the development of a menopause and, if this is so, the high incidence of CHD in the control group is not unexpected. A recent Swedish study has confirmed that women with myocardial infarction have an earlier than expected menopause[7] and a premature menopause has also been shown to be a significant contributory factor in women under 45 years who develop CHD[8].

Parity

An earlier study suggested that there is an increased incidence of coronary heart disease in women who have had multiple pregnancies and that there is a higher parity rate in women who have CHD[9] (Table 15.2). Whether this has anything to do with repeated pregnancies or not is speculative, since the correlation could equally relate to the increased amount of work and responsibility taken on by these women. In this respect, it is interesting that there has been a report showing that women who develop CHD have had more spontaneous abortions than paired controls[10] implying that the high CHD rate has little to do with the hyperlipidaemia of pregnancy.

Table 15.2 Parity and coronary heart disease[9]

	Coronary patients over 45 years	
	Total number	Number with four or more pregnancies
Hospital controls	439	135
Coronary group	439	170
	Healthy women over 45 years	
	Total number	Number with coronary disease
Three pregnancies or less	450	18
Four pregnancies or more	316	23

Risk factors

There are three major risk factors which have been associated with the development of CHD in men. These are cigarette smoking (particularly when in excess), hyperlipidaemia and hypertension. When CHD develops in women under the age of 45, these three major risk factors are also prominent and only 26% of a total of 145 women with proven CHD under the age of 45 did not show one of these[8] (Table 15.3). With the exception of cigarette smoking, which was more prominent in women who developed myocardial infarction, the prevalence of these factors was the same whether angina or myocardial infarction developed. Of course, other risk factors are also associated with the premature development of CHD and these particularly include a family history of CHD and premature menopause, as discussed above. Diabetes mellitus appears to be a less common associated condition than often thought.

What then does the menopause do to the three major risk factors? This is a question which ought to be easy to answer to-day but more evidence is required.

The first point to make is that there are no known secular changes in cigarette smoking around the menopause. It seems unlikely that non-smokers will start to smoke at that time, nor is there any reason to suppose that cigarette smoking becomes particularly heavy then. But recently, it has been shown from a retrospective autopsy survey that the mean age of coronary deaths in menopausal women is inversely related to the number of cigarettes which they smoke[11].

Table 15.3 Prevalence of each major risk factor in 81 patients with myocardial infarction and 64 with angina[8]

Risk factors	*Myocardial infarction patients* (%)	*Angina patients* (%)	(%)
Major			
Hypercholesterolaemia (≥ 270 mg/100 ml)	48	44	46
Diastolic hypertension (≥ 100 mmHg)	39	28	34
Cigarettes (≥ 20/day)	43	19	32
Total	79	69	74
Minor			
Premature menopause	22	17	20
Oral contraceptive	14	2	8
Obesity alone (≥ 15% standard)	4	6	5
Diabetes mellitus	2	3	3
Abnormal oral GTT result*	2	2	2
No evident predisposing factor	9	14	11

* GTT (Glucose Tolerance Tests) were undertaken in 94 women

Hyperlipidaemia does occur around and following the menopause. This has been known for a number of years[9] and has recently been emphasized again[6] (Table 15.4). The post-menopausal rise in plasma cholesterol and triglycerides can be considerable and may amount to as much as 20% of pre-menopausal values. It should be remembered that there is a regular menstrual cyclical change in plasma cholesterol levels and that the plasma cholesterol concentration can be as much as 15% lower at ovulation compared with the concentration in the middle of the luteal phase 5 or 6 days later[12].

There is no change in systolic or diastolic blood pressure around the menopause[13] and it has been stated[14] that 'menopausal hypertension would seem to have been an entity fabricated by imaginative minds out of the psychoneurotic and vascular events of the menopause'. This view has received support recently from a Swedish study[6] (Table 15.4). Yet hypertension is an important risk factor with regard to the premature development of CHD and the dominant male/female ratio is eliminated in its presence. This may explain the almost equal male/female ratio for CHD in negroes in the southern United States[15], where hypertension is common in women.

There is insufficient evidence to allow any conclusions about the effect of the menopause on the incidence of insulin-dependent diabetes.

Table 15.4 Blood pressure and serum lipids in 50-year old women[6]

	Pre-menopausal women (185)	*Post-menopausal women* (148)
Systolic BP (mmHg)	140 *	135
Diastolic BP	88	88
Serum cholesterol (mg/100 ml)	266	286 **
Serum triglyceride (mg/100 ml)	1·16	1·34 *

Oral contraceptives and effects of estrogens

Oral contraceptives constitute a negligible hazard in healthy women without risk factors under the age of 40. But there is a definite additional risk in women already at risk—that is to say those who smoke to excess, have hyperlipidaemia or hypertension. The risk is related to the duration of oral contraceptive treatment and it is reversed with withdrawal of oral contraceptives, implying that the increased risk is almost certainly thrombotic. These observations have been derived from the three recent studies[16–18]. Ethinyl estradiol and conjugated equine estrogens (Premarin) have both been shown to increase venous thromboembolism when given to men with coronary heart disease[19–21]. There was also an increased incidence of fatal heart attacks in the Coronary Drug Project. The doses of Premarin used were two: a dose of 5 mg daily had to be discontinued after $1\frac{1}{2}$ years while a dose of 2·5 mg was continued for a period of 5 years. The results are summarized in Table 15.5. It has recently been suggested by Coope *et al.*[22] that naturally occurring estrogens (1·5 mg Premarin daily) have as great a thrombotic risk as synthetically occurring estrogens.

Table 15.5 Vascular events in men with one or more previous myocardial infarcts treated with an estrogen [20, 21]

	1·5 years study		*5 years study*	
Complication	*Premarin* 5 mg/d (1101 men)	*Placebo* (2789 men)	*Premarin* 2·5 mg/d (1119 men)	*Placebo* (2788 men)
Coronary death	6·0	4·8	14·7	14·7
Non-fatal myocardial infarct	6·2 *	3·2	11·4	11·4
PE/thromboembolism	3·5 *	1·3	4·7 *	2·9

We do not at present have sufficient information to reach any conclusion about the safety or adverse effects of hormone replacement therapy either using naturally occurring or synthetic estrogens. It is probable, however, that they will be associated with an increased risk of vascular thrombosis in women who already have such a risk. It may take many years for this to become evident and it must be appreciated that the time scale for the development of CHD is very different from that of many other conditions. Even if an increased thrombotic tendency is induced, it is unlikely to lead to the development of myocardial ischaemia or infarction until or unless there is considerable coronary atherosclerosis.

My prediction is, then, that an increase will be seen in CHD deaths in women in their middle and late 50s in a few years time, if hormone replacement therapy becomes widespread. It will probably be particularly evident in those who smoke to excess and those who have a family history of CHD. It follows, if this is correct, that hormone replacement therapy should not be given even now in 1975—to such women. We should not wait for a change in national statistics before giving this selective advice.

Summary

There has been a dramatic increase in CHD death rate over the last 15 years in women aged 35–44 and over the last 4 or 5 years in women aged 45–54 years. These changes can, speculatively, be related to an increased incidence of cigarette smoking and possibly also to the more widespread use of oral contraceptives in middle-aged women.

Oral contraception increases the risk of myocardial infarction in women who are already at risk.

A premature menopause favours the early development of CHD.

There is an increase in serum lipids but not in blood pressure following the menopause.

It is predicted that hormone replacement therapy is likely to increase the heart attack rate and it is advised that it should not be given to women who smoke to excess and have a family history of CHD.

References

1. Heyden, S. (1971). Ischaemic heart disease in women. In G. Schettler and G. S. Boyd (eds.) *Atherosclerosis* p. 289
2. Todd, G. F. (1972). Statistics of smoking in the United Kingdom, Tobacco Research Council
3. Armstrong, A., Duncan, B., Oliver, M. F., Julian, D. G., Donald, K. W., Fulton, M., Lutz, W. and Morrison, S. L. (1972). Natural history of acute coronary heart attacks. A community study. *Br. Heart J.*, **34,** 67
4. Oliver, M. F. and Boyd, G. S. (1959). Effect of bilateral ovariectomy on coronary artery disease and serum lipid levels. *Lancet*, **ii,** 690
5. Sznajderman, M. and Oliver, M. F. (1963). Spontaneous premature menopause, ischaemic heart disease and serum lipids. *Lancet*, **i,** 962
6. Ritterband, A. B., Jaffe, I. A., Densen, P. M., Magagana, J. F. and Reed, E. (1963). Gonadal function and the development of coronary heart disease. *Circulation*, **27,** 237
7. Bengtssan, C. (1973). Ischaemic heart disease in women. *Acta Med. Scand. Suppl.*, 549
8. Oliver, M. F. (1974). Ischaemic heart disease in young women. *Br. Med. J.*, **4,** 253
9. Oliver, M. F. (1960). Sex factors In: L. McDonald (ed.) *Pathogenesis and Treatment of Occlusive Vascular Disease* p. 124 (London: Pitman)
10. Winkelstein, W., Stencheber, M. A. and Lilienfeld, A. M. (1958). Occurrence of pregnancy abortion and artificial menopause among women with coronary artery disease: A preliminary study. *J. Chronic Dis.*, **7,** 273
11. Spain, T. M., Seigal, H. and Bradess, V. A. (1973). Women smokers and sudden death *JAMA*, **224,** 1005
12. Oliver, M. F. and Boyd, G. S. (1953). Changes in the plasma lipids during the menstrual cycle. *Clin. Sci.*, **12,** 217
13. Hamilton, M., Pickering, G. W., Roberts, J. A. F. and Sowry, G. S. C. (1954). The aetiology of essential hypertension. I. The arterial pressure in the general population. *Clin. Sci.*, **13,** 11
14. Pickering, G. (1968). *High Blood Pressure* (London: J. & A. Churchill)
15. Furman, R. H. (1971). Endocrine factors in atherogenesis. G. Schettler and G. S. Boyd (eds.) p. 375, *Artherosclerosis*
16. Radford, D. and Oliver, M. F. (1973). Oral contraceptives and myocardial infarction *Br. Med. J.*, **2,** 428

17. Mann, J. I., Vessey, M. P., Thorogood, M., Doll, R. (1975). Myocardial infarction in young women with special reference to oral contraceptive practice. *Br. Med. J.*, **2,** 241
18. Mann, J. I. and Inman, W. H. W. (1975). Oral contraceptives and death from myocardial infarction. *Br. Med. J.*, **2,** 245
19. Oliver, M. F. and Boyd, G. S. (1961). Influence of reduction of serum lipids on prognosis of coronary heart disease: A five year study using oestrogen. *Lancet*, **ii,** 499
20. Coronary Drug Project (1970). Initial findings leading to modifications of its research protocol, Coronary Drug Project Research Group, *JAMA*, **214,** 1303
21. Coronary Drug Project (1973). Findings leading to discontinuation of the 2.5 mg/day estrogen group. Coronary Drug Project Research Group, *JAMA*, **226,** 652
22. Coope, J., Thomson, J. M. and Paul, L. (1975). Effects of 'natural oestrogen' replacement therapy on menopausal symptoms and blood clotting. *Br. Med. J.*, **3,** 139

16

The effects of ethinyl estradiol and conjugated equine estrogens on plasma lipids in oophorectomized women

C. H. Bolton

Introduction

There have been reports[1, 2] on the increased risk of both arterial and venous thrombosis in patients taking combined estrogen/progestogen oral contraceptives, and the synthetic estrogen has been particularly implicated[3]. Other workers have noted differences in behaviour between natural and synthetic estrogens[4].

In this study we have attempted to compare some metabolic effects of ethinyl estradiol (a synthetic estrogen) and Premarin (conjugated equine estrogens) given in doses considered to be of equivalent biological activity, to a group of oophorectomized women.

Serum lipid levels, notably cholesterol and triglycerides, have been considered[5, 6] risk factors in the development of arterial disease. Whether or not this risk is related to that derived from taking synthetic estrogen preparations is an open question.

We have measured these lipids, together with certain haemostasis-related parameters which may be relevant to the risk of venous thrombosis. We compared the estrogenicity of the preparations used by measuring the serum luteinizing hormone levels.

Patients and methods

Seventeen women took part in the study, the nature of which was fully explained to them. The mean age was 40 (range 32–46). They had all been oophorectomized for non-malignant conditions, seven within 90 days of starting the study, the rest more than 90 days previously. Seven of the women were taking an estrogen preparation before the study started, but the remainder were on no treatment.

The women were prescribed in random sequence ethinyl estradiol 20 μg or 50 μg daily, or Premarin 0·625 mg or 1·25 mg daily. Each regime was given for 3 months before changing to the next phase. After each course patients attended the out-patients clinic having fasted overnight. They were patients attended out-patients clinic having fasted overnight. They were weighed, questioned as to symptoms and blood was taken for lipid, haematological and LH analyses.

A control group comprised eight women who had been oophorectomized for more than 90 days and were not on hormonal replacement therapy.

Total serum cholesterol and triglycerides were measured by standard methods[7, 8] and lipoprotein electrophoresis was carried out on agarose gel[9]. Fibrinolysis was measured by the dilute clot lysis time[10], fibrinogen by the

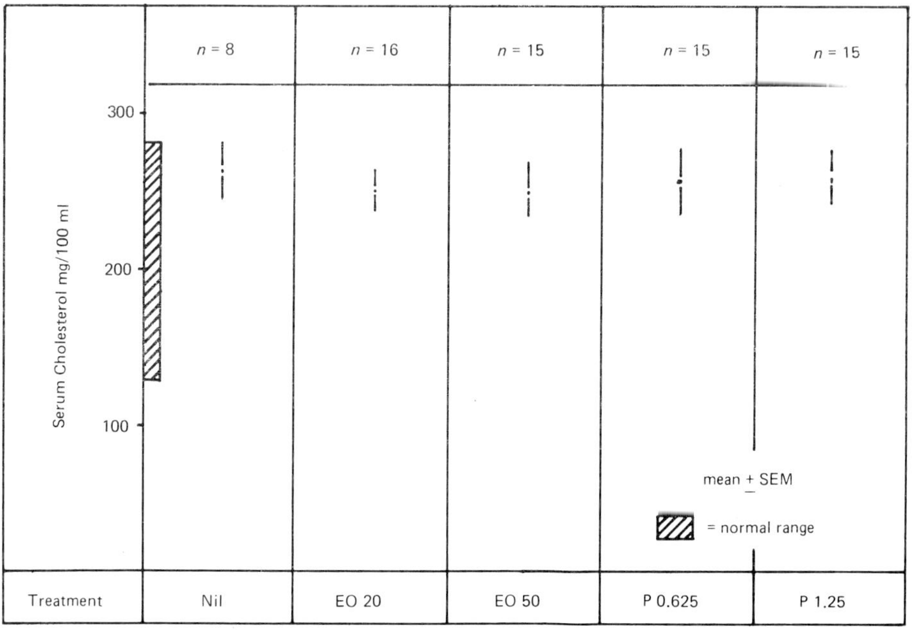

Figure 16.1 Serum cholesterol levels on the different estrogen regimes EO 20, EO 50 = ethinyl estradiol 20 μg, 50 μg daily P 0·625, P 1·25 = Premarin 0·625 mg, 1·25 mg daily. No significant differences between results—$p > 0{\cdot}05$. From Bolton *et al.*, *Clinical Endocrinology*, 1975, **4**, 131, courtesy of Blackwell Scientific Publications

clot weight method[11] and platelet adhesiveness by a modification of Borchgrevinck's method[12]. Activated partial thromboplastin time was measured by Eastham's method[13]. Serum LH was measured by a double antibody radioimmunoassay method.

Student's '*t*' test was used to compare mean values.

Results

The four estrogen preparations appeared to be similarly effective in relieving symptoms such as hot flushes, etc. Side effects were minimal and preferences were approximately equally distributed between ethinyl estradiol and Premarin. Body weight in all women remained unchanged throughout the study.

Serum cholesterol (Figure 16.1) showed no significant change on any of the treatments, the mean level in the untreated group being 259 mg/100 ml (6·73 mmol/l).

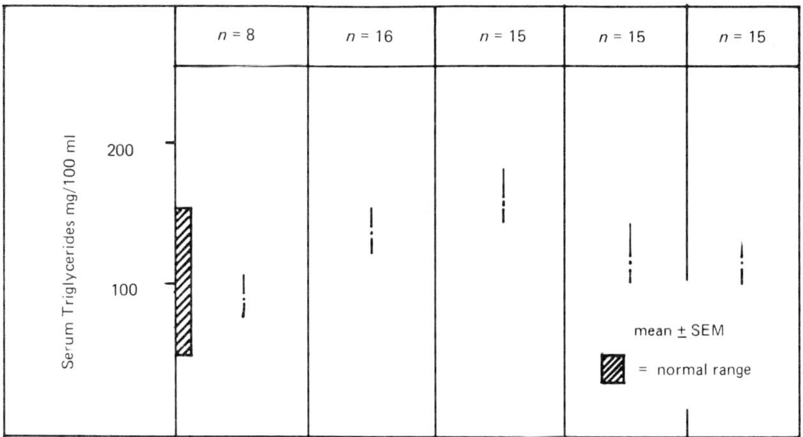

Treatment	Nil	EO 20	EO 50	P 0.625	P 1.25
Sign. vs. Nil	–	0.02	0.005	NS*	NS*
vs. E020		–	NS*	NS*	NS*
vs. E050			–	0.025	0.02
vs. P 0.625				–	NS*
vs. P1.25					–

Figure 16.2 Serum triglyceride levels on the different estrogen regimes. Abbreviations as in Figure 16.1. N.S. = $p > 0{\cdot}05$. From Bolton *et al.*, *Clinical Endocrinology*, 1975, **4**, 131, courtesy of Blackwell Scientific Publications

Table 16.1 Haemostasis related parameters in oophorectomized subjects

Regime	*Nil*	*EO* (20 μg)	*EO* (50 μg)	*P* (0·625 μg)	*P* (1·25 μg)
DCL★ (h)					
(m ± SD)	4·82 ± 2·31	5·51 ± 2·26	6·16 ± 1·81	5·38 ± 2·67	5·42 ± 1·75
n	9	15	11	16	15
Plasma fibrinogen (mg/100 ml)					
(m ± SD)	302·4 ± 65·5	290·6 ± 47·7	288·1 ± 61·7	293·9 ± 67·2	291·4 ± 58·7
n	8	12	11	15	13
Adhesive platelet count ($\times 10^3$/cu.mm)					
(m ± SD)	64·66 ± 44·80	77·81 ± 33·78	87·86 ± 29·55	77·37 ± 32·62	81·73 ± 30·33
n	9	16	15	16	15
APPT★★ (s)					
(m ± SD)	37·44 ± 3·92	36·77 ± 4·01	36·57 ± 3·43	37·50 ± 4·84	37·75 ± 4·30
n	9	15	15	16	15

★ Dilute clot lysis time
★★ Activated partial thromboplastin time
All changes N.S. ($p > 0·05$)

The mean serum triglyceride level (Figure 16.2) in the untreated group was 86·5 mg/100 ml (0·98 mmol/l). This was significantly raised by ethinyl estradiol 20 μg and 50 μg to 137 mg/100 ml (1·55 mmol/l) and 157 mg/100 ml (1·77 mmol/l) respectively. Premarin, 0·625 mg and 1·25 mg did not give a significant rise (112 mg/100 ml–1·26 mmol/l and 113 mg/100 ml–1·27 mmol/l respectively).

Lipoprotein electrophoresis revealed an intensified pre-β band when serum triglyceride levels were greater than approximately 160 mg/100 ml (1·81 mmol/l).

There were no significant changes in the haemostasis-related parameters (Table 16.1).

The mean serum LH (Figure 16.3) in untreated patients was 6·68 mU/ml. Ethinyl estradiol 20 μg (5·44 mU/ml) and 50 μg (3·23 mU/ml) and Premarin

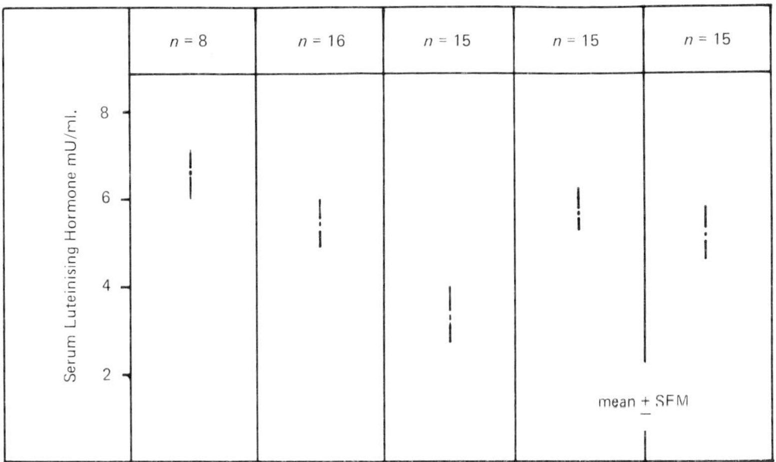

Treatment	Nil	EO 20	EO 50	P 0.625	P 1.25
sign. vs. Nil	–	0.05	0.001	NS*	0.05
vs. EO 20		–	0.001	NS*	NS*
vs. EO 50			–	0.001	0.01
vs. P 0.625				–	NS*
vs. P 1.25					–

Figure 16.3 Serum luteinizing hormone levels on the different estrogen regimes. Abbreviations as in Figure 16.1. N.S. = $p > 0·05$. From Bolton *et al.*, *Clinical Endocrinology*, 1975, **4**, 131, courtesy of Blackwell Scientific Publications

1·25 mg (5·11 mU/ml) caused significant reductions in serum LH levels. Ethinyl estradiol 50 μg daily caused significantly greater depression of serum LH levels than either ethinyl estradiol 20 μg or Premarin 1·25 mg.

Discussion

The choice of estrogen for replacement in an estrogen deficiency state or total estrogen lack can present some difficulties. Most commercially available synthetic products are based on either ethinyl estradiol or mestranol, or the non-steroidal diethylstilbestrol. The most widely used 'natural' product is without doubt the complex conjugated equine estrogen preparation commercially available as Premarin (Ayerst). More recently other products which claim to have 'natural' properties have become available, e.g. Harmogen (Abbott), Progynova (Schering), Hormonin (Carnrick).

There has been a long-standing debate on the relative merits of synthetic versus natural estrogen therapy, and quite apart from any clinical differences, which are often minimal, the comparative biochemical effects have been studied in some depth.

Much of the original work on the metabolic effects of synthetic estrogens was done in premenopausal women on oral contraceptives, to a large extent by Wynn and associates[14, 15]. Biochemically, oral contraceptive therapy presents some problems not only because of differing dose levels and differing durations of therapy, but, perhaps not least, because of interaction with the patient's own endogenous estrogens. The last of these difficulties can to a large extent be overcome by taking as a patient group post-menopausal women, in whom endogenous estrogen secretion is minimal. Whether the menopause is spontaneous or surgical has perhaps no direct relevance at this stage.

The oral contraceptive work has shown that there are slight to moderate increases in serum cholesterol and a slight increase in phospholipid. Perhaps most significant however, Wynn has shown a marked rise in serum triglycerides, and moreover, that this rise can be related almost directly to the amount of estrogen present in the preparation[15]. This hypertriglyceridaemic effect seems to be common to all synthetic estrogens.

Oophorectomy, *per se*, has an effect on serum lipids. For some reason, a functioning ovary seems to have a controlling influence on lipids. Whether or not this is related to the postulated protection enjoyed by women against the ravages of atherosclerotic heart disease is perhaps an open question. Snadjerman and Oliver[16] have indicated that post-menopausal susceptibility to ischaemic heart disease may be paralleled by increase in serum lipids.

Elevations in serum lipids may be related to the time of oophorectomy.

Aitken[17] for instance has shown that, if oophorectomy takes place before the age of 43, serum cholesterol may rise, but if after 43, there will probably be no rise. Estrogen replacement in those women with mestranol (20–40 μg daily) produced a fall in cholesterol and a rise in triglycerides.

Conjugated equine estrogens have been used in a group of myocardial infarcts[18, 19] but have also been used in the post-menopausal situation. Robinson[20] found that serum cholesterol levels were depressed and triglycerides slightly increased after 3 months' therapy with Premarin 0·625 mg and 1·25 mg daily. In a very comprehensive study Furman *et al.*[21], studying the effects of both estrogens and androgens, showed that conjugated equine estrogens in large doses invariably produced an increase in phospholipids and triglycerides, and variable effects on cholesterol. Indeed they quote: 'Serum triglycerides (VLDL) are a sensitive indication of estrogen administration—more than raised phospholipid, α-lipoprotein or a decreased cholesterol/phospholipid ratio'.

Our results confirm in principle the result of Stokes and Wynn[15], and Aitken *et al.*[17], in that synthetic estrogens were shown to produce marked rises in serum triglycerides, roughly related to the estrogen content. The administration of Premarin in both doses used in our study (0·625 mg and 1·25 mg daily) produced no significant elevation of triglycerides. We did not demonstrate any depression of serum cholesterol levels on any of the four treatment regimes. This confirms Utian's[22] work in Cape Town. Boyd[23] also had previously indicated that a hypolipidaemic dose was often 100 times higher than an estrogenically effective dose.

The effects of oral contraceptive therapy on clotting factors[24] and platelet function[25], and their relevance to thrombosis have been discussed at some length. Poller and his co-workers[26] have recently described changes in some clotting factors on Premarin therapy. We examined some factors related to haemostasis in our group of women and found no significant change on any of the four treatment regimes.

The comparison of estrogenic potency of different estrogen preparations is a major problem. The doses we have used have been regarded as equivalent[27–29], but other workers[30–32] in comparing Premarin with ethinyl estradiol have used different assay systems and arrived at different conclusions. We assessed estrogenicity by comparing serum LH levels on the different preparations. We found that ethinyl estradiol 50 μg was considerably more effective than Premarin at either dose. On none of the four regimes, however, did the LH revert to pre-menopausal levels.

On the basis of these results it would seem therefore that the elevation of serum triglycerides given by ethinyl estradiol cannot only be attributed to the estrogenic potency of the doses used. It would seem that there is a qualitative difference between (1) synthetic, (2) 'natural' exogenous, and (3) endogenously secreted estrogens.

The mechanism of the hypertriglyceridaemic effect is not established in full. The observed decrease in lipoprotein lipase activity[33, 34] on estrogens has been shown not to be connected with raised serum triglycerides. Perhaps a more logical explanation would be increased hepatic synthesis[14, 35] of the apoproteins present in VLDL—the major triglyceride carrier.

This points the direction in which future work on the effects of hormones on lipids might be directed—a study of the apoproteins and their changes under various stimuli. It would seem that until a more complete picture emerges based on such changes, information on metabolism will be difficult to clarify.

Acknowledgments

The work described in this paper was a combined effort. The author is grateful to all his colleagues and technicians in the Department of Medicine, Bristol Royal Infirmary for their considerable contributions.

References

1. Collaborative Study (1973). Oral contraception and increased risk of cerebral ischemia or thrombosis. *New Eng. J. Med.*, **288**, 871
2. Inman, W. H. W. and Vessey, M. P. (1968). Investigations of deaths from pulmonary, coronary and cerebral thrombosis and embolism in women of child-bearing age. *Brit. Med. J.*, **ii**, 193
3. Inman, W. H. W., Vessey, M. P., Westerholm, B. and Engelund, A. (1970). Thromboembolic disease and the steroidal content of oral contraceptives. A report to the Committee on Safety of Drugs. *Brit. Med. J.*, **ii**, 203
4. Elkeles, R. S., Hampton, J. R. and Mitchell, J. R. A. (1968). Effect of oestrogens on human platelet behaviour. *Lancet*, **ii**, 315.
5. Kannel, W. B., Castelli, W. P., Gordon, T. and McNamara, P. M. (1971). Serum cholesterol, lipoproteins and the risk of coronary heart disease: The Framingham Study. *Ann. Intern. Med.*, **74**, 1
6. Carlson, L. A. and Bottinger, L. E. (1972). Ischaemic heart disease in relation to fasting values of plasma triglycerides and cholesterol. *Lancet*, **i**, 865
7. Robertson, G. and Cramp, D. G. (1970). An evaluation of cholesterol determinations in serum and serum lipoprotein fractions by a semi-automated fluorimetric method. *J. Clin. Pathol.*, **23**, 243
8. Kessler, G. and Lederer, H. (1966). Fluorimetric measurements of triglycerides. *Automation in Analytical Chemistry* (Editor: L. T. Skeggs) p. 341 (New York: Mediad Inc.)
9. Noble, R. P. (1968). Electrophoretic separation of plasma lipoproteins in agarose gel. *J. Lipid Res.*, **9**, 693

10. Fearnley, G. R. and Tweed, J. M. (1953). Evidence of an active fibrinolytic enzyme in the plasma of normal people with observations of inhibition associated with the presence of calcium. *Clin. Sci.*, **12,** 81
11. Fearnley, G. R. and Chakrabarti, R. (1966). Fibrinolytic treatment of rheumatoid arthritis with phenformin plus ethyloestrenol. *Lancet*, **ii,** 757
12. Borchgrevinck, C. (1960). A method for measuring platelet adhesiveness *in vivo*. *Acta Med. Scand.*, **168,** 157
13. Eastham, R. D. (1962). An improved plasma recalcified clotting test and its modification as a simple rapid heparin retarded clotting test. *J. Clin. Pathol.*, **15,** 86
14. Wynn, V., Doar, J. W. H., Mills, G. L. and Stokes, T. (1969). Fasting serum triglyceride, cholesterol and lipoprotein levels during oral contraceptive therapy. *Lancet*, **ii,** 756
15. Stokes, T. and Wynn, V. (1971). Serum lipids in women on oral contraceptives. *Lancet*, **ii,** 677
16. Snadjerman, M. and Oliver, M. F. (1963). Spontaneous premature menopause, ischaemic heart disease and serum lipids. *Lancet*, **i,** 962
17. Aitken, J. M., Lorimer, A. R., McKay Hart, D., Lawrie, T. D. V. and Smith, D. A. (1971). The effects of oophorectomy and long-term Mestranol therapy on the serum lipids of middle-aged women. *Clin. Sci.*, **41,** 597
18. Stamler, J., Pick, R., Katz, L. N., Pick, A., Kaplan, B. M., Berkson, D. M. and Century, D. (1963). The effectiveness of estrogen therapy on myocardial infarction in middle-aged men. *J. Amer. Med. Assoc.*, **183,** 632
19. Marmorsten, J., Moore, F. J., Hopkins, C. E., Kuzma, O. T. and Werner, J. (1962). Clinical studies of long-term estrogen therapy in men with myocardial infarction. *Proc. Soc. Exp. Biol. Med.*, **110,** 400
20. Robinson, R. W. and LeBeau, R. J. (1965). Effect of conjugated equine estrogens on serum lipids and the clotting mechanism. *J. Atheroscl. Res.*, **5,** 120
21. Furman, R. H., Alaupovic, P. and Howard, R. P. (1967). Effect of androgens and estrogens on serum lipids and the composition and concentrations of serum lipoproteins in normolipemic and hyperlipidemic states. *Prog. Biochem. Pharmacol.*, **2,** 215
22. Utian, W. H. (1970). Cholesterol, coronary heart disease and estrogens. *Ph.D. Thesis*, University of Cape Town
23. Boyd, G. S. (1963). Hormones and cholesterol metabolism. *Biochem. Soc. Symp.*, **24,** 79
24. Leading Article (1972). Blood clotting and the Pill. *Brit. Med. J.*, **iv,** 378
25. Bolton, C. H., Hampton, J. R. and Mitchell, J. R. A. (1968). Effect of oral contraceptive agents on platelets and plasma phospholipids. *Lancet*, **i,** 1336
26. Coope, J., Thompson, J. M. and Poller, L. (1975). Effects of 'natural oestrogen' replacement therapy on menopausal symptoms and blood clotting. *Brit. Med. J.*, **iv,** 139
27. Israel, S. L. (1967). In: *Diagnosis and Treatment of Menstrual Disorders and Sterility*, 5th Edn. p. 41. (New York: Hoeber Medical Division, Harper and Row)
28. Yannone, M. E. (1967). The use of hormones in the menopause. *J. Iowa Med. Soc.*, **57,** 1099
29. Kistner, R. W. (1967). Feminine for ever? An evaluation of therapy during the peri-menopause. *Med. Sci.*, **18,** 42
30. Rudel, H. W. and Kincl, F. A. (1966). The biology of anti-fertility steroids. *Acta Endocrinol.*, **51,** Suppl. 105
31. Schalch, D. S., Parlow, A. F., Boon, R. C., Reichlin, S. and Lee, L. A. (1968).

Measurement of human luteinising hormone in plasma by radioimmunoassay. *J. Clin. Invest.*, **47**, 665

32. Wise, A. J., Gross, M. A. and Schalch, D. S. (1973). Quantitative relationships of the pituitary–gonadal axis in post-menopausal women. *J. Lab. Clin. Med.*, **81**, 28
33. Hazzard, W. R., Spiger, M. J., Bagdade, J. P. and Bierman, E. L. (1969). Studies on the mechanism of increased plasma triglyceride levels induced by oral contraceptives. *New Eng. J. Med.*, **280**, 471
34. Adams, J. H., Mitchell, J. R. A. and Soppitt, G. D. (1970). Effect of oral contraceptives on lipoprotein lipase activity and platelet stickiness. *Lancet*, **ii**, 333
35. Rössner, S., Larsson-Cohn, U., Carlson, L. A. and Boberg, J. (1971). Effects of an oral contraceptive agent on plasma lipids, plasma lipoproteins, the intravenous fat tolerance and post-heparin lipolytic activity. *Acta Med. Scand.*, **190**, 301

17

The effect of synthetic and natural estrogens on glucose tolerance, plasma insulin and lipid metabolism in post-menopausal women

T. Pyörälä

In recent years estrogens, either alone or with progestins in a sequential dosage schedule, have been introduced in the hormonal substitution treatment of post-menopausal women. Synthetic estrogen–progestin combinations given for contraceptive purposes are known to cause certain metabolic alterations (for a recent review see, e.g. Spellacy[1]). These include an increase in the fasting plasma insulin level and an increase in the plasma insulin response after glucose load. An increase in the serum triglyceride level is found almost without exception in women taking oral contraceptives. Alterations in serum cholesterol levels are less consistent.

In the following paper we shall give a review of the effects of synthetic and natural estrogens on the carbohydrate and lipid metabolism in post-menopausal women.

Carbohydrate metabolism

Synthetic estrogens

Buchler and Warren[2] administered stilbestrol or mestranol combined with norethynodrel to 14 menopausal women and found that the results of oral glucose tolerance tests became abnormal in 11 instances, whereas those of intravenous tests were all within normal limits. di Paola and associates[3] gave mestranol as a single agent to castrated and post-menopausal women in daily doses of 40 μg and 80 μg, either continuously or in periodic cycles of 15 to

20 days. Oral glucose tolerance tests after previous administration of prednisone were performed before starting the therapeutic programme and later every 3 months for a period of 12 months. An increase in the prevalence of abnormal tests was observed during the first 3 months, but later these abnormalities disappeared.

Danowski and associates[4] administered 25 μg quinestrol (ethinyl-estradiol-3-cyclopentyl ether) to 11 climacteric women; eight of them completed 6 months of treatment. They showed that quinestrol did not alter the blood glucose responses to oral glucose load. The insulin response to glucose seemed to be lower during quinestrol therapy.

We have investigated the effects of sequential therapy with ethinyl estradiol and megestrol acetate on carbohydrate metabolism[5]. The series comprised 16 post-menopausal women aged 41–58 years. Six of them were obese—their relative body weight was more than 120%. In all cases studies of vaginal smears revealed low estrogen indices. Before the beginning of the therapy an oral glucose tolerance test was performed—the glucose dose was 1 g per kg of body weight. Blood glucose was determined by the *o*-toluidine method from capillary blood and plasma insulin was determined by the radioimmunological method from venous blood.

After these studies sequential therapy was begun. Each treatment cycle started with a 16-day period during which ethinyl estradiol was given alone at a daily dosage of 25 μg. Thereafter followed a period of 7 days of combined treatment with 25 μg of ethinyl estradiol and 0.5 mg of megestrol acetate daily, and finally a 5-day period of placebo tablets, after which a new treatment cycle began.

Oral glucose tolerance tests and plasma insulin determinations were performed again during the second or third treatment cycle at the end of its estrogen period. The reason for this was that in a previous study on the sequential contraceptive treatment with the same estrogen and progestin components[6], we found that the decrease of glucose tolerance was most clearly evident in this phase and that even some improvement of glucose tolerance occurred during the last period of the treatment cycle, in which estrogen and progestin were given simultaneously. In 12 cases these studies were repeated after the patients has been treated for 11 to 14 months and in nine cases after 18 to 30 months' therapy.

As shown in Table 17.1 and Figure 17.1 the glucose tolerance showed a slight change in studies performed during the second or third cycle. Fasting blood glucose was slightly lower during treatment than before it and this change was even statistically significant. The area-index of the glucose tolerance test did not change significantly (Table 17.1). In studies made during the 11th to 14th and the 18th to 30th treatment cycles, the results of glucose

Table 17.1 The effect of sequential ethinyl estradiol + megestrol treatment on the results of Oral Glucose Tolerance Test (OGTT)

	Blood glucose levels during OGTT (mg/100 ml) Mean ± SD (Mean Δ ± SD)*					*Area of OGTT* Mean ± SD (Mean Δ ± SD)*
	0 min	30 min	60 min	90 min	120 min	
Before treatment (n = 16)	85·7 ± 8·8	134·7 ± 18·3	112·6 ± 14·1	99·4 ± 13·3	84·1 ± 11·2	431·5 ± 45·0
After 3–4 months (n = 16)	78·9 ± 6·7 (− 7·4 ± 11·1)	136·6 ± 14·2 (+ 1·9 ± 13·6)	117·8 ± 16·4 (+ 5·2 ± 11·9)	105·0 ± 13·9 (+ 7·9 ± 8·8)	95·3 ± 15·0 (+ 11·2 ± 14·2)	446·4 ± 46·3 (+ 14·2 ± 30·4)
p-value	< 0·02	N.S.	N.S.	< 0·01	< 0·01	N.S.
After 11–14 months (n = 12)	79·9 ± 11·8 (− 7·8 ± 13·2)	122·3 ± 23·3 (− 14·0 ± 23·7)	115·4 ± 16·1 (+ 5·8 ± 14·9)	105·3 ± 15·5 (+ 3·8 ± 12·8)	90·2 ± 13·0 (+ 5·1 ± 15·1)	428·0 ± 56·1 (− 6·3 ± 45·8)
p-value	N.S.	N.S.	N.S.	N.S.	N.S.	N.S.
After 18–30 months (n = 9)	79·3 ± 11·5 (− 4·7 ± 14·2)	133·1 ± 22·2 (− 1 ± 18·2)	115·6 ± 20·2 (2·9 ± 13·8)	105·4 ± 13·4 (6·7 ± 12·5)	90·7 ± 14·7 (7·4 ± 12·6)	439·1 ± 63·7 (9·8 ± 45·4)
p-value	N.S.	N.S.	N.S.	N.S.	N.S.	N.S.

* Compared with the corresponding values before treatment

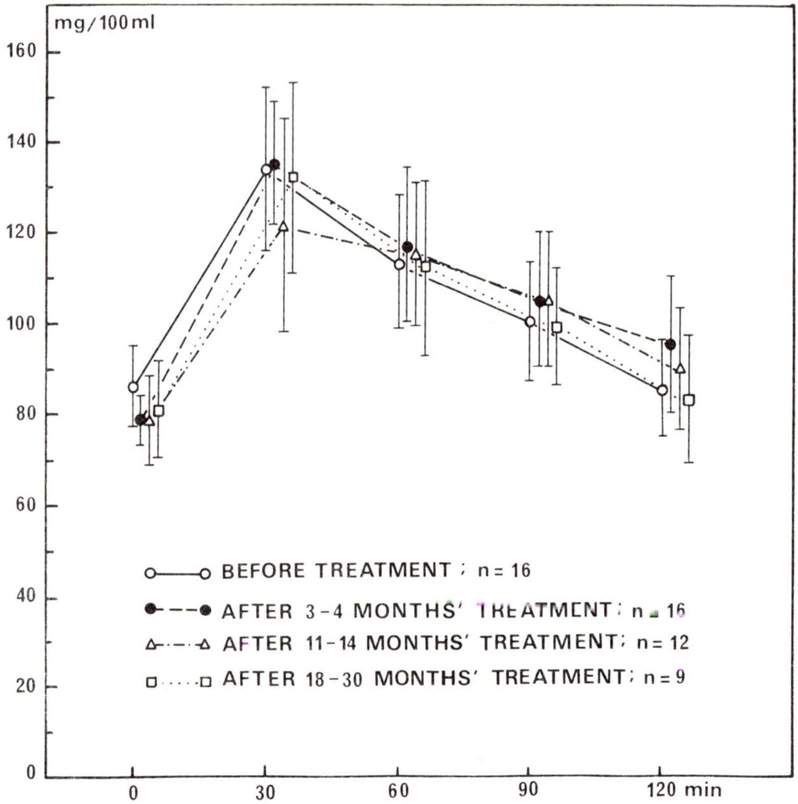

Figure 17.1 Mean blood glucose levels (mg/100 ml) during an oral glucose tolerance test performed before and after 3–4, 11–14 and 18–30 months of treatment with sequential ethinyl estradiol + megestrol

tolerance tests did not differ from those made during the control period.

Plasma insulin levels during glucose tolerance tests are shown in Table 17.2 and Figure 17.2. After two or three treatment cycles the fasting plasma insulin levels and the insulin response during glucose tolerance tests did not differ from those observed during the control period.

The so-called insulinogenic index—that is the ratio of the area under the insulin response curve to the area under the glucose tolerance curve—was also calculated. After 11–14 months' treatment the plasma insulin response, defined by the area under the insulin response curve, was slightly but

Table 17.2 The effect of sequential ethinyl estradiol + megestrol treatment on plasma insulin response during Oral Glucose Tolerance Test (OGTT)

	Plasma insulin levels during OGTT (μU/ml) Mean ± SD (Mean Δ ± SD)*				*Insulin area* Mean ± SD (Mean Δ ± SD)*	*Insulinogenic index* Mean ± SD (Mean Δ ± SD)*
	0 min	30 min	60 min	120 min		
Before treatment	11·6 ± 5·6	67·2 ± 38·9	51·2 ± 37·8	31·2 ± 21·8	181·0 ± 90·1	0·429 ± 0·200
(n = 13)						
After 3–4 months	9·4 ± 6·6	55·2 ± 24·9	57·2 ± 33·5	33·4 ± 18·7	179·2 ± 83·6	0·402 ± 0·168
(n = 13)	(−0·5 ± 7·8)	(−11·0 ± 31·9)	(+5·9 ± 35·7)	(+2·2 ± 11·2)	(−1·2 ± 57·0)	(−0·027 ± 0·139)
p-value	N.S.	N.S.	N.S.	N.S.	N.S.	N.S.
After 11–14 months	12·0 ± 9·3	46·3 ± 24·8	48·4 ± 29·6	27·1 ± 15·4	151·9 ± 68·9	0·359 ± 0·159
(n = 11)	(−1·1 ± 6·0)	(−18·1 ± 25·4)	(−7·3 ± 32·6)	(−6·9 ± 14·1)	(−36·4 ± 54·1)	(−0·084 ± 0·119)
p-value	N.S.	$< 0·05$	N.S.	N.S.	$< 0·05$	N.S.
After 18–30 months	11·3 ± 4·5	49·3 ± 31·1	38·6 ± 20·9	24·6 ± 10·9	137·4 ± 66·2	0·301 ± 0·126
(n = 7)	(0·29 ± 5·53)	(−25·9 ± 50·2)	(6·7 ± 36·2)	(1·4 ± 10·5)	(−14·2 ± 70·0)	(−0·051 ± 0·142)
p-value	N.S.	N.S.	N.S.	N.S.	N.S.	N.S.

* Compared with the corresponding values before treatment

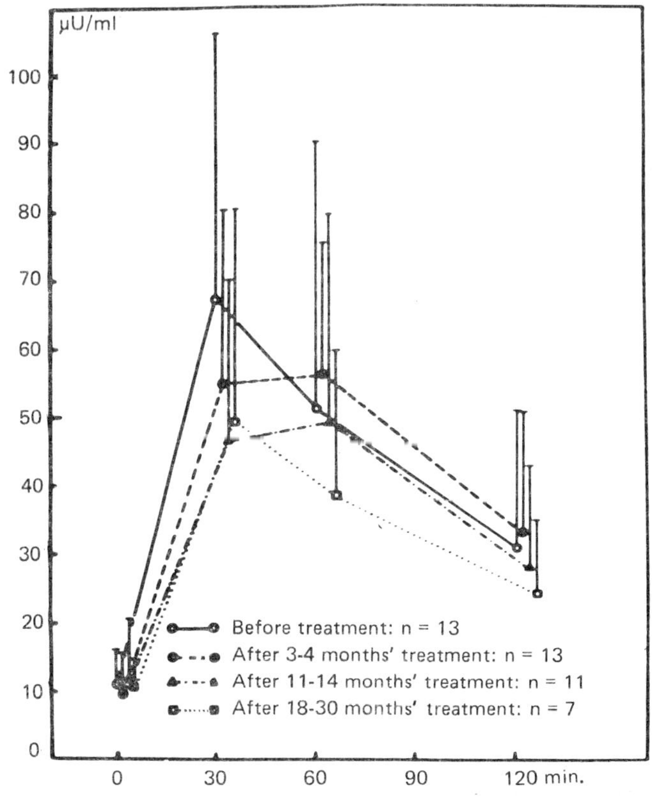

Figure 17.2 Mean plasma insulin levels (µUnits/ml) during an oral glucose tolerance test performed before and after 3–4, 11–14 and 18–30 months of treatment with sequential ethinyl estradiol + megestrol

Table 17.3 The effect of estradiol valerate treatment on the results of Oral Glucose Tolerance Test (OGTT)

	Blood glucose levels during OGTT (mg/100 ml) Mean ± SD (Mean Δ ± SD)*					*Area of OGTT* Mean ± SD (Mean Δ ± SD)*
	0 min	30 min	60 min	90 min	120 min	
Before treatment (n = 8)	86·75 ± 8·75	135·50 ± 24·95	120·62 ± 29·21	107·88 ± 29·71	86·12 ± 24·75	450·44 ± 88·30
After 3–4 months	83·12 ± 7·51	129·88 ± 19·45	120·75 ± 21·42	106·25 ± 16·02	84·88 ± 9·42	440·25 ± 51·96
(n = 8)	(− 3·62 ± 9·12)	(− 5·62 ± 16·16)	(1·38 ± 16·19)	(− 1·62 ± 23·57)	(− 1·25 ± 25·79)	(− 10·19 ± 57·41)
p-value	N.S.	N.S.	N.S.	N.S.	N.S.	N.S.
After 8–12 months	80·17 ± 10·83	121·67 ± 26·52	112·67 ± 16·00	109·00 ± 13·18	92·17 ± 16·80	429·50 ± 53·05
(n = 6)	(− 6·00 ± 13·18)	(− 19·50 ± 29·47)	(− 11·00 ± 24·48)	(− 2·83 ± 22·92)	(2·00 ± 16·17)	(− 35·33 ± 82·67)
p-value	N.S.	N.S.	N.S.	N.S.	N.S.	N.S.

* Compared with the corresponding values before treatment

significantly lower than before treatment. However, the insulinogenic index did not differ significantly from the pretreatment value. The same applied for results after 18–30 months' treatment.

Natural estrogens

Goldman and Ovadia[7] administered 1·25 mg of Premarin to 30 post-menopausal patients. The control group was composed of 32 women in the post-menopausal period. There were ten patients with a history suggestive of pre-diabetes in the test group and seven in the control group. Intravenous glucose tolerance tests were done before treatment, after 3 months' therapy and 3 months after estrogens were discontinued. The mean *k* value in 30

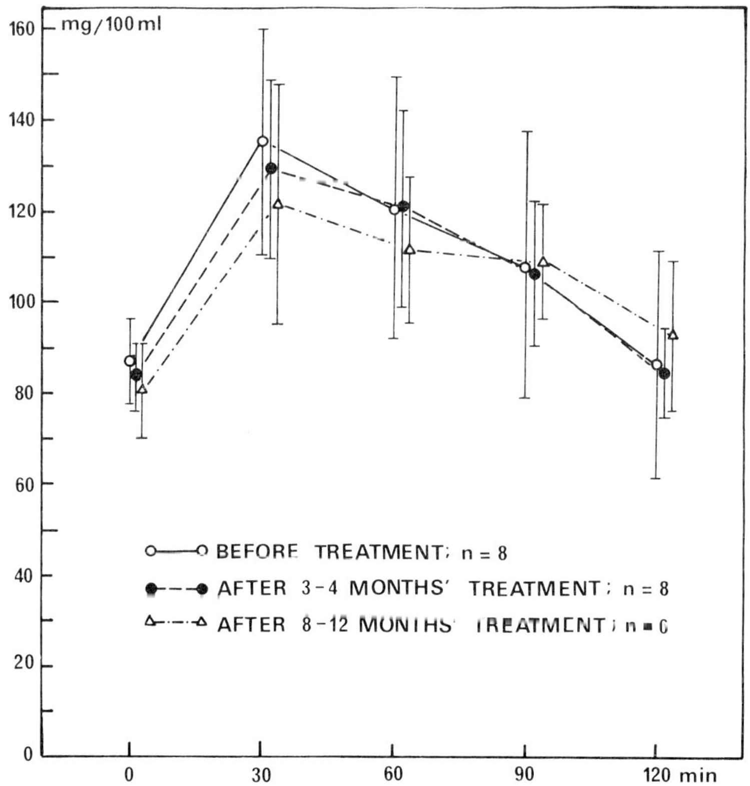

Figure 17.3 Mean blood glucose levels (mg/100 ml) during an oral glucose tolerance test performed before and after 3–4 and 8–12 months of treatment with estradiol valerate

Table 17.4 The effect of estradiol valerate treatment on plasma insulin response during Oral Glucose Tolerance Test (OGTT)

	Plasma insulin levels during OGTT (μU/ml) Mean ± SD (Mean Δ ± SD)*				*Insulin area* Mean ± SD (Mean Δ ± SD)*	*Insulinogenic index* Mean ± SD (Mean Δ ± SD)*
	0 min	30 min	60 min	120 min		
Before treatment (n = 8)	14·75 ± 13·74	47·0 ± 36·61	47·12 ± 34·11	34·0 ± 39·73	159·3 ± 122·9	0·335 ± 0·207
After 3–4 months	10·0 ± 5·07	38·88 ± 22·56	41·50 ± 31·00	23·50 ± 18·61	129·5 ± 78·4	0·288 ± 0·154
(n = 8)	(−4·75 ± 10·07)	(−8·12 ± 18·86)	(−5·62 ± 15·74)	(−10·50 ± 22·12)	(−29·8 ± 51·9)	(−0·048 ± 0·062)
p-value	N.S.	N.S.	N.S.	N.S.	N.S.	< 0·05
After 8–12 months	9·17 ± 5·60	34·50 ± 20·94	37·33 ± 19·25	27·0 ± 19·63	121·3 ± 65·4	0·283 ± 0·133
(n = 6)	(−8·0 ± 13·84)	(−16·33 ± 22·79)	(−14·18 ± 20·87)	(−14·33 ± 29·94)	(−57·3 ± 79·9)	(−0·078 ± 0·122)
p-value	N.S.	N.S.	N.S.	N.S.	N.S.	N.S.

* Compared with the corresponding values before treatment

women in the post-menopausal group was 1·74 before, 1·45 at the end of, and 1·68 three months after cessation of estrogen administration. It showed a significant decline following estrogen therapy. In pre-diabetic women in this group, the decline in *k* was more marked (1·73 to 1·23). In the control group, there was no significant decrease in *k* (1·72 to 1·71), when intravenous glucose tolerance tests were repeated after 3 months.

We have studied the effect of estradiol valerate on glucose tolerance and plasma insulin response in eight post-menopausal women aged 41–53 years[6]. Each treatment cycle consisted of 20 days of estradiol valerate treatment at daily doses of 2 mg, and this was followed by an interval of 8 days. An oral glucose tolerance test, and plasma insulin determinations were carried out before the treatment and again repeated after 3–4 months' treatment. The results are presented in Table 17.3 and Figure 17.3. Estradiol valerate treatment did not cause any significant changes in blood glucose values during oral glucose tolerance tests.

Plasma insulin response tended to become slightly smaller during the treatment (Table 17.4 and Figure 17.4). After 3–4 months' therapy the insulinogenic index was significantly lower than before treatment (Table 17.4).

Lipid metabolism

Synthetic estrogens

Stokes and Wynn[8] have shown that fasting serum triglyceride levels increase with estrogen content in women taking the combined oral contraceptives, mestranol and ethinyl estradiol having identical effects at the same dose. Both mestranol and ethinyl estradiol did not have any definite effect on serum cholesterol levels.

Aitken and his associates[9] studied the effect of mestranol, 20–40 μg daily, in a series of 40 oopherectomized women, randomized into two groups. One of them received mestranol and the other placebo tablets for one year. Mestranol treatment was found to cause a significant decrease of serum cholesterol level and a significant rise of serum triglyceride level.

Our own results by sequential substitution therapy (ethinyl estradiol 25 μg, 16 days, and ethinyl estradiol 25 μg + megestrol 0.5 mg, 7 days) in post-menopausal women[5] are presented in Table 17.5. There was no definite change in serum cholesterol level. The triglyceride level showed a significant increase in the 2nd to 3rd treatment cycle and this change seemed to persist even after 18 to 30 months' treatment. Also the free fatty acid level showed a rising trend during treatment, but the individual variation was wide.

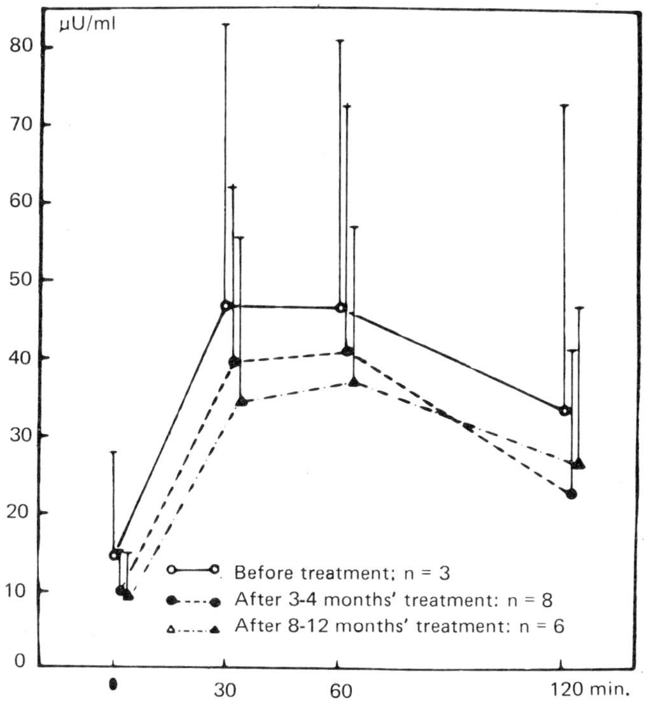

Figure 17.4 Mean plasma insulin levels (μUnits/ml) during an oral glucose tolerance test performed before and after 3–4 and 8–12 months of treatment with estradiol valerate

Natural estrogens

Robinson and Lebeau[10] have studied the effect of 1·25 mg or 2·5 mg of conjugated equine estrogens in 40 post-menopausal women and found a decrease in total cholesterol including beta-lipoprotein cholesterol, but an increase in alpha-lipoprotein cholesterol, phospholipids and triglycerides.

Furman and associates[11] studied the effect of 6 weeks' administration of equilin sulphate (10 mg/day) and conjugated equine estrogens 2·5–15 mg/day and found an increase in alpha- and VLD-lipoprotein lipids. Since alpha-lipoproteins are rich in phospholipid and VLD-lipoproteins are rich in

Table 17.5 The effect of sequential ethinyl estradiol + megestrol treatment on serum lipid levels

		Before treatment	*After 2–3 months*	*After 11–14 months*	*After 18–30 months*
Cholesterol (mg/100 ml)	Mean ± SD	277·7 ± 45·1 (n = 15)	263·3 ± 54·6 (n = 14)	274·5 ± 68·0 (n = 11)	255·0 ± 45·0 (n = 8)
	Mean Δ ± SD*		−12·7 ± 34·5	−16·3 ± 36·8	−7·1 ± 23·4
	p-value		N.S.	N.S.	N.S.
Triglycerides (mg/100 ml)	Mean ± SD	96·7 ± 50·2 (n = 12)	131·4 ± 50·9 (n = 12)	147·6 ± 78·3 (n = 8)	152·6 ± 81·3 (n = 7)
	Mean Δ ± SD*		+34·6 ± 31·5	+47·8 ± 68·6	+77·8 ± 64·9
	p-value		< 0·01	< 0·01	< 0·05
Free fatty acids	Mean ± SD	713·7 ± 141·8 (n = 15)	776·1 ± 210·0 (n = 13)	927·2 ± 275·6 (n = 11)	762·8 ± 152·3 (n = 7)
(mg/100 ml)	Mean Δ ± SD*		95·6 218·7	+244·2 ± 372·8	+43·7 ± 128·9
	p-value		N.S.	< 0·01	N.S.

* Compared with the corresponding values before treatment

Table 17.6 The effect of estradiol valerate treatment on serum lipid levels

		Before treatment	*After 3–4 months*	*After 8–12months*
Cholesterol (mg/100 ml)	Mean ± SD	267·5 ± 26·5 (n = 8)	249·0 ± 30·2 (n = 8)	236·0 ± 22·1 (n = 6)
	Mean Δ ± SD*		− 15·9 ± 13·8	− 26·7 ± 26·2
	p-value		< 0·05	< 0·01
Triglycerides (mg/100 ml)	Mean ± SD	136·1 ± 33·0 (n = 8)	132·6 ± 33·8 (n = 8)	146·7 ± 31·7 (n = 6)
	Mean Δ ± SD*		− 3·5 ± 32·7	8·7 ± 33·2
	p-value		N.S.	N.S.
Free fatty acids	Mean ± SD	557·5 ± 174·0 (n = 8)	576·3 ± 218·6 (n = 8)	532·5 ± 170·9 (n = 6)
	Mean Δ ± SD*		18·8 ± 82·9	− 32·5 ± 102·3
	p-value		N.S.	N.S.

* Compared with the corresponding values before treatment

triglyceride, the net result, as far as serum lipids are concerned, was an increase in the levels of both phospholipid and triglyceride. They did not find any significant change in serum cholesterol level.

Widholm and associates[12] investigated the effect of sequential administration of conjugated equine estrogen (2 mg) and megestrol acetate (2·5 mg) on the lipid metabolism. They noticed a significant decrease of total cholesterol, but no change in the triglyceride level.

Daxemüller and associates[13] reported that the administration of estriol succinate (2 mg/day) did not cause any definite change in serum cholesterol and total lipid levels in women treated for 3 years.

In our own study with estradiol valerate (2 mg) the serum cholesterol showed a significant decrease after 3–4 months' treatment and this trend persisted after 8–12 months' treatment (Table 17.6)[14]. This treatment did not cause any significant changes in serum triglyceride and free fatty acid levels.

Discussion

Synthetic estrogens given at a low dosage apparently do not have any clinically significant effect on the carbohydrate metabolism. The same applies to natural estrogens.

As to the effects of the estrogens on serum lipids, the results are more controversial; summary of these results is given in Table 17.7. Both the synthetic and natural estrogens have in most studies induced a slight decrease of serum cholesterol level. Discrepancies between the results of different studies in this respect may in part be due to differences in the initial composition of the series in regard to age, initial serum cholesterol level, etc. It may also be of importance, whether oophorectomized women or women with the natural menopause have been treated, since Aitken and associates[9] have shown that age trends of serum cholesterol are different in these two groups of post-menopausal women; the younger aged, oophorectomized women tend to have higher serum cholesterol levels than women with intact ovaries.

An increase of serum triglyceride levels has been a consistent finding in women taking contraceptive pills containing synthetic estrogens. Kekki and Nikkilä[15] have shown in their studies on triglyceride kinetics that both the rate of production and the removal of serum triglyceride are increased by synthetic estrogens. However, the removal is enhanced less and thus the net result is an increase of the serum triglyceride level. Observations on the effects of synthetic estrogens on triglyceride levels in post-menopausal women are similar to the findings in younger women taking contraceptives; a persistent rise of serum cholesterol level occurs during treatment with synthetic estrogens.

Observations concerning the effects of natural estrogens on serum triglyceride level are controversial. In one of these studies no definite change of triglyceride was found[12], but in the other two an increase of serum triglyceride was observed. In our own study[14] with estradiol valerate no definite change was found in serum triglyceride level.

Table 17.7 Summary of the results of studies on the effects of synthetic and natural estrogens on serum lipids in post-menopausal women

Compound and dosage	*Authors*	*The effect on serum lipids* Cholesterol	Triglycerides
Synthetic estrogens			
Ethinyl estradiol 25 μg	Pyörälä and associates[5]	↔	↑
Mestranol 20–40 μg	Aitken and associates[9]	↓	↑
Natural estrogens			
Conjugated equine estrogens 2·5–15 mg	Furman and associates[11]	↔	↑
Conjugated equine estrogens 1·25–2·5 mg	Robinson and Lebeau[10]	↓	↑
Conjugated equine estrogens 2 mg	Widholm and associates[15]	↓	↔
Estradiol valerate 2 mg	Pyörälä and associates[10]	↓	↔
Estriol succinate 2 mg	Daxelmüller and associates[13]	↔	—

In conclusion, the treatment of post-menopausal women with small doses of synthetic or natural estrogens appears to be safe with respect to carbohydrate metabolism. More studies, however, are needed on their effects on plasma lipids. Their possible serum cholesterol lowering effect and their possible adverse effect on triglyceride metabolism in post-menopausal women should be explored in larger controlled studies taking initial characteristics of the study population more carefully into account. A comparison between various estrogens is also needed and an attempt should be made to carry out such studies employing dosages of different estrogens which are equivalent in their estrogenic activity.

References

1. Spellacy, W. N. (1974). Metabolic effects of oral contraceptives. *Clin. Obstet. Gynecol.*, **17**, 53
2. Buchler, D. and Warren, J. C. (1966). Effects of estrogen on glucose tolerance. *Am. J. Obstet. Gynecol.*, **95**, 479
3. di Paola, G., Robin, M. and Nicholson, R. (1970). Estrogen therapy and glucose tolerance test. *Am. J. Obstet. Gynecol.*, **107**, 124
4. Danowski, T. S., Kenny, F. M., Wilson, H. R., Sabeh, G., Sunder, J. H. and Corredor, D. G. (1970). Biochemical, endocrine and other indices during quinestrol therapy. *Clin. Pharmacol. Ther.*, **11**, 260
5. Pyörälä, T., Pyörälä, K. and Lampinen, V. (1968). Glucose tolerance during sequential oral contraceptive treatment and during post-menopausal estrogen progestin treatment. (Abstract). *Scand. J. Clin. Invest.*, **101**, 26
6. Pyörälä, K., Pyörälä, T. and Lampinen, V. (1967). Sequential oral contraceptive treatment and intravenous glucose tolerance. *Lancet*, **ii**, 776
7. Goldman, J. A. and Ovadia, J. L. (1969). The effect of estrogen on intravenous glucose tolerance in women. *Am. J. Obstet. Gynecol.*, **103**, 172
8. Stokes, T. and Wynn, W. (1971). Serum lipids in women on oral contraceptives. *Lancet*, **i**, 677
9. Aitken, J. M., Lorimer, A. R., McKay Hart, D., Lawrie, T. D. and Smith, D. A. (1971). The effects of oophorectomy and long term mestranol therapy on the serum lipids of middle-aged women. *Clin. Sci.*, **41**, 597
10. Robinson, R. W. and Lebeau, R. J. (1965). Effect of conjugated equine estrogens on serum lipids and the clotting mechanism. *J. Atheroscler. Res.*, **5**, 120
11. Furman, R. H., Alaupovic, P. and Howard, R. P. (1967). Effects of androgens and estrogens on serum lipids and the composition and concentration of serum lipoproteins in normolipemic and hyperlipemic states. *Prog. Biochem. Pharmacol.*, **2**, 215
12. Widholm, O., Timonen, S., Vartiainen, E. and Procopé, B-J. (19vv). Effects of conjugated equine estrogen on serum lipids. (In preparation).
13. Daxelmüller, L., Lauritzen, Ch. and Heilbrunn, A. (1974). Therapie des klimakterischen Syndroms mit Östriol-Succinat. *Zeitschrift für Therapie*. Verlag von Duncker & H[illegible]blot, Berlin, **1**, 14
14. Pyörälä, K., [illegible]rälä, T. and Weintraub, D. (1971). Glucose tolerance, plasma insulin and [illegible] in postmenopausal women during estradiol valerate treatment. (Abstract). *VI Annual Meeting of the Scandinavian Society for the Study of Diabetes*, April 15–17, Sandefjord.
15. Kekki, M. and Nikkilä, E. A. (1971). Plasma triglyceride turnover during use of oral contraceptives. *Metabolism*, **20**, 878

Discussion on Section D:

Lipid Metabolism

Chairman: *Mr T. M. Coltart*

Dr Robert Greenberg (Community Psychiatrist, London): If I remember rightly, Finland is top of the league in coronary artery disease. To what extent therefore does Dr Pyörälä's work have general application, and do his findings shed any light on why Finland is top of the league. At the other end of the scale, Japan is among the three lowest in the league. Have either Professor Oliver or Dr Pyörälä looked at these national figures in relation to what they have been saying, and do they know of anything which might shed any light on why Japan is bottom of the league.

Dr Oliver made reference to the number of pregnancies in relationship to atherosclerosis. Many years ago a very interesting study was done in Denmark on immigrants from Eastern Europe which showed that those women already had a much higher incidence of coronary disease than the men, and it was attibuted to the greater degree of economic and physical stress of the women in that group. Could pregnancy be one of the stress factors?

Professor M. F. Oliver (Physician, Edinburgh): I should not like to enter into that one. These epidemiological studies are of about 15 years standing, and there is no obvious answer to why these national differences exist. There are, for example, striking differences between England and Wales and Scotland. We have the misfortune in Scotland of having double the attack rate, and mortaility rate from coronary artery disease. The standardized mortality ratio of death rate for coronary heart disease just south of London and for East Anglia is half the death rate for the South-West and Scotland—and I do not necessarily mean the conurbation of Glasgow. So it is not urbanism, it is the rural districts as well. The gradients in certain countries are quite astounding. The gradient in Norway is very large and also between East and West Finland. Karelia in East Finland where many studies are taking place now, has probably the highest attack rate of all. When it comes to coronary disease in women, there is still the gradient, although it appears to be less, between England and Wales, or Southern England, for example, and Scotland. Possibly this is because there is less coronary heart disease anyway in younger women, and it may be that this is simply a false statistic in that we do not have sufficient women to be sure how large the gradient is.

The questioner also asked about pregnancies and the relationship to atherosclerosis. I deliberately, having thrown up the data, rather sidestepped it, because I do not understand it, but it has come out in several studies. It is also true of Arab immigrants coming into Israel, in exactly the same way as we heard described for Denmark. It is obvious that the poorer the population in general, the more pregnancies there are, which may be why the affluence index of coronary heart disease is reversed in women. There is a higher coronary heart disease rate in the lower income groups who have more pregnancies. This comes out very clearly in relation to the negro in the southern parts of the United States, for the male to female differences that I showed for the U.K. do not apply in the U.S. Southern negro—it is almost a one to one attack rate. Why they are more hypertensive is not clear but it has been suggested that more pyelitis is present, and they have more pregnancies.

Mr E. S. Saunders (Gynaecologist, London): Most of the lecturers at the Symposium have reported their results on estrogen administered by the oral route. Oral application of medicines goes back for centuries, but the hormone has to go through the stomach and intestines to the liver which is a complicated chemical factory and completely changes the molecular composition of the hormone. The hormone causes toxic effects

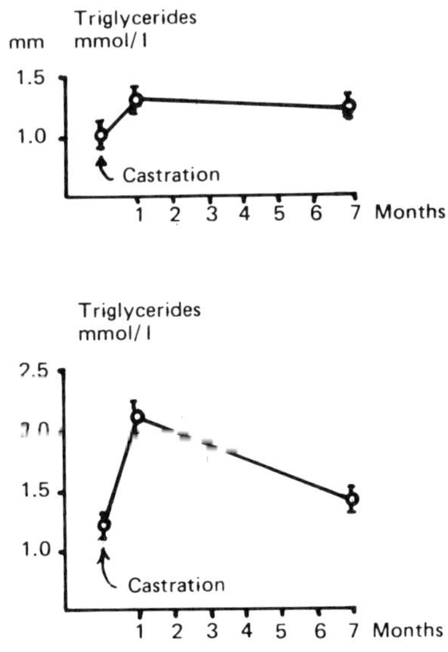

Figure 1 (top) The effect of bilateral oophorectomy on serum triglycerides. (bottom) The effect of peroral estradiol valerate therapy on serum triglycerides

on the liver, and even tumours. Hepatomas have been reported following administration of oral contraceptives. Therefore attempts have been made to bypass the liver and the intestinal route by using implants of hormones. The method is simple, and I have been using it for the last 20 years, and whilst I have seen cases of thrombosis after oral contraceptives, I have never seen any thrombosis following the use of thousands of implants.

Professor L. Rauramo (Gynaecologist, Turku): I have some results of our investigations—previously unpublished—on lipids in castrated women with and without estrogen replacement therapy. We have divided a group of 150 castrated women into three groups of about 50 persons in each. One group served as controls, the second group received estradiol valerate (Progynova) 2 mg/day and the third group had estriol succinate (Synapause) 2 mg/day.

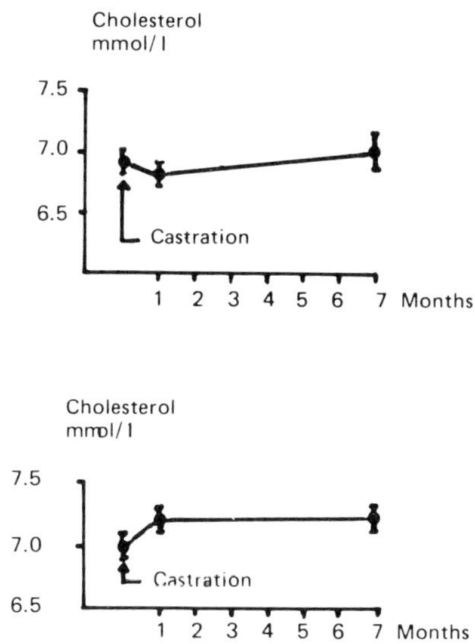

Figure 2 (top) The effect of bilateral oophorectomy on serum cholesterol. (bottom) The effect of peroral estradiol valerate therapy on serum cholesterol

In the estradiol valerate group there would seem to be a slight rise in triglycerides after castration but these changes are not significant (Figure 1). Similarly there do not appear to be any significant changes in cholesterol levels after 6 month's therapy. (Figure 2). After castration, the phospholipids remain about the same in the control group; there is some tendency for them to rise on estradiol valerate therapy but again nothing statistically significant (Figure 3).

The study with estradiol valerate was over half a year, but we made a 3-year study with estriol succinate, and some changes in the lipid levels of the control group can be

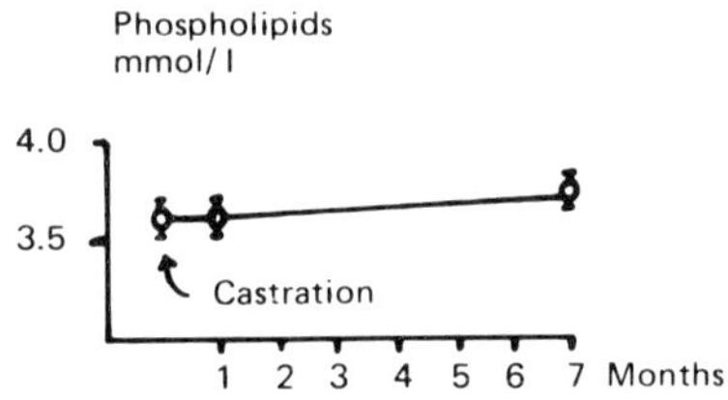

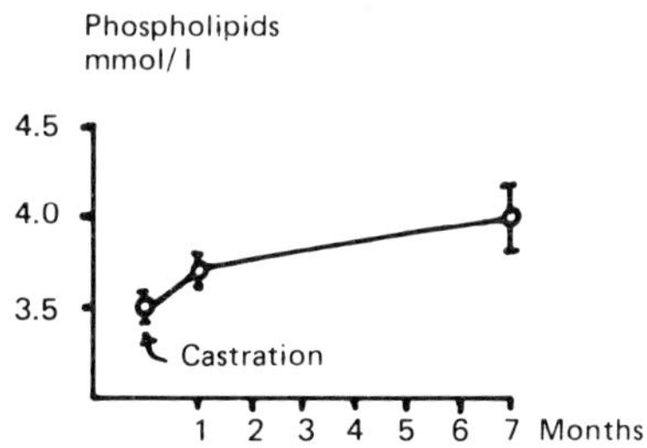

Figure 3 (top) The effect of bilateral oophorectomy on serum phospholipids. (bottom) The effect of peroral estradiol valerate therapy on serum phospholipids

observed after 3 years. The slight rise in cholesterol 1 month after oophorectomy becomes very marked after 3 years, whereas triglycerides and phospholipids do not change significantly (Figure 4). Serum cholesterol levels in the estriol succinate treated cases remain constant for about 18 months, but thereafter there is a statistically significant fall which is sustained for the remainder of the 3 years (Figure 5). No changes in serum triglycerides were found after 3 years therapy with estriol succinate (Figure 6) and although the phospholipids show a tendency to rise slightly, the changes found are not statistically significant.

Professor V. Wynn (Human Metabolism, London): Professor Oliver showed a slide on the heart attack rate in women, with age. The graph was a dead straight line. How does he argue from that that there is a post-menopausal increase in the heart attack rate? My concept of a post-menopausal rise of heart attack rate would imply that the line should rise in some form of exponential manner.

Professor M. F. Oliver: Probably the slide flashed on to the screen rather fast. What it is showing is that the proportionate rise in coronary artery disease in patients between 45 and 54 years is the same as that between 55 and 64 years and that there is a linear relationship. In men, however, the increase between 45 to 54 is greater than that between 55 and 64 years, while women start with a lower rate and rise more quickly. If the figure was to be taken into an earlier age group, then the exponental rise which Professor Wynn expected to see would become apparent.

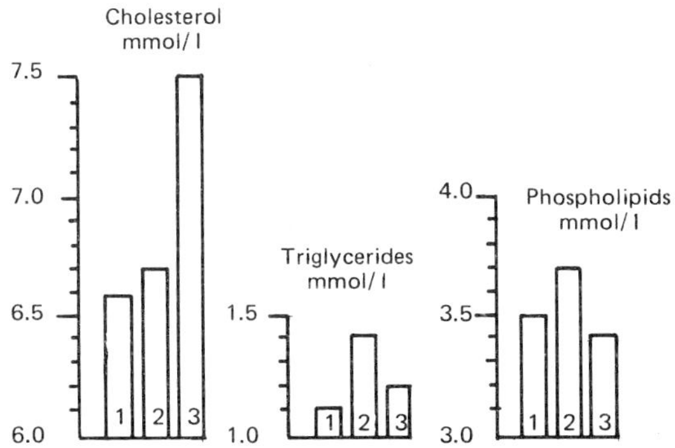

Figure 4 The effect of bilateral oophorectomy on serum cholesterol, triglycerides and phospholipids (no hormone therapy). 1. Before castration. 2. 1 month after castration 3. 3 years after castration

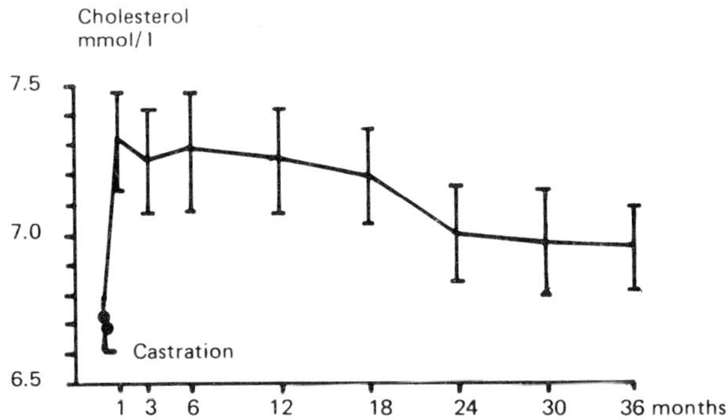

Figure 5 The effect of peroral estriol succinate therapy on serum cholesterol

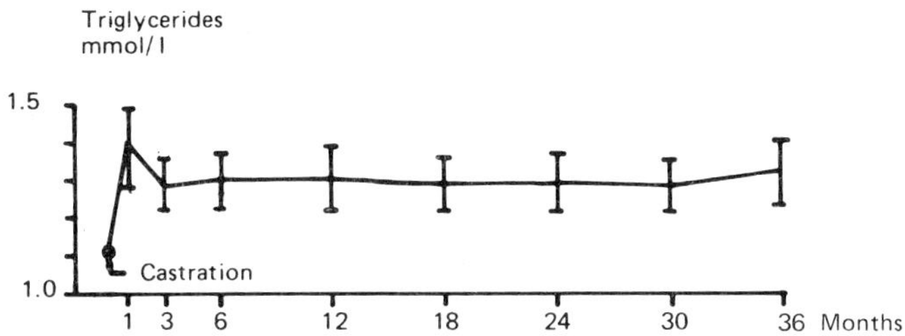

Figure 6 The effect of peroral estriol succinate therapy on serum triglycerides

Professor C. Lauritzen (Gynaecologist, Ulm): If I understood him correctly, Professor Oliver's general conclusion was that estrogens increase the risk of coronary atherosclerosis and myocardial infarction, particularly in those patients who are cigarette smokers and who have a familial disposition. I find that conclusion too general. Such conclusions have added much in the past to an undue discrimination against estrogens. The material to which the Professor referred is only applicable to conjugated estrogens, oral medication, and in doses of 2.5 mg and 5 mg, not in the doses which are used therapeutically 0·6 and 1·25 mg, and ethinyl estradiol as high as 100 and 200 micrograms. Is there any evidence about therapeutic dosages of conjugated estrogens, 0·625 mg and 1·25 mg, or with estradiol valerate in oral medication. We have heard something about estriol and estriol succinate. Is there any knowledge of or experience with long-term investigations into the risks of the last-named compound? Secondly, is there any evidence on parenteral medication? I want to stress the point already put by Mr Saunders. Oral medication may not be the best means of application for hormones because these compounds go direct to the liver where they stimulate reactions which may become pathological.

Lastly, evidence should be cited from the Boston Collaborative Drug Surveys—or about twelve hospitals in the Boston area who have shown that with doses of 0·625 mg and 1·25 mg of conjugated estrogens no thromboembolic episodes have been noted in the group taking the medication, although there have been eleven such episodes among the controls.

Professor M. F. Oliver: The word 'conclusion' has proved confusing. I was concluding my talk. I am in no position to conclude with regard to the use of hormone replacement therapy. I merely drew a parallel between a number of situations which looked to me, as a cardiologist, somewhat disconcerting, and drew a warning as to what I think may well take place. I would be quite surprised, on the evidence that we have, if there were not an increase in coronary heart attack in women who smoke heavily, who have a family history of coronary heart disease and who go on to hormone replacement therapy, but I think that it will take a number of years to show. One has to bear in mind information on venous thromboembolism which is much better documented than anything in the Boston Drug Survey*, which has all sorts of problems in the selection of the population. We cannot possibly suggest that estrogens and the oral contraceptive do not increase venous thromboembolism in 1975. The evidence is very clear about that, and it is also fairly clear about arterial thrombosis too, or at least that is my standpoint.

In all the long-term studies that have been done, the information that there is an increased thrombotic risk is not evident for about 3 or 4 years. That may be because of the vast populations that have to be studied to achieve statistical significance. I hope that Mr Saunders's remark on parenteral estrogens indicates that studies are being made on many many hundreds of women otherwise they are useless. In the world of coronary heart disease, we are concerned with a timescale which is quite different from the timescale that many others think of for it takes 30 to 35 years for us to develop our coronary heart disease. We do not have raised lipids until we are aged about 15, and

* Boston Collaborative Drug Surveillance Program. (1974). *N. Engl. J. Med.*, 290, 15

we do not get coronary heart disease until we are 45 or 50. The timescale with which we are concerned is entirely different to that of most diseases and short-term observations about the lack of thrombosis when this or that hormonal replacement therapy is given do not impress me.

Professor Lauritzen is right in indicating that I only referred to 2·5 mg Premarin, because no studies have been done with smaller doses in terms of vascular thrombosis. A study would have to be established in something like 850 patients, with a further 850 in a control group, and treated for 5 years, which is a big undertaking. The first requirement for a clinical trial is to have a grandson old enough to carry it on!

Section E

CALCIUM METABOLISM

Chairman: G. V. P. CHAMBERLAIN

18

Post-menopausal changes in calcium and phosphorus metabolism

C. E. Dent

The current interest in what is often called 'post-menopausal osteoporosis' dates from the work of the Albright group[1] as subsequently carried on by and reported in the important paper by Henneman and Wallach[2]. This latter paper claimed that height loss, used as an indication of increasing vertebral body collapse from oestoporosis, could be prevented if women at the beginning of their menopause were given estrogen, the untreated controls all losing height. This investigation suffered from insufficient height measurements, and has lost importance even more because nobody has since published observations which have confirmed these findings. It is surprising also that more recent investigators have rarely used simple height measurements, which are highly specific for their purpose, but have favoured often very complicated histological, radiological and radioactive techniques of less proved value.

Measurements of the heights of large samples of the normal population show that loss of height begins around 40 years of age and progresses faster with increasing age, especially in women, with no clear exacerbation at the average age of menopause. Further studies related to time of menopause as distinct from chronological age would still be worth doing for there is still no clear proof that the menopause as such causes osteoporosis, and even less that sex hormones can avert it. However, it must be stressed that many clinicians, and this is our experience too, have noted that severe osteoporosis may follow years after artificial ovari- and orchid-ectomy in relatively young subjects but that this is by no means a common occurrence.

Biochemical methods are of little use in furthering our knowledge of this subject. All plasma levels are normal, while urine calcium excretion may be raised in the early phases of the disease. Calcium balances, troublesome to perform, are helpful as the partition of calcium excretion is nearly always abnormal with 24-hour faecal calcium excretion usually only a little less than 24-hour dietary intake. This has led some to suggest that this malabsorption of calcium may be the primary cause of the disease. However, if more absorption is encouraged by giving high doses of vitamin D, or circumvented by giving repeated calcium infusions by vein, this extra calcium is not retained but is lost in the urine. This would not be expected if simple calcium deficiency was the cause of the disease. A difficulty with interpreting calcium balance studies arises because the disease develops only slowly over years and the inevitable negative balance may only be 30 mg or so of calcium per day which is not measurable with accuracy by the method. Likewise if a curative treatment were to be found one would hardly expect the ensuing positive balances to be more than 30 mg or so, again beyond reach of the technique. The same criticism applies of course to all alternative methods of determining the amount of calcium going in or out of the skeleton. Total body calcium measurements claimed to be accurate to 3–5%, sound very useful until it is realized that this refers to 30–50 g of calcium in the kilogram or so of skeletal calcium. To retain a modest 30 g of calcium at a positive balance of 30 mg a day would require 1000 days, so follow up of patients on possibly curative regimes would require years to pass before they could be properly assessed by total body (or limb) calcium determinations using modern techniques such as neutron activation.

The effects of male and female sex hormones given separately or together and in various synthetic and natural forms have been extensively studied and reported in the medical literature, usually with ambiguous and often with contradictory results. Only one clear finding has seemed to stand the test of time and that is that in patients having a more acute onset of osteoporosis, who usually have a high calcium excretion in urine as well as in the faeces, the administration of sex hormones does usually lower the urine calcium and makes the balance less negative, but it never makes it positive as if arrest of the process rather than its reversal is all that is within our power by this means. This of course takes us back to where Henneman and Wallach left off in 1957, and stresses the urgent need for more studies to confirm or deny their work in a longer and more detailed study, perhaps including also a sufficient number of patients who have had early artificial menopause.

More general aspects of osteoporosis have been covered in more detail by the author in other publications[3, 4]. The more recent literature deals with treatment trials using many other drugs such as calcitonin, 1-α-hydroxycholecalciferol, parathyroid hormone and fluoride, the wide variety of these, each acting on bone in quite different ways, showing better than I can describe, our therapeutic despair in dealing with a very common important and intractable disease. In my opinion there is no real evidence yet that any of these newer methods are at all effective, in spite of many claims to the contrary. Therefore when the clinical pressure is so great as to demand some form of treatment I still fumble with sex hormones which at least have some theoretical justification.

References

1. Albright, F. and Reifenstein, E. C. (1948). *The Parathyroid Glands and Metabolic Bone Disease* (Baltimore: Williams & Wilkins)
2. Henneman, P. H. and Wallach, S. (1957). *Arch. Intern. Med.*, **100,** 715
3. Dent, C. E. and Watson, L. (1966). *Postgrad. Med. J.*, Oct. Suppl., 583
4. Dent, C. E. (1968). Osteoporosis, *Thule Internat. Symp. Ageing of Connective & Skeletal Tissues*, 261. (Stockholm: Norkiska Bokhandels)

19

Osteoporosis and its relation to estrogen deficiency

J. M. Aitken

The concept, that vertebral crush fractures in women were a direct consequence of the menopause, was first expounded by Fuller Albright over 30 years ago[1]. Albright's simple hypothesis proposed an aetiological association between loss of ovarian function and the development of osteoporosis in women. Subsequent metabolic balance studies indicated that both estrogen and androgen therapy would be effective in the treatment of post-menopausal osteoporosis[2]. Reifenstein[3] went on to make a number of sweeping assumptions by a process of extrapolation and claimed that sex hormone therapy given to post-menopausal women with established osteoporosis would effectively increase skeletal mass by 30% after only 5 years of treatment. However, with the advent of more precise methods for the quantification of skeletal mass[4–7], it soon became clear that at best estrogen therapy merely prevented further post-menopausal skeletal wasting[8, 9], and unless androgens were given in virilizing dosage[10] they proved to be ineffective in the treatment of osteoporotic women[11]. It was not surprising therefore that over the past decade considerable doubt has been cast upon Albright's original hypothesis. There still existed however a substantial body of circumstantial evidence that ovarian function was in some way tied up with skeletal mass in women, in so far as the ovarian weight of non-pregnant women is greatest between the ages of 30 and 40 years[12], at which time the 24-hour urinary estrogen excretion shows a similar pattern of change[13] (Figure 19.1) and bone mass reaches a maximum value in the female population at about the age ot 35 years[14] (Figure 19.2). In view of these uncertainties and unfounded suppositions, we endeavoured to re-examine the relationship between ovarian function, estrogens and skeletal homeostasis.

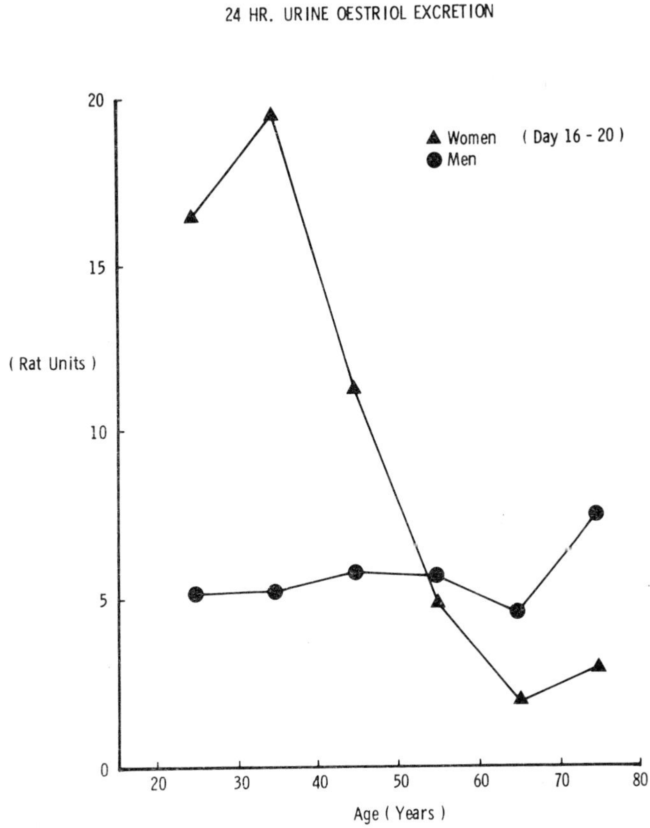

Figure 19.1 Relationship between urinary estrogen excretion and age. After Pincus *et al.* (1954)[13]

Oophorectomy and osteoporosis

We decided to study only women who had undergone hysterectomy with or without bilateral salpingo-oophorectomy for non-malignant disease, at a time when they were still having regular menstrual periods; the most common cause for operation being dysfunctional uterine bleeding[15]. Assessment of bone mass was made by X-ray densitometry using the metacarpal as the bone density reference site[6], and the results were expressed as percentile values by reference to the normal female population data of Smith *et al.*[14]

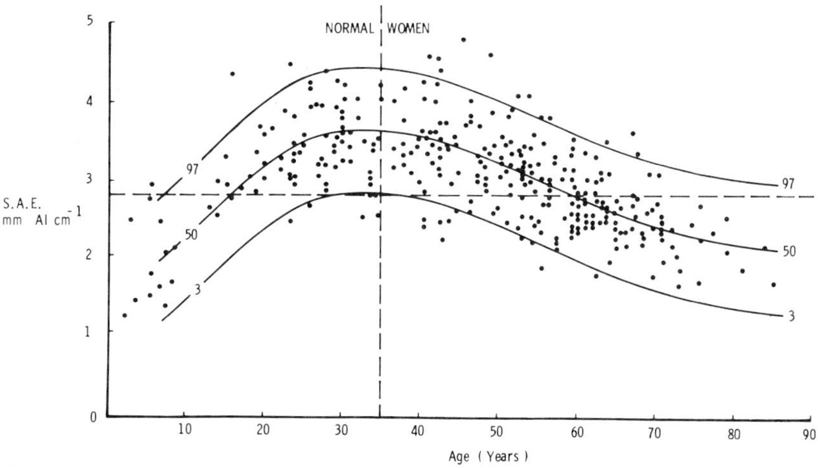

Figure 19.2 Relationship between the Standardised Aluminium Equivalent (SAE) of the third metacarpal and age in women. The 3rd, 50th and 97th percentile lines have been drawn through the data. After Smith *et al.* (1969)

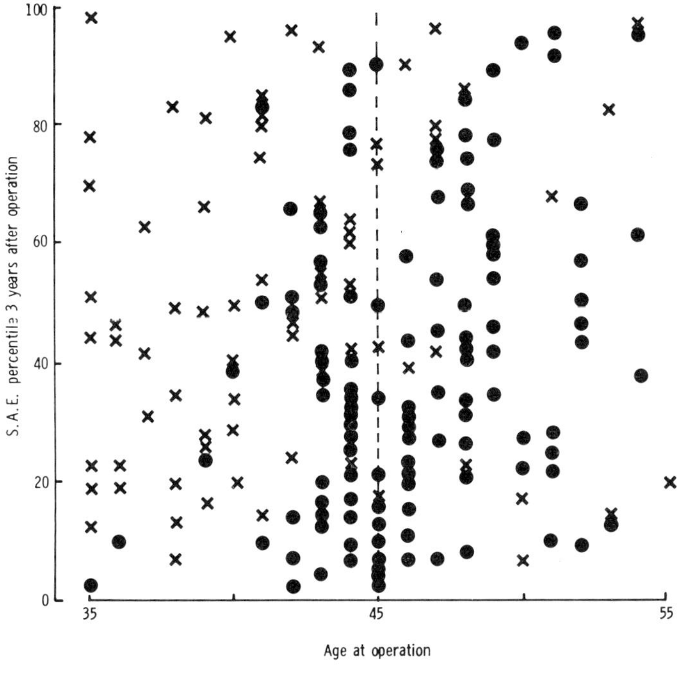

Figure 19.3 Effect of oophorectomy on metacarpal mineral content percentile value when assessed 3 years after operation. ×, hysterectomy alone; ●, hysterectomy and oophorectomy

(Figure 19.2). We found that whereas oophorectomy after the age of 45 years had no apparent effect on subsequent bone mineral loss with age, oophorectomy before the age of 45 years, especially where the operation had been performed before the age of 40 years, was associated with the premature development of a significant degree of osteoporosis (Figure 19.3 and 19.4).

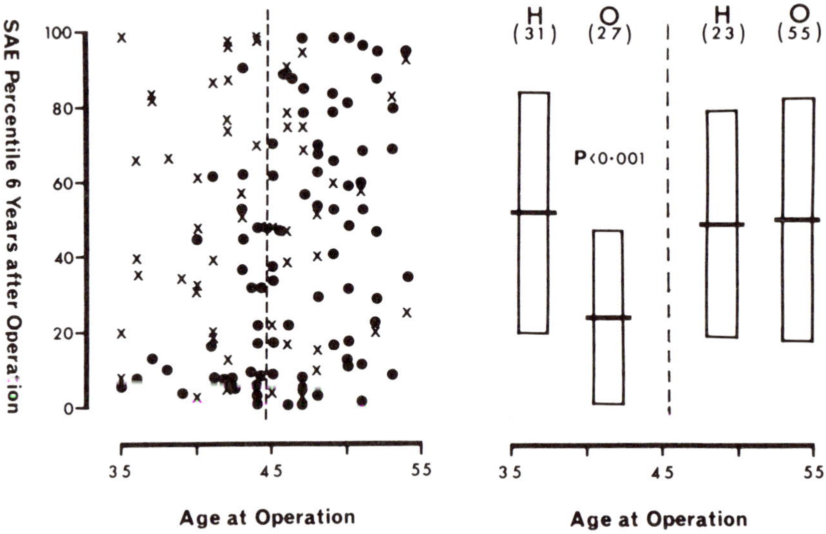

Figure 19.4 Effect of oophorectomy on metacarpal mineral content percentile value when assessed 6 years after operation. ×, hysterectomy alone; ●, hysterectomy and oophorectomy. On the right are the means ± 1 SD of the SAE percentile value of women operated upon before and after the age of 45 years. Numbers of patients in parentheses. H, Hysterectomy alone; O, hysterectomy and oophorectomy

Estrogen therapy after oophorectomy

The rate of loss of bone mineral after oophorectomy was then assessed by gamma ray photonabsorptiometry[7], again using the metacarpal as the skeletal reference site. The women studied were given either 20 μg mestranol tablets or placebo tablets, and bone density measurements were made at yearly intervals thereafter. Broadly speaking three separate groups of women were studied according to the time that had elapsed between oophorectomy and the start of treatment—the time intervals being, 2 months, 3 years and 6 years after operation. Some of the women in the 3-year post-oophorectomy group also had measurements of serum and urinary calcium, by atomic absorption spectrophotometry, plasma and urinary cortisol by fluorimetry and differential protein binding respectively, and plasma 17-hydroxy androgens (17OHA) and sex hormone binding globulin (SHBG) by standard methods[17].

Duration of estrogen deprivation and skeletal responsiveness

The effect of mestranol therapy when started within 2 months of oophorectomy is shown in Figure 19.5. There was a rapid fall in bone mass within

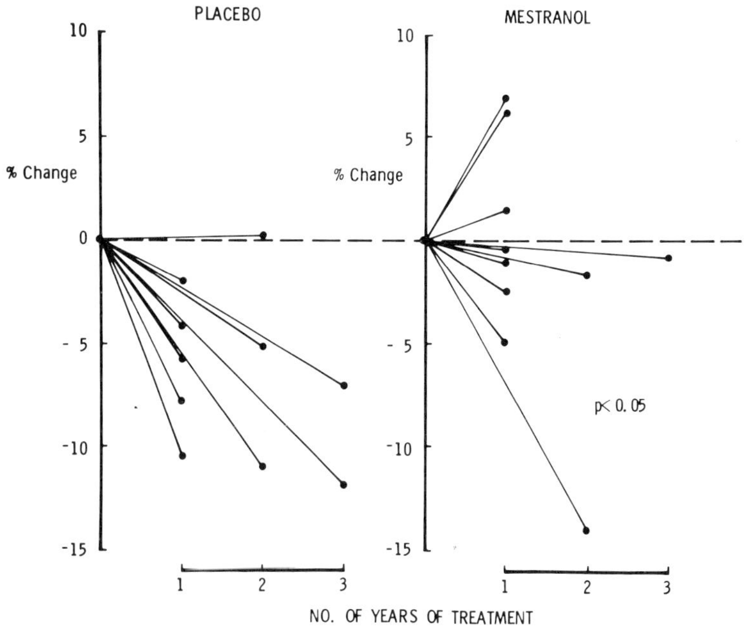

Figure 19.5 Effect of mestranol therapy on metacarpal mineral content when treatment first started within 2 months of oophorectomy

2 months of operation in the placebo treated group, whereas the estrogen treated women experienced no significant mean change in bone mass. When mestranol was started after 6 years of estrogen deprivation both groups of women lost bone mass at a similar rate irrespective of treatment (Figure 19.6). When mestranol was first started 3 years after oophorectomy, there was a significant increase in bone mass in the estrogen treated group as opposed to a small mean fall in bone mass in the placebo group (Figure 19.7).

It is clear therefore that the response of the post-menopausal skeleton is critically related to the duration of estrogen deprivation, with estrogen appearing to lose its osteotrophic action within 6 years of the menopause, but where no more than 3 years of estrogen deficiency has elapsed subsequent estrogen therapy not only appears to prevent further bone mineral loss, but in those women who have already become somewhat osteoporotic there may be a significant increase in bone mass[16].

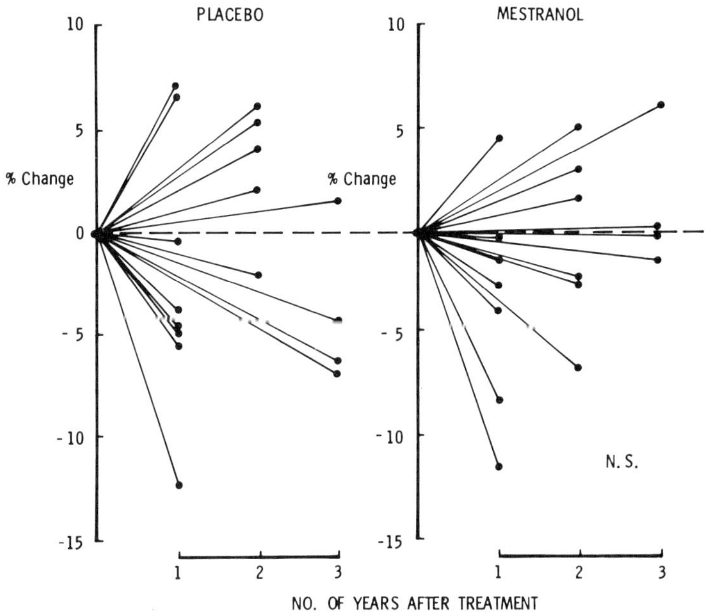

Figure 19.6 Effect of mestranol therapy on metacarpal mineral content when treatment first started 6 years after oophorectomy

Endogenous androgens and osteoporosis

Twenty-four placebo-treated and 13 mestranol-treated women from the 3-year post-oophorectomy group had measurements of plasma 17OHA and SHBG performed[17]. Plasma 17OHA levels were similar in both groups of women, but as expected the estrogen-treated women had significantly higher SHBG levels ($P < 0{\cdot}001$). It was of especial interest to find that in the placebo-treated women the 17OHA/SHBG ratio was inversely related to the rate of bone mineral loss ($r = -0{\cdot}40$), such that whereas six out of seven women with values $> 0{\cdot}2$ lost bone mineral, only seven out of 17 women lost bone mineral where the 17OHA/SHBG ratio was $< 0{\cdot}2$. Since women with a high 17OHA/SHBG ratio have higher free androgen levels and commonly show signs of virilization[17], this suggests that in women, contrary to the claims of Reifenstein[3], an excess of circulating androgens would appear to be associated with the development of post-menopausal osteoporosis.

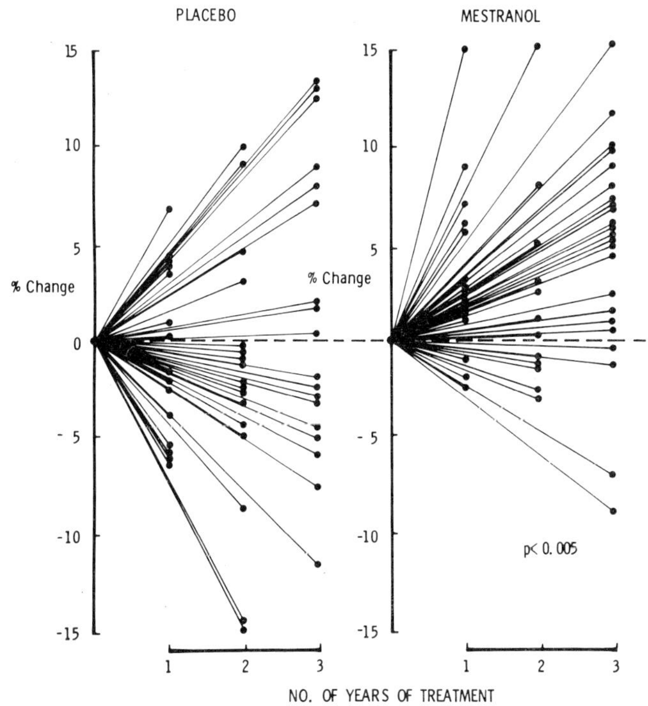

Figure 19.7 Effect of mestranol therapy on metacarpal mineral content when treatment first started 3 years after oophorectomy

Changes in serum and urinary calcium

In the 3-year post-oophorectomy mestranol-treated women there was an overall small mean fall in serum calcium and a significant fall in urinary calcium excretion[18], but these changes were not linearly related to the associated change in bone mass (Figure 19.8). It has furthermore been shown that even where a significant fall in bone mineral content occurs, as in the 6-year post-oophorectomy mestranol-treated group, a similar degree of hypocalcaemia and hypocalciuria was to be found[19].

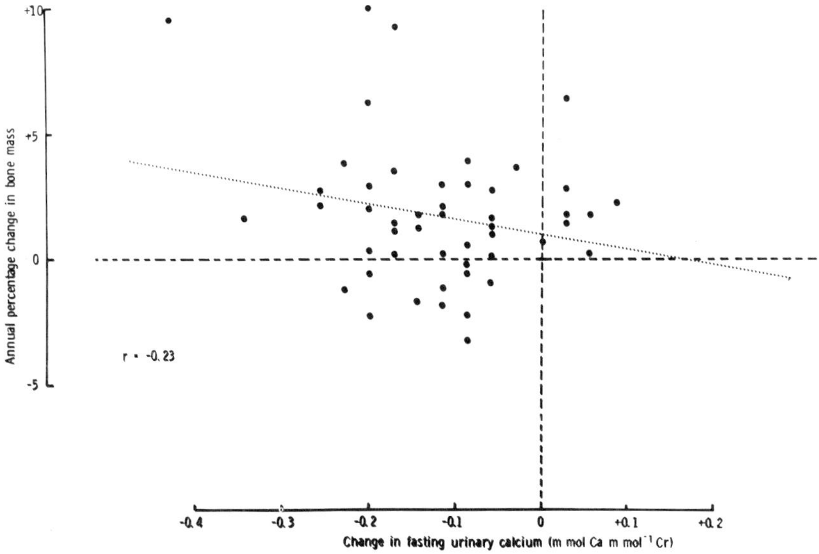

Figure 19.8 Relationship between the change in urinary calcium excretion after mestranol treatment for 1 year, and the associated change in metacarpal mineral

Hypercorticism and estrogen therapy

It has long been known that the exhibition of estrogens to normal women is associated with a significant rise in plasma cortisol binding globulin (CBG) and hence total plasma cortisol concentration rises. We confirmed this observation in oophorectomized women given small doses of mestranol[20], but we were surprised to find that those women with the higher plasma cortisol values whilst on estrogens, tended to lose bone mineral (Figure 19.9). These findings suggest that estrogen induced hypercortisolaemia is not solely the result of an increase in plasma CBG concentration. This hypothesis was further supported by the observation that in mestranol-treated women urinary free cortisol excretion, although within the normal range, also showed an inverse relationship with skeletal response to estrogen.

As a result of this investigation, we suggested that in certain circumstances the measurement of the plasma 09.00 h fasting fluorigenic cortisol level may be helpful in avoiding excessive estrogen dosage and maintaining the osteotrophic response at an optimum level.

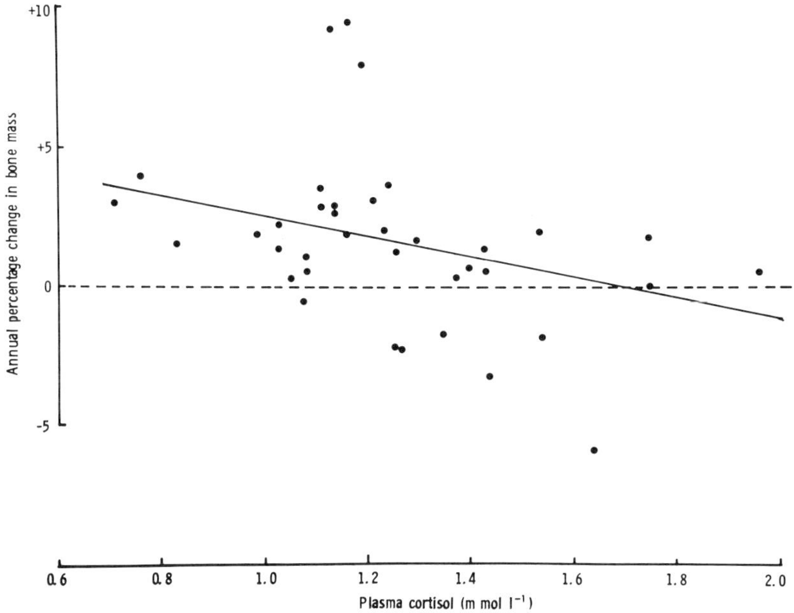

Figure 19.9 Relationship between fasting plasma 09.00 h cortisol in the 3-year post-oophorectomy mestranol treated women and the associated change in metacarpal mineral content

Vasomotor symptoms and estrogen dosage

It is tempting, in post-menopausal women with flushes and sweating, to use the abolition of such symptoms as an index of the adequacy of estrogen dosage. We examined this possibility and our findings are shown in Figure 19.10). It can be seen that whereas most women taking 10 μg mestranol daily retained their vasomotor symptoms, there were about 8% of women taking as much as 40 μg mestranol daily who still had flushing and sweating. However the optimum osteotrophic response was obtained in those women taking about 20 μg mestranol daily where the prevalence of vasomotor symptoms was 17%. Hence it would appear unwise to increase the dose of estrogen until flushes and sweating have completely disappeared, since by so doing a number of women will be deprived of the important osteotrophic effect[16].

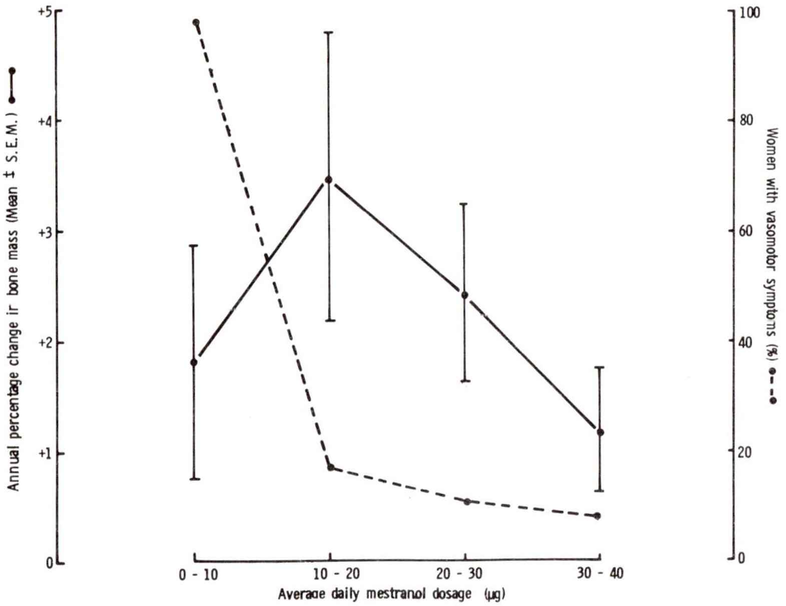

Figure 19.10 Effect of estrogen dosage on prevalence of vasomotor symptoms after oophorectomy and associated bone mineral response. Means ± SEM

Conclusions

Oophorectomy after the age of 45 years in pre-menopausal women does not carry an increased risk of subsequent osteoporosis, but oophorectomy before the age of 45 years is attended by a significant reduction in bone mass, and such patients require the early administration of ovarian hormone therapy if the premature development of osteoporosis is to be prevented. Mestranol is a convenient cheap estrogen and its administration for periods of up to 3 years has not to date been associated with any important adverse reactions. The optimum dose of mestranol would appear to be about 20 μg daily, but we would recommend that estrogen treatment should be discontinued during the first 7 days of each calendar month. There is at present no precise information on the osteotrophic equivalence between mestranol and either ethinyl estradiol or conjugated equine estrogens (Premarin), and therefore until the appropriate studies have been performed *in vivo* in women one can only make an intuitive guess at the respective dose equivalence. Excessive estrogen dosage in women should be avoided since there is no evidence that increasing the dose to the limits of tolerance is associated with an increase in osteotrophic action, and commonly this practice will lead to an inferior skeletal response. Monitoring the plasma 09.00 h fasting fluorigenic cortisol level may be helpful in avoiding excessive estrogen dosage, and where the cortisol level exceeds 45 μg/dl the dose of estrogen should be reduced. The not uncommon pharmaceutical practice of adding small doses of androgens to sex hormone preparations for the climacteric patient should be strongly discouraged, since we present evidence herein that endogenous androgens would appear to hasten rather than retard the development of post-menopausal osteoporosis.

Acknowledgments

This work was carried out in the University Department of Medicine at the Western Infirmary, Glasgow and was supported by a personal grant from the Scottish Hospital Endowments Research Trust. Messrs. G. D. Searle, High Wycombe, gave us generous financial support and supplied the mestranol and placebo tablets. Drs. D. M. Hart and R. Lindsay gave invaluable clinical assistance.

References

1. Albright, F., Smith, P. H. and Richardson, A. M. (1941). Postmenopausal osteoporosis; its clinical features. *J. Amer. Med. Ass.*, **116,** 2465
2. Albright, F. (1947). The effect of hormones on osteogenesis in man. *Recent Progr. Hormone Res.*, **1,** 293
3. Reifenstein, E. C. (1957). The relationships of steroid hormones to the development and management of osteoporosis in aging people. *Clin. Orthoped.*, **10,** 206
4. Barnett, E. and Nordin, B. E. C. (1960). The radiological diagnosis of osteoporosis: a new approach. *Clin. Radiol.*, **11,** 166
5. Cameron, J. R. and Sorenson, J. (1963). Measurement of bone mineral *in vivo*: An improved method. *Science*, **142,** 230
6. Anderson, J. B., Shimmins, J. and Smith, D. A. (1966). A new technique for the measurement of metacarpal density. *Brit. J. Radiol.*, **39,** 443
7. Shimmins, J., Smith, D. A., Aitken, M., Anderson, J. B. and Gillespie, F. C. (1972). The accuracy and reproducibility of bone mineral measurements *in vivo*. (b) Methods using sealed isotope sources. *Clin. Radiol.*, **23,** 47
8. Davis, M. E., Strandjord, N. M. and Lanzl, L. H. (1966). Estrogens and the aging process. *J. Amer. Med. Ass.*, **196,** 219
9. Meema, H. E. and Meema, S. (1968). Prevention of postmenopausal osteoporosis by hormone treatment of the menopause. *Canad. Med. Ass. J.*, **99,** 248
10. Partridge, J. W. Boling, L., De Wind, L., Sheldon, M. and Kinsell, L. W. (1953). Metabolic and clinical effects of methylandrostenediol in human subjects. *J. Clin. Endocrinol.*, **13,** 189

11. Gordan, G. S., Picchi, J. and Roof, B. S. (1973). Antifracture efficacy of long-term estrogens for osteoporosis. *Trans. Ass. Amer. Physicians*, **86,** 326
12. Lauritzen, C. (1972). Endocrinology of the menopause and the postmenopausal period. In: P. E. Lebech, K. Ulrich, A. Helles (eds.). *Klimakteriet*, p. 17. (Kobenhavn: Frederiksberg Bogtrykkeri)
13. Pincus, G., Romanoff, L. P. and Carlo, J. (1954). The excretion of urinary steroids by men and women of various ages. *J. Gerontol.*, **9,** 113
14. Smith, D. A., Anderson, J. B., Shimmins, J., Speirs, C. F. and Barnett, E. (1969). Changes in metacarpal mineral content and density in normal male and female subjects with age. *Clin. Radiol.*, **20,** 23
15. Aitken, J. M., Hart, D. M., Anderson, J. B., Lindsay, R., Smith, D. A. and Speirs, C. F. (1973). Osteoporosis after oophorectomy for non-malignant disease in premenopausal women. *Brit. Med. J.*, **2,** 325
16. Aitken, J. M., Hart, D. M., Lindsay, R. and MacDonald, E. B. (1974). Oestrogen dosage in the treatment of postmenopausal osteoporosis. *Medikon International*, **8,** 3
17. Anderson, D. C. (1974). Sex-hormone-binding globulin. *Clin. Endocrinol.*, **3,** 69
18. Aitken, J. M., Hart, D. MacKay and Smith, D. A. (1971). The effect of long-term mestranol administration on calcium and phosphorus homeostasis in oophorectomized women. *Clin. Sci.*, **41,** 233
19. Aitken, J. M., Hart, D. M. and Lindsay, R. (1973). Oestrogen replacement therapy for the prevention of osteoporosis after oophorectomy. *Brit. Med. J.*, **3,** 515
20. Aitken, J. M., Hall, P. E., Rao, L. G. S., Hart, D. M. and Lindsay, R. (1974). Hypercortisolaemia and lack of skeletal response to oestrogen in postmenopausal women. *Clin. Endocrinol.*, **3,** 167

Discussion on Section E:

Calcium Metabolism

Chairman: *Mr G. V. P. Chamberlain*

Dr P. Bye (Schering Chemicals, Sussex): Neither Professor Dent, nor Dr Aitken, has drawn any attention to the role of the bone matrix in osteoporosis. They have both talked about it as though it was solely a problem of calcium metabolism. Perhaps Professor Dent referred to it briefly when talking about the simplicity of treating osteomalacia, which is a pure calcium deficiency. In osteoporosis the loss of bone matrix is equally important and accounts, perhaps, for some of the confusing findings in Professor Dent's calcium motabolism studies.

I should also like to suggest to Dr Aitken that his finding of cortisol levels showing a relationship to bone loss might have had nothing to do with sex binding globulin, or similar problems, and might simply reflect the effect of cortisol itself on collagen. It has been shown by various workers (Nordin, B. E. C., Gallagher, J. C., Aaron, J. E., and Horsman, A. (1975). 'Estrogens in the Post-menopause' *Frontiers Hormone Res.*, Vol. 3, p. 131, (Basel: Karger), that there is increased hydroxyproline loss after the menopause, that hydroxyproline is a breakdown product of collagen, and that the administration of estrogens will reduce the loss of hydroxyproline. It has also been shown recently that estrogens increase the linkages in collagen thus tending to stabilize it (Henneman, Dorothy, H. (1973). 'Effect of ostrogen and growth hormone on collagen in endocrinology'. Ed. Scow, R.D. Excerpta Medica.). The problem needs to be recognized.

Professor C. E. Dent (Physician, London): I accept what has been said about matrix absolutely. This is my criticism of short-term calcium balance studies because one can easily calcify slightly under-calcified bones. All our bones are slightly under-calcified. One can always push in a bit more calcium, but not necessarily show that one has done the person any good, and this applies even in the longer term studies such as measuring the total calcium in the forearm. I do not know that anyone has ever shown that a bird, with all those bony trabeculi in its hollow bones, if given estrogens, would have stronger bones than before. I would rather suggest they were not. This is the difficulty, and this is why I feel that we are still in a primitive steam age clinical survey situation. We have had splendid hints from the second speaker as to what we should be doing, but until we can work on bone matrix properly, and as yet we cannot, we shall need long-term follow up for fragility of bones, which I think is due to imperfect matrix. We know that the matrix changes for example by polymerization of collagen, and cross-linking with age and so on. The stage is set.

Dr J. M. Aitken (Physician, Colchester): The real reason why one measures bone mineral content, as opposed to bone collagen content, is that one can measure bone mineral content *in vivo* without taking out a chunk of bone and assaying it. It has been suggested, by many observers, that the bone in osteoporotic patients is normal in its chemical composition and in its histological appearance, the only difference being that there is less of it than is found in the younger patient. The inference, therefore, is that if there is less bone mineral present, there will also be less bone matrix.

We have measured urinary hydroxyproline excretion in our patients, but again I should like to put in a word of caution, namely that we also found a fall in urinary hydroxyproline excretion in patients who were not showing a significant change in bone mineral content. The 6-year post-oophorectomy group who were given estrogen showed a fall in urinary hydroxyproline excretion. How that is brought about is another matter. The 3-year post-oophrectomy group treated with estrogens also show a fall in urinary hydroxyproline excretion, and many studies have also confirmed it. But—and this is the problem—does this really represent a turnover of collagen in the skeleton, or is it some quirk of metabolism—for example a bit more of the collagen being broken down into free hydroxyproline, which by and large is not excreted in the urine, as opposed to less of it being broken down, and liberated as peptides which appear in the urine and are assayed.

Dr R. C. Greenberg (Community Psychiatrist, London): The subject of osteoporosis and fractures happens to be far more important in the post-menopausal woman than would appear from the amount of space devoted to it in the programme. The incidence of drop attacks in women, a lot of which are due to changes in the cervical vertebrae, and fractures, rapidly increase, so that at between 60 and 70 years of age, 60% of women will fall, and one in four of those will fracture the neck of the femur. Can the Panel cast any light at all on some improvement of this very grave situation?

Professor C. E. Dent: I am afraid that I cannot. I accept that it is an important point. But one cannot say that a person has osteoporosis because she has fractured her forearm. It may be that women get these fractures more than men because they get drop attacks so much more easily. How can one tell that a fracture is pathological in a lady, when so many do have these drop attacks?

Dr J. M. Aitken: With the sort of study which is taking place in Glasgow, under the surveillance of Dr Hart and Dr Lindsay, then hopefully, in the course of the next 10 to 20 years, we shall be able to show that those patients who were estrogen treated—and we have made measurements before they have actually fallen down—have a lower incidence of fracture as a result of falling about. Until a sufficiently long-term prospective study has been done, one really cannot be certain about anything.

Mr. J. W. W. Studd (Gynaecologist, London): I find the work of Professor Nordin totally convincing, that estrogen therapy prevents, or significantly retards mobilization of bone in the metacarpals. My problem is that I am just a gynaecologist with just a passing knowledge of bones, and one of the world's authorities on osteoporosis, Professor Dent, finds Nordin's work less convincing than I do. What have I missed?

Professor C. E. Dent: The Leeds group have not published a single clinical paper on the treatment of osteoporosis and that is the only ultimate test. I try to be as scientific as I can, but I know that science is only the quick way of directing clinical research. Science gives one splendid ideas of what to do next, but one must end up with clinical proof, like in the Henneman and Wallach study* whether they fracture, whether they lose height, or get less pain, and so on, which can only be done in the long term. There has not been a single clinical paper from Leeds. What is particularly unconvincing is that they keep on changing their theories from high urinary calcium during the night to vitamin D deficiency, and so on. If it is due to vitamin D, why not try to cure them and put out a paper saying that they have got better by taking vitamin D? The other point is that in some of these scientific studies they show increases in calcification of the bone that are very large. In some of the ladies on their graphs they get a 15% increase in 3 or 4 years. I cannot believe that bone can be made at that speed in old age, because the known turnover rate is much less than that. It looks to me as though it is not normal bone formation but some other sort of calcification; some of Nordin's figures are impossible to accept as true bone formation, which goes back to the point about the matrix and the collagen, and whether by increasing calcium content we are making thing any better—in other words, whether the bones are any stronger at all.

Dr J. M. Aitken: Two points. First, any method that one uses, in our case gamma ray photon absorbteometry, has an error attached to it. For instance, some of our high results may well be errors. The trend which we found is probably reasonable, but amounted to something like an increase in bone mineral content of about 2% per year for a limited period of time. We have analysed the data in a different way by looking at how much bone our patients gained in the first year, second year, third year and fourth year of estrogen therapy, and there is no doubt at all that the 3-year post-oophorectomy group gained most bone mineral in the first year after treatment. In the second year it was rather less, and in the third year less still. In the fourth year they are plateauing. So in our opinion it is just a short burst of activity. Secondly, as far as Professor Nordin's figures are concerned, the biggest problem with his studies is that he does not really have any controls. I know that he is trying to persuade Dr Stanbury from Manchester to offer him some of his patients to act as controls; Dr Stanbury's patients are all 'controls', because he does not believe in treating any of them. But this is his present problem—he has no controls.

Dr L. Goldman (Medical Correspondent, London): Dr Aitken treated groups of patients for 3 years and 6 years with hormones. Can he be certain that those patients took their treatment for that time? I know of at least twenty published studies that

* Henneman, P. H. and Wallach, S. (1957). *Arch. Intern. Med.*, **100**, 715

say that after 3 months of medication between 30% and 50% of people default from taking their medication, and that has even been shown with tuberculosis patients. How can we be certain that his patients actually took their therapy every day? Secondly, I was interested to hear that Dr Aitken used mestranol, and would like to know why, partly because the Committee on the Safety of Drugs showed some years ago that mestranol seemed to be associated with a higher incidence of thromboembolism than ethinyl estradiol.

Dr J. M. Aitken: To answer the second question first, we used mestranol because that was the drug supplied to us by the drug firm who financed some of our studies, although they have no financial interest whatever as they have no products on the market for treating menopausal women. As far as thromboembolism is concerned, admittedly the number of patients we have studied is small. We have 300 to 400 patients now. The incidence of thromboembolic episodes comparing the mestranol-treated women with the placebo-treated women is no different, which conflicts with some of the retrospective studies that have been done by other people. We must remember that the information from the Committee on Safety of Drugs was initially obtained retrospectively.

As to whether we knew if the patients were taking their treatment, one of the last slides showed that a considerable number of patients were not taking the dose of estrogen that we suggested that they take. We assessed the dose taken by a card system whereby when the patient first came to the clinic she was given two bottles of tablets and a card, and she was instructed to return the card to the pharmacy when she was getting near the end of her tablets. The pharmacy then sent her another couple of bottles of tablets. That went on over the period of observation going on for something like 5 or 6 years. In this way we were able to assess—roughly speaking—how many tablets the patients were taking. We certainly cannot say whether the patients were taking the drugs regularly every day. Perhaps as I suggested in one of the slides they were taking it intermittently, and maybe those patients who were only taking between 10 and 20 micrograms/day were faring better than the other patients because they were taking it intermittently. I doubt very much that they took half a mestranol tablet every day.

Section F

SKIN

Chairman: I. L. CRAFT

20

The effect of estrogens on the skin

P. Shahrad and R. Marks

The menopause is not only the time of decreasing ovarian function it is also the time for the winding down of all biological functions. It is in the same period of life that the cumulative effects of chronic injury from solar irradiation become clinically evident. For these reasons it is totally unjustifiable to uncritically assume that a particular lesion or disorder of the skin in a menopausal woman is due to estrogen deficiency. In this paper it is planned to briefly review the main actions of estrogen on the various tissue components of the skin and distinguish them where appropriate from the effects of ageing and injury from the sun's ultraviolet light. In addition it is intended to present some preliminary results from our own studies of the effects of estrogens on the skin.

Skin as a target organ for estrogenic action

The skin is an important bearer of secondary sex characters and is a major target organ for estrogenic action. The distribution of body hair and subcutaneous fat and the characteristic feel of a woman's skin are all determined by a balance between estrogenic and androgenic action. Stumpf and his colleagues[1] found that epidermal nuclei, the nuclei of the dermal fibroblasts and the nuclei of the adnexal structures all incorporated tritiated estradiol to an appreciable degree when this was administered by injection to mice some hours previously. They used an autoradiographic technique and found that the accumulation of autoradiographic grains was more marked over basal epidermal nuclei but varied according to body site. Perineal skin seemed particularly active in taking up the estradiol. That skin actively metabolizes estrogens was shown by members of Hsia's group in Miami[2] who found that human infant foreskin had the ability to interconvert estradiol and estrone. They found that foreskin converted 47% of [^{14}C] estradiol to estrone in 5 hours while abdominal skin only converted 10% and vaginal mucosa changed even less. It has also been shown that hair follicle epithelium actively takes up estrogens and interconverts them to a degree dependent on the stage of the hair cycle[3].

Thus, the skin takes up and metabolizes estrogens but although there has been considerable work on estrogenic receptors in the uterus there has been little work to identify the specific protein receptor material for estrogen in the skin.

The effect of estrogens on the dermis

The fact that estrogenic substances profoundly influence dermal connective tissue becomes evident from the classical work of Zuckerman and his associates and others in this field[4, 5]. The perineal and neighbouring skin of some primates becomes swollen and discoloured during estrus and these same changes can be induced by the injection of physiological doses of estrogenic materials. Many experiments have since been performed demonstrating that the swelling is due to an increase in water and mucopolysaccharide content of the dermal connective tissue[6, 7]. More recently, Nina Grossman[8, 9] has demonstrated in mouse skin that there is a specific effect of estrogens on dermal acid mucopolysaccharides—particularly hyaluronic acid. This material may increase 7 or 8 times in concentration after administration of estrogenic compounds. This worker also found that there was a changed ratio of hyaluronic acid to its associated protein after estrogen treatment and this together with an increase in low molecular weight hyaluronic acid fractions was taken to indicate increased metabolism of hyaluronic acid. A positive correlation was also found between the amount of hyaluronic acid present and the dermal water content. This apparently specific effect of estrogens on dermal acid mucopolysaccharides may well have a therapeutic application for some conditions characterized by dermal atrophy.

Aside from promoting synthetic activity in the dermis there appears to be a slowing down of collagen degradation after injection of estrogens. Katz and Kappas[10] found a decreased urinary excretion of hydroxyproline peptides after injection of estrogens. In addition, Skosey and Damgaard[11] showed that the half life of collagen was increased by a factor of more than two. Fundamental alterations also take place in the synthesis and degree of polymerization and crosslinking of collagen fibres. Henneman[12] has shown that although there is a decrease in total skin mass and in soluble collagen in estrogen-treated animals, there is actually an increase in the amount of insoluble collagen present. This rather suggests that estrogens in some way increase the polymerization status of the collagen peptide chains and the amount of cross linking between the collagen chains.

The increase in hyaluronic acid content (and consequently water content), the decrease in collagen degradation, and the increase in the amount of insoluble collagen present add up to a fundamental effect of estrogens on dermal connective tissue. One word of general caution should be sounded at this particular point. Estrogenic action differs according to the species of animal considered, the particular skin site under consideration and as to whether physiological or pharmacological doses are administered. The effect of estrogen administration will also depend on the degree of estrogenic receptor saturation at that particular time.

Table 20.1 Radiological dermal thickness after estriol succinate administration

Patient	*Dermal thickness (mm)*		
	Initially	*1 month*	*3 months*
1	0·79	0·89	0·74
2	0·75	0·85	0·80
3	0·77	0·83	–
4	0·78	0·90	0·91
5	0·80	0·88	–
Mean	0·78	0·87	0·82
± S.D.	0·02	0·03	0·08

The skin of menopausal patients is reputedly improved in texture and appearance following estrogen therapy. Certainly in our experience the skin does seem to increase in thickness radiologically. We are at present involved in a study in which women about to undergo oophorectomy in the course of operative treatment for prolapse are given estriol succinate 2 mg twice daily. As part of this study dermal thickness measurements have been made radiologically using our modification of a radiological method first devised by Black[13, 14]. This technique is extremely useful as it is accurate, reproducible, cheap and non-invasive. Thus far we have examined five women in this study and have results for dermal thickness at 1 and 3 months. Essentially there has been a significant increase in dermal thickness after 1 month and smaller and non-significant increase after 3 months (Table 20.1).

It must be said that the administration of these compounds although causing some increase in dermal thickness is most unlikely to fundamentally alter the facial appearance of any woman. Most of the wrinkling that one sees is due to the ravages of the sun in the shape of a particular and characteristic degenerative condition of the upper dermis termed elastotic degeneration[15]. It is termed 'elastotic' because the curious homogenized and faintly basophilic connective tissue that patchily replaces the papillary and upper dermis takes on the staining properties of elastic tissue. There is in addition a gradual diminution of dermal substance and loss of dermal resilience during old age which is partially due to loss of mucopolysaccharide and partially due to an increase in the amount of cross linkage present in the collagen. It is most unlikely that administration of estrogens can do more than slightly increase the amount of water and mucopolysaccharide present and it is by no means certain that dermal connective tissue retains the same response to estrogens in old age.

The effect of estrogens on the epidermis

The literature on this subject is a veritable quagmire and is full of contention. The epidermis tends to become thinner with increasing age—in both sexes In addition it has been shown by Baker and Blair[16] that the rate of epidermal cell proliferation decreases in old age.

It should not be assumed therefore that decreased epidermal thickness or decreased mitotic rate is due to the estrogen withdrawal of menopause. Earlier studies such as those of Hooker and Pfeffer[17]and Burrows[18] demonstrated epidermal thinning after 1–2 months treatment of small mammals with estrogens. However, Bullough[19] noted epidermal thickening at first and only later epidermal thinning; Ebling[20] noted a similar sequence of events. More recently detailed studies by Punnonen[21] have been published. This worker investigated the effect of castration and of estriol succinate or estradiol valerate oral therapy in 167 patients. He studied the epidermal thickness planimetrically and the autoradiographic labelling indices of the epidermis after the intracutaneous injection of tritiated thymidine. He found that the epidermis became thinner the longer the time from castration—7 months after castration the epidermis was significantly thinner in 55% when compared to the preoperative biopsies. After both forms of estrogen therapy the epidermis thickened and the labelling indices increased. To quote his final paragraph: 'In not a single case did estrogen therapy exert an atrophying effect on the epidermis and no inhibition of mitoses was observed. It seems evident from this study that peroral estrogen therapy is capable of causing epidermal proliferation. Atrophy of the epidermis can thus be prevented in this way and atrophy that has already originated can be eliminated. . . .' The therapeutic implication contained in the last paragraph should be accepted cautiously in the light of results published by workers from other centres. Our own preliminary findings employing adult male skin *in vitro* and using pharmacological doses of estrone suggest that estrogens can depress growth and metabolism. The method that we employ is based on that described by Marks, Fukui and Halprin[22] and involves the removal of thin sheets of skin consisting predominantly of epidermis with a Castroviejo Keratotome. Normal healthy adult male volunteers have been used and the skin removed has been divided into rectangular fragments and then incubated for 24 hour periods in nutrient medium containing estrone. During the last 4 hours of incubation either tritiated thymidine or tritiated proline was added to the medium. The incorporation of the precursor materials was determined by 'counting' extracts of the incubated explants in a scintillation counter. The activity of each explant is expressed in terms of the area of the explant from which it was derived and per hour of incubation. The results that we have obtained so far can be seen in Table 20.2.

Table 20.2 Incorporation of tritiated materials by human skin explants in the presence of large doses of estrone

Tritiated precursor used	*Dose of estrone* (μg/ml)	*Number of expts*	*Counts** ± S.D.	% *change*
Thymidine	0	7	10·1 ± 3·5	—
Thymidine	20	5	6·1 ± 2·8	65·6
Thymidine	50	6	6·0 ± 4·4	59·2
Thymidine	100	6	3·8 ± 4·0	39·7
Proline	0	2	366·3	—
Proline	20	2	296·8	81·0

* Mean corrected counts per minute per sq. mm of skin per hour

Even though the concentrations employed were enormous in physiological terms, the results do indicate that the estrone had a depressant effect on thymidine incorporation (reflecting epidermal DNA synthesis) and proline incorporation (reflecting epidermal protein synthesis).

We are also involved in the investigation of the effect of oral estrogen therapy on epidermal growth in the same group of patients about to undergo oophorectomy discussed previously in relation to dermal thickness. An autoradiographic technique is used on tissues removed 1 hour after the intracutaneous injection of tritiated thymidine. At the time of writing we have only the results in three patients before and after 3 months of estriol succinate treatment and can only hesitantly say that we cannot confirm the trend noted by Punnonen[21].

It is perhaps worth noting that some other epithelial tissues show depression of mitotic activity in the presence of estrogens. An example is the reversible mitotic delay in Hela cells *in vitro* evoked by estradiol described by Rao[23].

It seems that the action of estrogens on epidermis is not all straightforward and clearly much more work is necessary in this area before any firm conclusions can be reached.

Estrogens and pigmentation

Estrogens have an undeniable and profound series of effects on skin pigmentation. Snell and Bischitz found that in castrated guinea pigs the administration of estrogens caused melanocytes to increase in numbers and to become larger and more active[24]. Similar changes were noted by the same workers in human abdominal skin during pregnancy[25] though whether these changes were entirely the result of increased levels of circulating estrogens during pregnancy or enhanced melanocyte stimulating hormone levels from the pituitary is unknown. Clinically, the histological changes described by Snell and Bischitz are mirrored by the slight overall increase in skin pigmentation, the development of 'the mask of pregnancy' or 'Melasma' and the darkening of the infra-umbilical skin in the midline (linea nigra). The contraceptive pill may also cause melasma[26].

Effect of estrogens on sweat glands, hair follicles and sebaceous glands

Sweat glands

The rate of sweating from eccrine sweat glands is greater per unit stimulus for men than for women though whether estrogens are responsible or not cannot be said with certainty. Apocrine glands are mainly found in the axillae and in the pubic region though they are also occasionally found on the scalp and even the face. They are larger than eccrine glands and empty their viscid secretion into hair follicles. It is generally believed that it is the bacterial decomposition of apocrine secretion that is responsible for body odour. It is also thought that the apocrines have a sexual function and that their activity is cyclical. There is some evidence that administration of sex steroids affects apocrine gland function in animals but none in man. Wales and Ebling[27], found for example, that in rabbit some types of apocrine gland are smaller and less active in estradiol treated than in testosterone treated animals.

Sebaceous glands

In general terms androgens stimulate and estrogens depress sebaceous glands. Women have a lesser rate of sebum secretion than men. At one time there was a vogue for the treatment of acne patients with estrogens but the side effects made this unpopular and at the present time pharmaceutical houses are looking for effective anti-androgens instead. In 1973, Ebling[28] noted that in the castrated rat implanted with testosterone both estrogen and cyproterone acetate decreased sebum secretion but interestingly when both were given together they had an additive effect. On the basis of these findings it was suggested that the two compounds had different points of action. Ebling believed that the increased sebum secretion seen after androgen administration was due to increased sebaceous cell production and increased lipid secretion by each cell whereas estrogen may merely antagonize one of these actions. Estrogens have also been found to reduce the uptake of testosterone by sebaceous gland analogues in rats and mice and to inhibit the conversion of testosterone to dehydrotestosterone in the glands[29]. Some estrogens produce epidermal thickening and sebaceous gland hypertrophy in the guinea pig nipple[30] showing that the target organ as well as the stimulus must be considered before predicting a particular tissue response.

Hair

Most secondary sexual hair is under androgenic control. Thus change from a vellus hair to a terminal hair can be induced by intracutaneous injection of testosterone in most body sites. Administration of estrogens tends to cause depression of hair growth. However, there is evidence that estrogens are actively taken up and metabolized by the hair follicle and presumably therefore have a role to play in the physiology of hair growth.

Conclusion

Clearly estrogens have profound actions on the skin whose components actively bind and metabolize these hormones. We are at the beginning of some understanding of their mode of action and in the future we may be able to utilize their actions in the treatment of patients with a variety of skin disorders.

References

1. Stumpf, W. E., Madhabananda, S., and Joshi, S. G. (1974). Oestrogen target cells in the skin. *Experentia*, **30,** 196
2. Frost, P., Weinstein, G. D. and Hsia, S. L. (1966). Metabolism of oestradiol and oestrone in human skin. *J. Invest. Dermatol.*, **46,** 584
3. Rampini, E., Davis, B. P., Moretti, G. and Hsia, S. L. (1971). Cyclic changes in the metabolism of oestradiol by rat skin during the hair cycle. *J. Invest. Dermatol.*, **57,** 75
4. Zuckerman, S. J. (1938). Oestrogen threshold of the uterus of the rhesus monkey. *Endocrinology*, **22,** 142
5. Ogston, A. G., Philpott, J. St. L. and Zuckerman, S. S. (1939). Observations related to swelling of sexual skin in rhesus monkeys. *J. of Endocrinology*, **1,** 231
6. Durran-Reynolds, F., Bunting, H. and Wagenen, G. Van. (1950). Studies on the sex skin of *Macaca mulatta. Ann. New York Acad. Sci.*, **52,** 1006
7. Rienits, K. G. (1960). The acid mucopolysaccharides of the sexual skin of apes and monkeys. *Biochem. J.*, **74,** 27
8. Grosman, N., Hvidberg, E. and Schou, J. (1971). The effect of oestrogenic treatment on the acid mucopolysaccharide pattern in skin of mice. *Acta Pharmacol. Toxicol.*, **30,** 458
9. Grosman, N. (1973). Studies on the hyaluronic acid protein complex, the molecular size of hyaluronic acid and the exchangeability of chloride in skin of mice before and after oestrogen treatment. *Acta Pharmacol. Toxicol.*, **33,** 201
10. Katz, F. H. and Kappas, A. (1968). Influence of estradiol benzoate and oestriol on urinary excretion of hydroxproline in man. *J. Lab. Clin. Med.*, **71,** 65
11. Skosey, J. L. and Damgaard, E. (1973). Effect of oestradiol benzoate on degradation of insoluble collagen of rat skin. *Endocrinology*, **93,** 311
12. Henneman, D. H. (1971). Effect of oestradiol-17 on collagen biosynthesis, degradation and reutilization *in vivo. Biochem. Biophys. Res. Commun.*, **44,** 326
13. Black, M. M. (1969). A modified radiographic method for measuring skin thickness. *Br. J. Dermatol.*, **81,** 661
14. Marks, R. Dykes, P. and Roberts, E. (1975). The measurement of corticosteroid induced dermal atrophy by a radiological method. *Arch. Dermatol. Res.*, **253,** 93
15. Lever, W. F. (1967). Histopathology of the Skin. Fourth Edition. (Philadephia: J. B. Lippincott Company).
16. Baker, H. and Blair, C. P. (1967). Cell replacement in the human stratum corneum in old age. *Br. J. Dermatol.*, **80,** 367
17. Hooker, C. W. and Pfeffer, C. A. (1943). Effect of sex hormones on body growth, skin, hair and sebaceous glands in rats. *Endocrinology*, **32,** 69
18. Burrows, H. (1945). In: *Biological Actions of Sex Hormones*. p. 239. (Cambridge: Cambridge University Press)
19. Bullough, H. F. (1947). Epidermal thickness following oestrone injection in the mouse. *Nature (London)*, **159,** 101
20. Ebling, F. J. (1953). Some effects of oestrogen on epidermis. *J. Endocrinol.*, **9,** XXX
21. Punnonen, R. (1972). Effect of castration and peroral oestrogen therapy on the skin. *Acta Obstet. Gynaecol. Scand. Suppl.* 21
22. Marks, R. Fukui, K. and Halprin, K. (1971). The application of an *in vitro* technique to the study of epidermal replication and metabolism. *Br. J. Dermatol.*, **84,** 453
23. Rao, P. N. (1969). Oestradiol induced mitotic delay in Hela cells: reversal by calcium chloride and putrescine. *Exp. Cell Res.*, **57,** 230

24. Bischitz, P. G. and Snell, R. S. (1960). A study of the effect of ovariectomy, oestrogen and progesterone on the melanocytes and melanin in the skins of female guinea pigs. *J. Endocrinol.*, **20,** 312
25. Snell, R. S. and Bischitz, P. G. (1963). The melanocytes and melanin in human abdominal wall skin, a survey made a different ages in both sexes and during pregnancy. *J. Anat. (London)*, **97,** 361
26. Resnik, S. (1967). Melasma induced by oral contraceptive drugs. *J. Am. Med. Ass.*, **199,** 601
27. Wales, N. A. M. and Ebling, F. J. (1971). The control of the apocrine glands of the rabbit by steroid hormones. *J. Endocrinol.*, **51,** 763
28. Ebling, F. J. (1973). The effects of cyproterone acetate and oestradiol upon testosterone stimulated sebaceous activity in the rat. *Acta Endocrinologica*, **72,** 361
29. Sansone-Bazzano, G., Reisner, R. M. and Bassano G. (1972). A possible mechanism of action of oestrogen at the cellular level in a model sebaceous gland. *J. Invest Dermatol.*, **59,** 299
30. Maggiora, A. Reiffers, J., Bujard, E. and Jadassohn, W. (1968). The action of oestrogens on the sebaceous glands of the guinea pigs nipple. *Experentia*, **24,** 1262

21

Effect of castration and peroral estradiol valerate and estriol succinate therapy on the epidermis

L. Rauramo

The effect of estrogens on the skin has been studied in numerous animal experiments. The results have been extremely diversified. In general, the studies have shown increased mitotic activity in the epidermis, even though some scientists have also established obstruction of mitosis. The effect of local estrogen therapy on the human skin has also been studied and has been found to have a generally stimulating effect on the ageing skin[1]. Today, peroral estrogen therapy has become important to an increasing extent in the treatment of post-climacteric women. Nevertheless there exist very few publications about the effects of this type of estrogen therapy on the skin besides a few studies published during the last few years[2–5].

Material and methods

The effect of estradiol valerate therapy on the thickness of the epidermis was studied in 52 women and the effect of peroral estriol succinate in 61 patients, all of whom had been castrated 1 month before the institution of therapy. These patients were given 2 mg estradiol valerate (Progynova) or 2 mg estriol succinate (Synapause) daily. The mean age of the patients was 42 years and 49 years respectively, the youngest being 36 years and the oldest 64 years. Incorporation of epidermal [^{3}H]thymidine was studied in 15 women in both groups.

54 patients whose mean age was 47 years acted as a control group, the youngest being 36 and the oldest 58. The thickness of the epidermis was

studied in 47 cases, and epidermal [^{3}H]thymidine incorporation in 14 cases. All these patients had continued menstruating until surgery was performed. The patients generally developed climacteric symptoms post-operatively and the medication for all the patients in this group was 30 mg of oxazepam daily. This drug is a benzodiazepine derivative and has no hormonal effect. Oxazepam therapy was started 1 month after castration.

Skin biopsies were taken 1, 4 and 7 months post-operatively, that is, at the institution of therapy and after 3 and 6 months of estrogen or oxazepam therapy. The biopsies were taken from the sides of the thigh, 15 cm above the lateral femoral epicondyle. New biopsies were always taken about 10 mm from the previous site. The local anaesthetic used was 3 ml of 1% lignocaine hydrochloride. The skin biopsy specimens were fixed immediately in 10% neutral formalin for 24 hours. Histological sections (7 μm thick) perpendicular to the surface were prepared and stained with Harris's haematoxylin–eosin.

Planimetry was employed for the evaluation of the epidermal thickness. The histological specimen was projected at a magnification of 80× and boundaries of the epidermis along the upper surface of the stratum granulosum were carefully plotted on paper. The stratum corneum was therefore

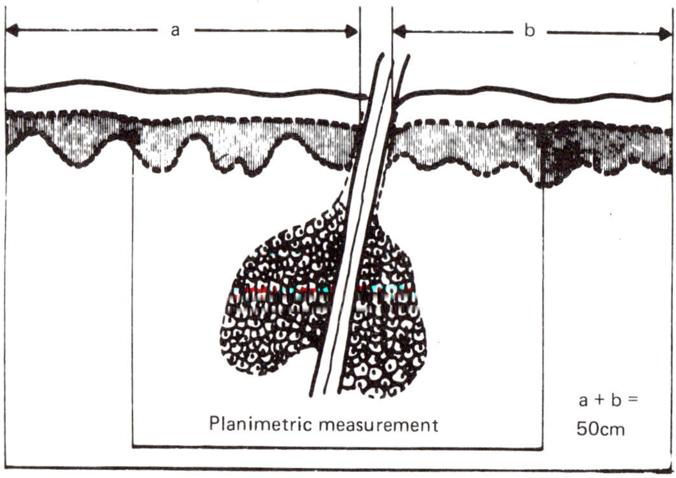

Figure 21.1 Evaluation of epidermal thickness (see text)

not included. The resulting upper surface length was measured from each plotted section by a map tracer (length of upper surface 50 cm in the projection field); all the values obtained were thus mutually comparable. The surface areas were measured with an Aristo planimeter. Five sections were measured at five to six 7 μm intervals to represent each skin specimen (Figure 21.1).

For the study of [³H]thymidine incorporation, the biopsy specimens were taken post-operatively at the intervals mentioned above. The specimens were in fact always taken at the same time of the day (between 14.00 and 16.00 hours). Tritiated thymidine (TRK 61, specific activity > 10 Ci/mM, Amersham) was used for the study. 5 μCi diluted in 0·2 ml of physiological saline were injected subepidermally. The biopsy specimens were taken after an incorporation period of 60 minutes. The anaesthetic used was again 1% lignocaine hydrochloride. The samples were fixed immediately in 10% neutral formalin for 24 hours and 7 μm histological sections were prepared. The slides were coated with Kodak NTB-3 liquid emulsion, exposed for 14 days, and then developed and stained with Harris's haematoxylin–eosin.

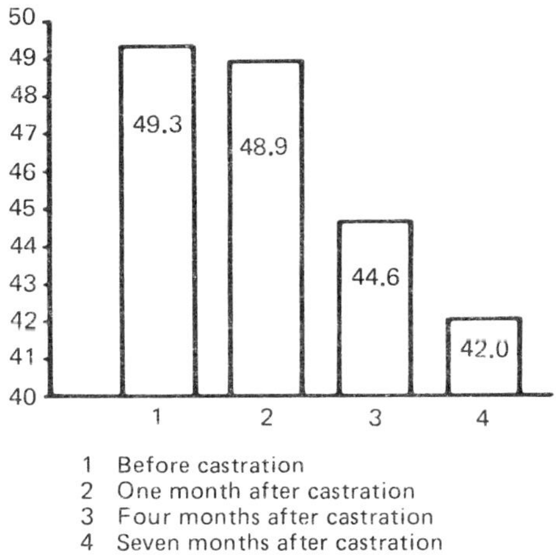

Figure 21.2 Effects of castration on epidermal thickness. Planimetric measurements

Results

In the control group the thickness of the epidermis one month after castration was significantly bigger ($p < 0{\cdot}01$) than 4 months and also 6 months after castration ($p < 0{\cdot}001$). The results are shown graphically in Figure 21.2.

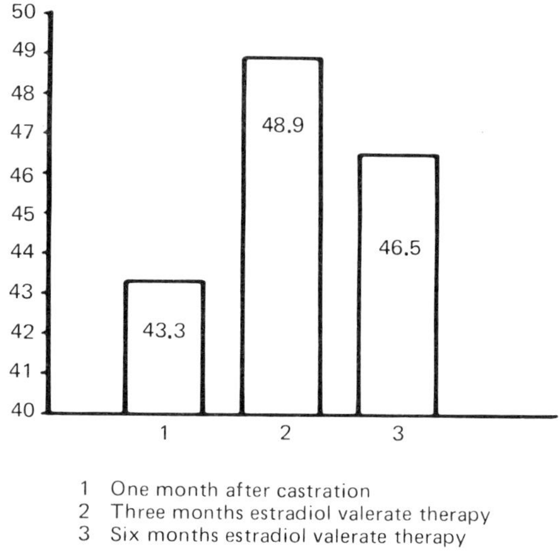

Figure 21.3 Effect of estradiol valerate on epidermal thickness, Planimetric measurements

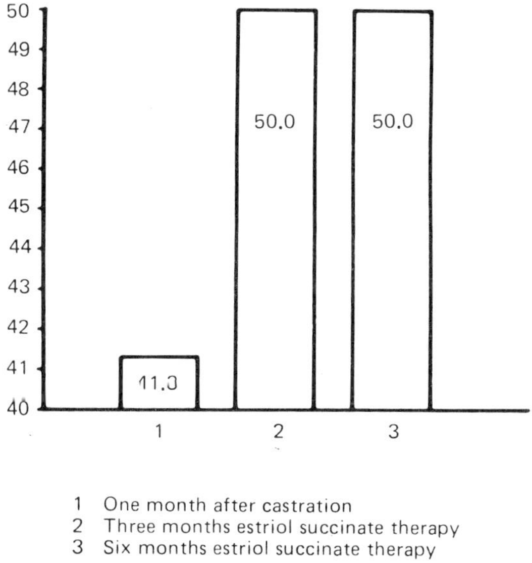

Figure 21.4 Effect of estradiol succinate on epidermal thickness. Planimetric measurements

After both estradiol valerate and estriol succinate therapy the thickness of epidermis was significantly bigger both after 3 months of therapy ($p < 0{\cdot}001$) and 6 months of therapy ($p < 0{\cdot}01$). Between the samples taken after 3 months of therapy or 6 months of therapy no significant differences were found. The results are shown in Figures 21.3 and 21.4.

Incorporation of epidermal [^{3}H]thymidine

In the control group the differences between the labelling indices 1 month after castration and 4 and 7 months after castration were not statistically significant (Figure 21.5).

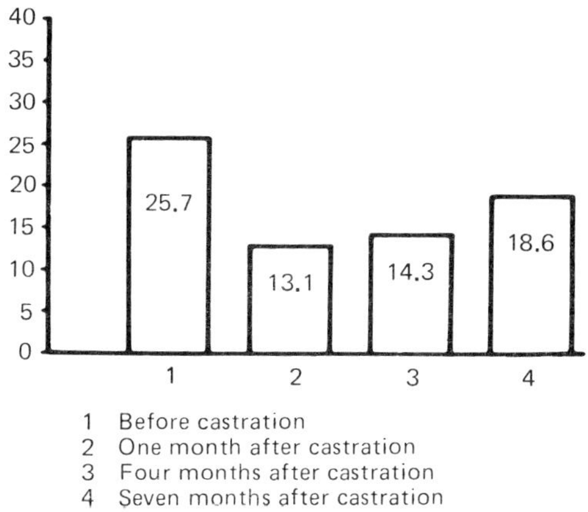

Figure 21.5 Effect of castration on epidermal [^{3}H]thymidine labelling index

The labelling indices were significantly higher ($p < 0{\cdot}001$) both after 3 and 6 months of estradiol valerate therapy than before the institution of therapy. There could not be seen any significant differences between a 3-month period of therapy and a 6-month period of therapy ($p > 0{\cdot}05$) (Figure 21.6).

The labelling indices after 3 and 6 months of estriol succinate therapy were also significantly higher ($p < 0{\cdot}01$) than before the institution of therapy (Figure 21.7).

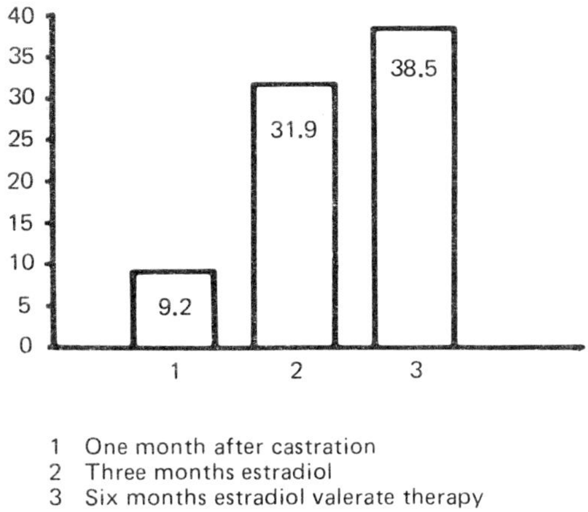

Figure 21.6 Effect of estradiol valerate on epidermal [^{3}H]thymidine labelling index

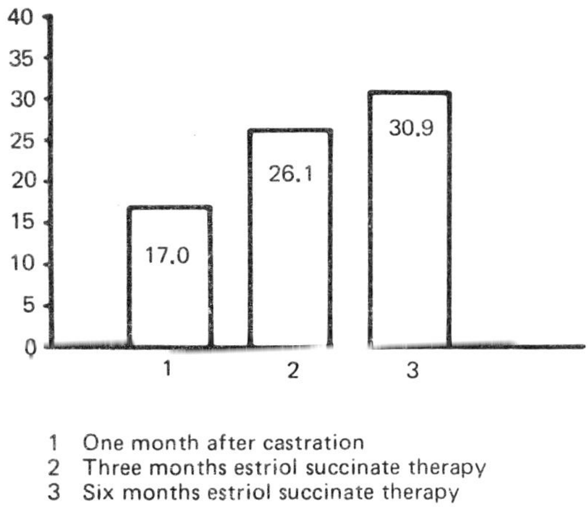

Figure 21.7 Effect of estriol succinate on epidermal [^{3}H]thymidine labelling index

Discussion

The epidermal specimens were compared planimetrically. The measurements thus obtained are comparable, because the measured distances of the upper surface of the stratum granulosum are equal in length. Biopsies were taken from sites approximately 10 mm apart. The thickness of the epidermis does not vary very much over this distance, but it is long enough not to affect specimens taken later. Tritiated thymidine was injected locally at the biopsy site. Christophers and Petzold[6] showed that the technique employed here was equal to the intravenous technique. It was shown by Bullough[7] that mitotic activity increases up to a distance of about 1 mm from the puncture edge. The histological specimens were, of course, taken as perpendicularly to the skin surface as possible, but an oblique section could not be avoided in every case. The average error is small, however, and at any rate by no means systematic.

After castration it could be established that the epidermis became considerably thinner during the next half-year period and that the number of mitosis remained relatively low. Estradiol valerate or estriol succinate therapy of both 3 months and 6 months duration caused the epidermis to thicken clearly and also the number of mitoses to increase considerably.

Also, other changes in the epidermis took place during estrogen therapy. These changes, for instance, in the elasticity and blood circulation, have been described in more detail by Aertgeerts[5]. As with Aertgeerts, these changes were not statistically significant, although it seemed to us that they did in fact occur. Of special interest is the question of the relation of hair and pubic hair to estrogen therapy. Some patients told us spontaneously that their already grey hair had started getting darker at the roots and that there was a clear improvement in the elasticity and loss of pubic hair. According to Aertgeerts a clear improvement of the elasticity of pubic hair took place in his patients during estrogenic therapy as well as some slight improvement in the colour of grey hair and grey pubic hair. Equally a slight improvement in pubic hair loss was noted.

As mentioned above we have not been able to show statistically the effect of estradiol valerate therapy on the hair and pubic hair, but on the other hand there seems to be no reason to doubt the spontaneous information from the patients in regard to the improvement of these details. Thus, it is possible that at least in some patients, estrogen therapy might have a favourable effect both on the hair and pubic hair.

The results show that estradiol valerate and estriol succinate therapy have in many ways a positive effect on the female skin after ovarian activity has ceased. These changes may be well suited to support the skin to

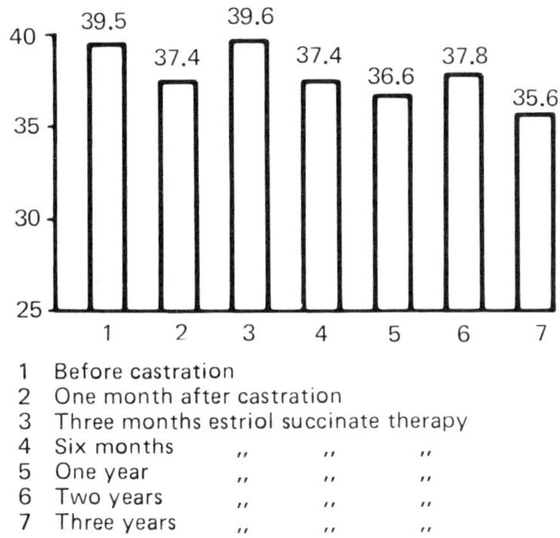

Figure 21.8 Effect of estriol succinate on epidermal thickness. Planimetric measurements

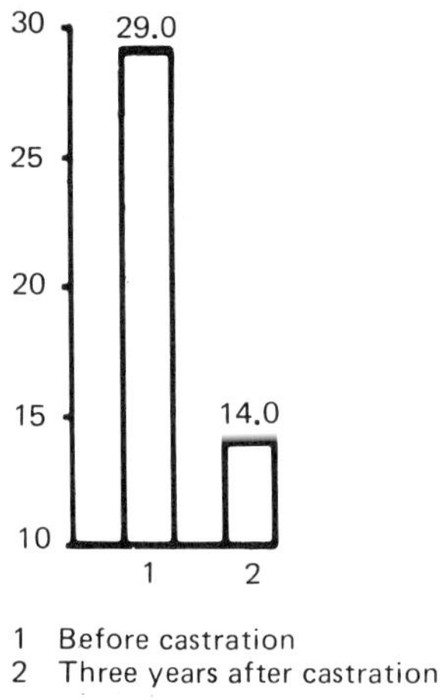

Figure 21.9 Effect of castration on epidermal [^{3}H]thymidine labelling index

endure external irritants, and thus to contribute to the patient's well-being.

We have also studied the long term effect of estriol succinate on the skin over 3 years. At present our material consists of only 18 patients in the estrogen and control groups, so it was not justifiable to draw any definite conclusions before the material had been analysed statistically. Anyhow it can be seen from Figures 21.8–21.10 and that there apparently is still some influence of estrogen therapy left after 3 years.

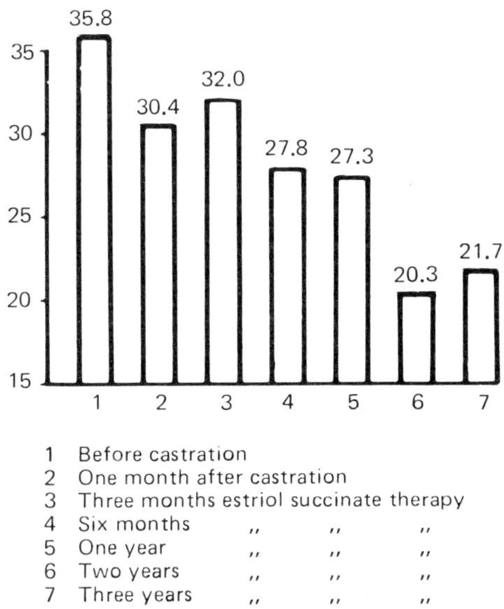

Figure 21.10 Effect of estriol succinate on epidermal $[^3H]$thymidine labelling index

However, when studying the effects of estradiol valerate and estriol succinate on the skin it has been our principal goal to find out whether it would be possible to prevent post-climacteric, degenerative changes more generally. Naturally, it would also have been very interesting to study with biopsy specimens the changes, for instance, in bones, muscles or blood vessels, but it was technically easier to take the test specimens from the skin. In our understanding, with regard to the effects of estrogens on the skin, the results confirm, that the degenerative changes occurring in tissues after the discontinuance of the ovarian activity could, to some extent, be prevented with estrogens for some time.

References

1. Goldzieher, M. A. (1946). The effects of estrogens on the senile skin. *J. Gerontol.*, **1**, 196
2. Rauramo, L. and Punnonen, R. (1969). Wirkung einer oralen Östrogentherapie mit Östriolsuccinat auf die Haut kastrierter Frauen. *Z. Haut. Geschlechtskr.*, **44**, 13, 463
3. Rauramo, L. and Punnone, R. (1971). Über die Wirkung peroraler Oestrogentherapie mit Oestradiolvalerat auf die Haut kastierter Frauen. *Arch. Gynäkol.*, **211**, 202
4. Punnonen, R. (1972). Effect of castration and peroral estrogen therapy on the skin. *Acta Obstet. Gynec. Scand.*, 5 suppl. **21**, 21
5. Aertgeerts, J. Influence d'un traitement oestrogene sur la peau de femmes menopausees ou castrees. *Brux-méd.*, 52 année· no 3, mars 1972
6. Christophers, E. and Petzold, V. (1969). Epidermal cell replacement. *Brit. J. Dermatol.*, **81**, 598
7. Bullough, W. S. (1955). Hormones and mitotic activity. *Vitamins, Hormones*, **13**, 261

22

The correlation of menopausal symptoms with cytohormonal status

H. Gordon

Vaginal cytology is a convenient and simple method of assessing the estrogen status in menopausal women.

The structure of the vaginal epithelium is dependent on the type and concentration of circulating sex hormones. In the absence of hormone stimulation, the vaginal epithelium becomes thin and atrophic, consisting only of a basal layer together with one or more layers of parabasal cells. In the presence of optimal amounts of unopposed estrogen, the epithelium becomes a 'mature' thick, multilayered structure with a well-developed superficial zone. In these two situations, the exfoliated cells reflect the state of the epithelium accurately.

In the former situation, there will be many parabasal cells, in the latter a high percentage of superficial cells with small pyknotic nuclei. The interpretation of the hormonal situation is much more complex if the epithelium has not reached its full maturation potential. This is a common pattern in menopausal women, where the majority of smears are composed mainly of intermediate cells with a few superficial cells and a low percentage of parabasal cells. This smear pattern reflects rather feeble estrogenic effect and possibly some increased androgen activity.

Initial survey

To document the cytohormonal status of post-menopausal women, we first analysed routine smears from women at least 1 year after the cessation

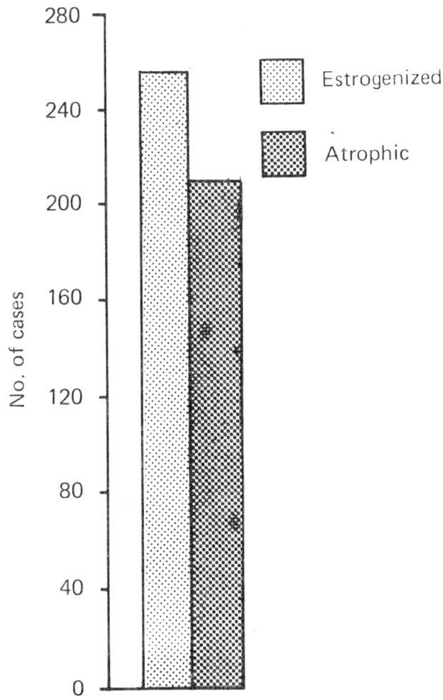

Figure 22.1 Cytological estrogen assessment in the post-menopause—all ages

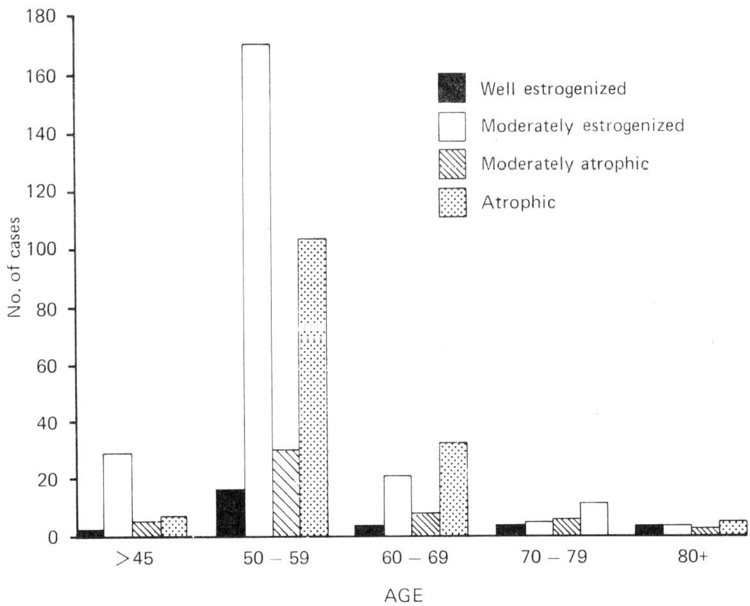

Figure 22.2 Cytological estrogen assessment in the post-menopause according to age

MENOPAUSAL CYTOLOGY SURVEY

Date ______________

FAMILY DOCTOR ______________ Patient No. ______________

PATIENT NAME ______________ Date of Birth ______________

Single ☐ Married ☐ Widowed ☐ Living with partner ☐ Divorced ☐ (Tick appropriate)

Patient's Occupation (previous or present) ______________

(ex) Husband's Occupation " ______________

Family problems YES ☐ NO ☐ Specify ______________

Is she still having intercourse YES ☐ NO ☐

Sex interest: Excellent ☐ Fair ☐ Poor ☐ Undetermined ☐

MENOPAUSAL YES ☐ NO ☐ Recent period irregularities YES ☐ NO ☐

LMP ______________ Comment ______________

PREVIOUS HISTORY: Has the patient had:–

Any breast disease YES ☐ NO ☐ Specify ______________

Bilateral Oopherectomy YES ☐ NO ☐ Date ______________

Hysterectomy YES ☐ NO ☐ Date ______________

Any endocrine disorders YES ☐ NO ☐ Specify ______________

TREATMENT

Oral contraceptives YES ☐ NO ☐ Oestrogens YES ☐ NO ☐ Other Hormones YES ☐ NO ☐

Formulation ______________ Duration ______________

OTHER MEDICATION (Especially Digitalis/Tranquillisers) YES ☐ NO ☐

Specify ______________

History of mental disease YES ☐ NO ☐

Specify ______________

Does the patient look her age ☐ Younger ☐ Older ☐ (Tick one)

BLOOD PRESSURE Systolic ______________ Diastolic ______________

WEIGHT Kg ______________ or Pounds ______________

ANY SYMPTOMS: (Disregard very mild, occasional symptoms)

Symptoms (List)	Severe	Mod	Mild	Duration

If severe, describe:–

____

CYTOLOGY	Atrophic	Slightly oestrogenised	Well oestrogenised
Date			
Date			

COMMENTS ______________

5.E6 106/20

Figure 22.3 Menopausal cytology survey questionnaire

of menstruation. These smears were received as part of the cytology service at Hammersmith, and came from gynaecological out-patients and from medical and surgical in-patients. Patients with gross vaginal inflammation, endocrine abnormality or those patients receiving hormone therapy, were excluded. The ages of the patients varied from 45–82 years, and the duration of amenorrhea from 1–35 years. Overall, more of these patients showed cytological evidence of estrogen effect than showed evidence of atrophy (Figure 22.1).

When the patients were grouped by age (Figure 22.2), it became evident that good estrogen effects persisted into old age in some women, and some young women showed cytological evidence of severe estrogen lack[1]. These findings were in agreement with the results of Meisel's Canadian study[2]. On the basis of these findings, we then proceeded to a prospective study of vaginal cytology in the perimenopausal years.

Material and methods

This study concentrated on normal women from general practices in the West London area, augmented by samples obtained at Well Woman Clinics at Hammersmith and Watford Hospitals. Any woman over 45 years was

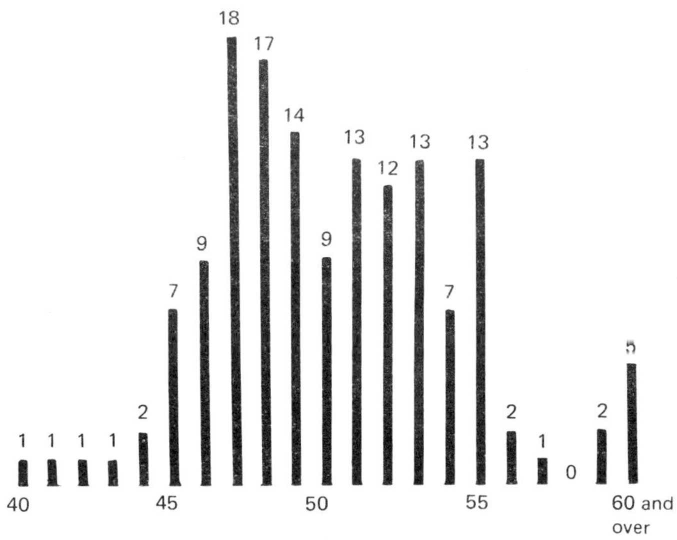

Figure 22.4 Result of smear test according to age in 148 women aged between 40 and 78

admitted to the study, as well as younger menopausal women with one or more years of amenorrhea. Samples were obtained by posterior fornix aspiration or by lateral vaginal wall scrape. By use of a questionnaire (Figure 22.3), we tried to correlate smear patterns with symptomatology and a variety of social, psychiatric and physical features.

Results

These studies have now been in progress for 6 months and to date we have received and analysed the smears of 148 women aged between 40 and 78. Figure 22.4 shows this age distribution, with a heavy concentration on the perimenopausal years. Indeed, nearly half the patients were still menstruating (Table 22.1).

Table 22.1 148 patients

70	menstruating	78	amenorrheic
27	regular menses	35	3 months to 2 years
43	irregular menses	43	longer than 2 years
Age range 44–55 mean 48·8		Age range 40–78 mean 52	

Table 22.2 Atrophic smears PB ≥ 5%

(30 women)		
No symptoms	14	
Hot flushes	10	(severe 4)
Other symptoms	13	(severe 2)
		Depression
		Dyspareunia
33·3%	Hot flushes	

Atrophic smears (defined as a parabasal cell count of 5% or more) were found in 30 women, of whom a third complained of hot flushes. The overall symptomatology is detailed in Table 22.2. Two smears were unsuitable for reporting; the remaining 116 women showed no evidence of atrophy. Their symptomatic complaints were not significantly different from the atrophic group (Table 22.3).

As hot flushes are widely considered to be related to estrogen lack, and other symptoms are harder to assess, it is important to note that the incidence of hot flushes did not differ significantly between the two groups (Table 22.4). When only severe hot flushes were considered, there was a wide variation in cytohormonal status, the symptom occurring in four women with markedly well estrogenized smears (Table 22.5).

If we now consider the 30 women with atrophic smears related to time since menopause (Figure 22.5), 13 women showed evidence of atrophic change within 2 years of the menopause—8 of these were either still menstruating or had been amenorrheic for less than a year.

Table 22.3 No atrophy (116 women)

No symptoms	54	
Hot flushes	49	(severe 19)
Other symptoms	18	(severe 4)
		Depression
42·3%	Hot flushes	

Table 22.4 Flushes related to cytology

	Atrophic 30		*No atrophy 116*	
Flushes	10	(33·3%)	49	(42·2%)
No symptoms	14	(40·7%)	54	(46·7%)
Differences not significant				

Table 22.5 Severe hot flushes (23 women)

		PB 5%	*K1 0–10*	*K1 10+*
Menstruating	6	0	4	2
Amenorrhea to 2 years	8	2	5	1
Amenorrhea over 2 years	9	2	6	1

In summary, we have shown no correlation between symptoms and cytohormonal status. Some women show good estrogen effects lasting well into old age whilst others have evidence of early atrophy.

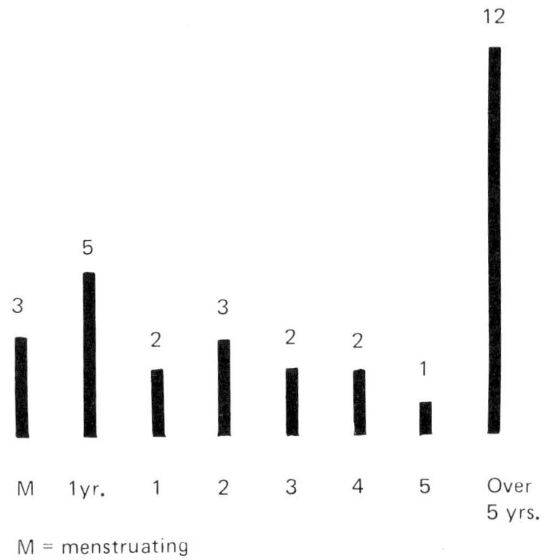

Figure 22.5 Result of 30 women with atrophic smears related to time since menopause

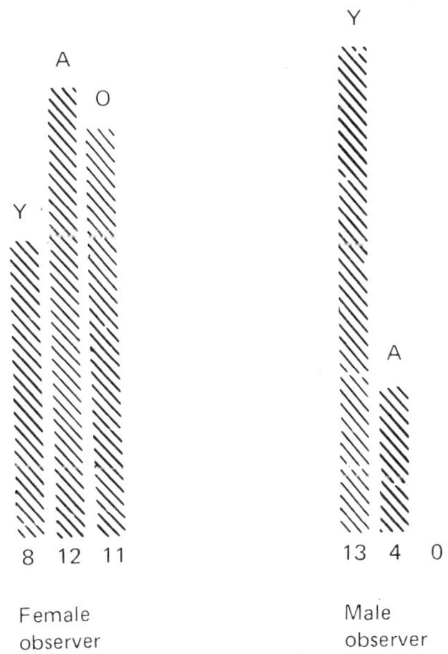

Figure 22.6 Assessment of age by sex of observer

We may suggest that the early atrophic group could be the same group who suffer medical ill effects such as osteoporosis—they may for example compare with the known high risk group of surgically castrated women. We can also speculate on the mode of action of estrogen replacement. In women with well estrogenized smears, does hormone replacement therapy act by placebo effect only or are we wrong in assuming that the vasomotor side effects of the menopause are hormone-dependent?

Other variables such as social class and coital habits may be of interest when more patients enter the study. We asked all doctors if the patients looked their age, older, or younger. It happens that in West London we knew the sex of the observer, and Figure 22.6 suggests an unexpected degree of chivalry in our male GPs, none of whom admitted that their patients looked older than their years.

References

1. Wachtel, E. (1975). Vaginal cytology after the menopause. In *Estrogens in the post-menopause. Front. Hormone Res.*, **3**, 63
2. Meisels, A. (1966). The menopause—a cytohormonal study, *Acta Cytol.*, **11**, 249

23

Cervical colposcopic changes associated with the menopause

A. E. Crompton

During the different epochs of female life the cervix undergoes a cycle of change which affects its size and appearance. These changes involve the stroma, the vasculature and the epithelium.

Colposcopic appearances are determined by the type of epithelium present and the underlying capillary patterns. Epithelial changes are enhanced by the application of dilute acetic acid which whitens and thickens atypical epithelium and produces a characteristic villous change in columnar epithelium. The degree of glycogenation is suggested by the application of aqueous iodine solution and blood vessels are brought into prominence by the interposition of a green filter into the optical system. In the teens the peripheral areas of the cervix are covered by a mature pink well-glycogenated squamous epithelium which is typically sharply demarcated from a circumoral zone of columnar-covered stroma (Figure 23.1). A lowering in the vaginal pH appears to be the first factor which stimulates the adhesion of the villi and the transformation of the columnar covering into a metaplastic squamous epithelium[1] (Figure 23.2). This process of transformation referred to as the dynamic phase of metaplasia by Coppleston[2], may initially progress relatively quickly especially after pregnancy until the only visible evidence of the previous columnar epithelium is the presence of small mucous retention cysts or Nabothian follicles. The early stage of active squamous metaplasia appears to be a vulnerable time when inimical influences may alter the process outlined above leading to the production of dysplastic squamous epithelium and ultimately in some of these patients to the development of cervical carcinoma. The association of this abnormal epithelial development with promiscuity in the teens has led to the implication of various agents in the initiation of cervical epithelial atypia such as spermatozoa[3], viruses[4], and *Chlamydia*[5].

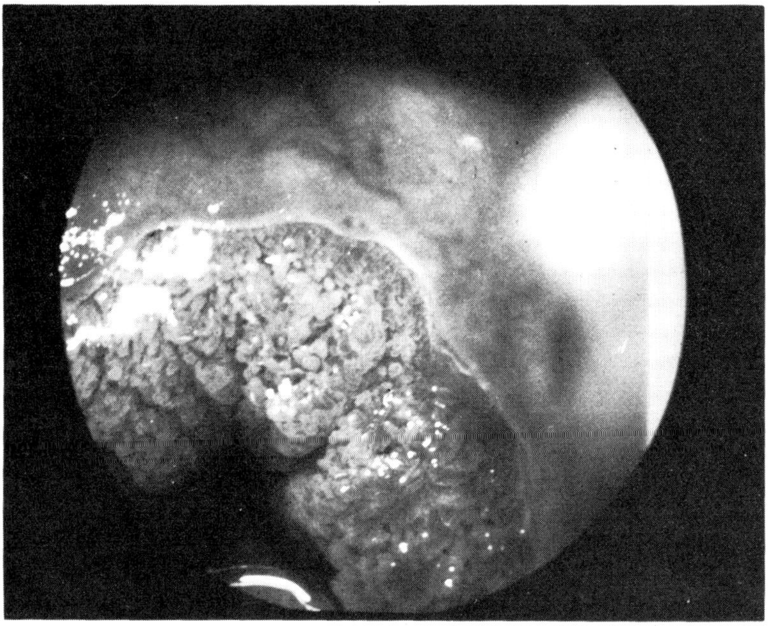

Figure 23.1 Cervix of nulliparous 18-year-old girl treated with 2% acetic acid showing the sharp squamo-columnar junction. (×4).

The transformation zone is therefore the area in which benign squamous metaplasia and many of the squamous epithelial atypia are located but in fixed specimens in the laboratory these areas often appear to lie within the lower endocervical canal. This is in part due to tissue fixation and differential shrinkage[6]. In life the use of a bivalve speculum tends to evert the lower part of the endocervical canal improving visualization.

The original squamo-columnar junction can be seen histologically by the position of the most distal gland underlying the metaplastic squamous epithelium. Colposcopically this area is demarcated by small retention cysts and differences in the colour and underlying vascular patterns of the epithelium. The usual appearances at different ages are shown in Figure 23.3.

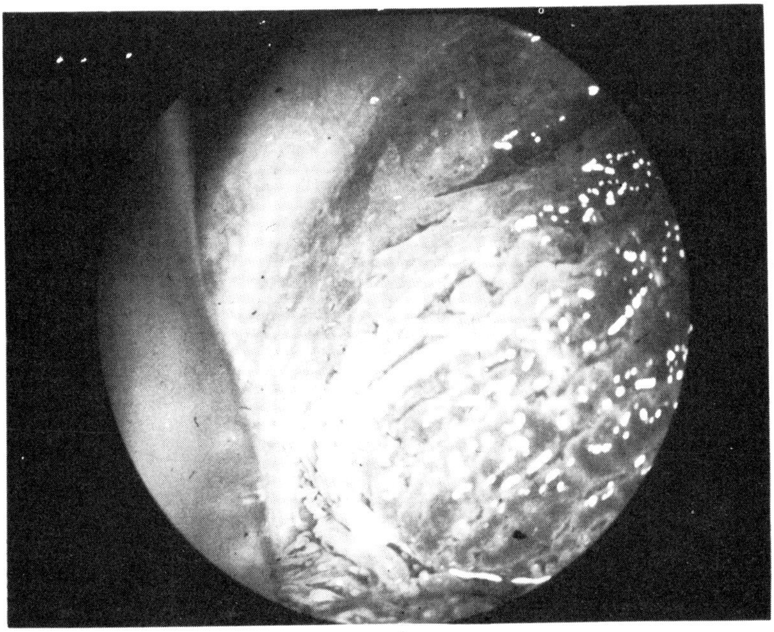

Figure 23.2 Early transformation zone. Ridge formation and metaplastic squamous epithelium can be seen

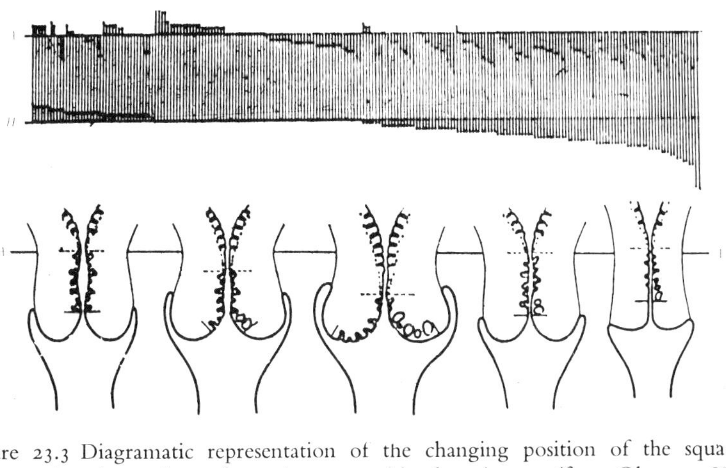

Figure 23.3 Diagramatic representation of the changing position of the squamo-columnar junction and transformation zone with advancing age (from Ober, 1958[9])

In a series of over 1000 colposcopic examinations the types of benign epithelial changes encountered are shown at different decades in Figure 23.4. The original squamous epithelium becomes the predominant visible finding after the menopause and transformation zones become less apparent as they tend to lie within the endocervical canal. Almost 20% of women still present with an ectopy in the forties though the percentage falls to less than 5% after fifty. The squamous epithelium both original and metaplastic becomes

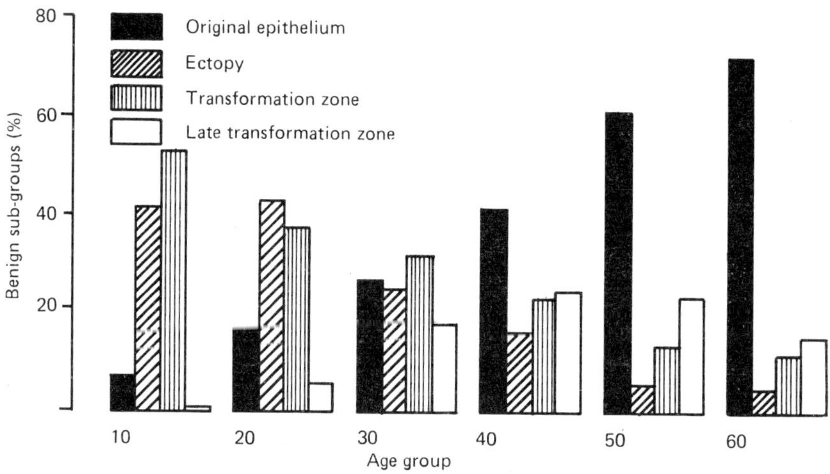

Figure 23.4 The variation in benign colposcopic appearances with advancing age

noticeably thinner after the menopause. This can be appreciated by the colposcopist because the sub-epithelial capillary network becomes readily visible through the thinned epithelium[8] (Figure 23.5). The exhibition of estrogens can similarly be seen to reverse this appearance. Because the epithelium is so much thinner the vessels are very easily traumatized so that even careful speculum examination can produce petechial haemorrhages or slight bleeding. Polyps are also much more frequently found in post-menopausal women presenting in the gynaecological clinic (Figure 23.6).

The degree of glycogenation of the squamous epithelium can be demonstrated by staining with Schiller's iodine solution. Before the menopause benign squamous epithelium stains a mahogany brown. Brett[7] has noticed that around the time of the menopause the intensity of this staining sometimes seems to increase. Usually within two or three years of the cessation of the periods the intensity of the colour change begins to fade. Interestingly this loss of glycogenation occasionally appears to be more marked on the posterior lip of the cervix rather than on the anterior lip. At least 10% of women show persistent glycogenation years after the menopause. It has been suggested that this is more likely to occur in women who have remained

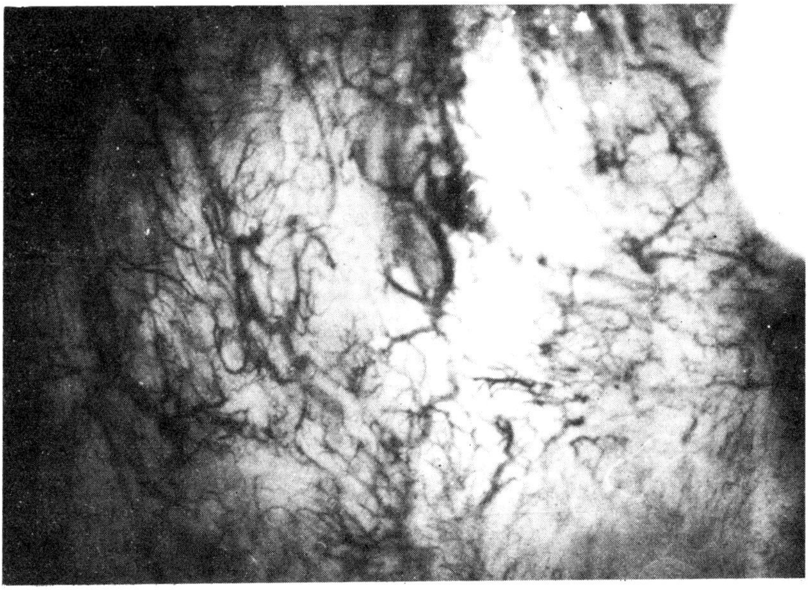

Figure 23.5 The sub-epithelial capillary network seen through the thinned post-menopausal cervical squamous epithelium

sexually active. Nevertheless the usual appearances after the application of iodine are of a uniform pale yellow epithelium in the post-menopausal woman.

In general the most important application of colposcopy is in the investigation of patients with abnormal cytology. This is particularly the case in young women especially if they have not completed their child-bearing career. Colposcopy is still useful in this respect in the post-menopausal woman but because of some loss of tissue elasticity, a tendency to upwards migration of the metaplastic area and a greater likelihood that the cervix will be stenosed from previous operative intervention, adequate visualization of the abnormal area is not always possible. Other diagnostic methods may have to be used such as endocervical curettage or diagnostic cone biopsy.

Summary

After the menopause the colposcope shows that the usual epithelial covering of the cervix is the original squamous epithelium which is typically thinner

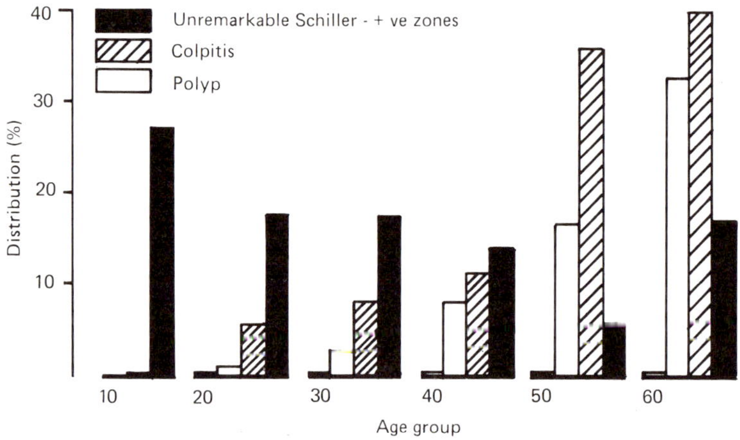

Figure 23.6 Increasing frequency of polyps and colposcopic colpitis (here including atrophic vaginitis) with increasing age in patients presenting as gynaecological out-patients

and lacks the degree of glycogenation seen in younger women. There is a tendency for the metaplastic squamous epithelium to recede within the endocervical canal. Though colposcopy remains a useful method for investigating the site of cervical epithelial atypia after the menopause the observer is sometimes limited by an inability to see the endocervical extent of any abnormal change present.

References

1. Walz, W. (1958). Über die Genese der sogenannten indirekten Metaplasie im Bereich des Müllerschen—Gang—Systems. *Z. Geburtsh. Gynakol.*, **151**, 1
2. Coppleson, M., Pixley, E. and Reid, B. (1971). *Colposcopy*. p. 70 (Springfield, Ill.: Charles C. Thomas)
3. Reid, B. (1966). The fate of the nucleic acid of sperm phaged by regenerating cells. *Aust. N.Z. Obstet. Gynaecol.*, **6**, 30

4. Naib, Z. M., Nahmias, A. H. and Josey, W. E. (1966). Cytology and histopathology of cervical Herpes simplex infection. *Cancer*, **19,** 1026
5. Crompton, A. C. (1971). *A Critical Evaluation of Colposcopy*. p. 120. (Manchester University: M.D. Thesis)
6. Przybora, L. A. and Plutowa, A. (1959). Histological topography of carcinoma in situ of the cervix uteri. *Cancer*, **12,** 263
7. Brett, J. and Coupez, F. (1960). *Colposcopie*, p. 216. (Paris: Masson et Cie)
8. Koller, O. (1963). *The Vascular Patterns of the Uterine Cervix*. (Oslo: University Press)
9. Kaufmann, C. and Ober, K. G. (1958)

Discussion on Section F: Skin

Chairman: *Mr I. L. Craft*

Professor C. Lauritzen (Gynaecologist, Ulm): What makes the skin look young? Certainly it is not the epidermal thickness, nor the number of mitoses. It is mainly due to three other factors. One is the degree of hyperaemia or perfusion which is known to be increased by estrogens. This can be measured by taking the temperature of the skin and by measuring the perfusion by xenon clearance. Secondly there is the degree of water retention. That has been mentioned, but it is an important point in connection with the succulence of the skin, or the tension of the surface of the skin. It is another factor which makes the skin look younger, and not only because of the increase of hyaluronidase, but also because there is an extra-cellular sodium retention in the skin. Thirdly, there is the alteration of carbohydrate metabolism, which I cannot go into now.

Dr Marks, according to one of his slides, gave a huge amount of estrone, 20 μg, to the skin. It is an incredibly high amount, and must be about 20 ml/kg, which I think is a highly toxic quantity.

Lastly, and referring to Dr Gordon's paper. We should not confuse a proliferation of the vaginal smear with an estrogenic effect. It is something quite different. This paper, and others, have shown that the vaginal smear is more or less useless as an indication of endogenous estrogen production.

Professor L. Rauramo (Gynaecologist, Turku): I agree with Professor Lauritzen. It would be important to study the vascularization of the skin, but we have not found any suitable methods of making precise measurements of this. The two parameters we chose were the ones that we could study exactly, and that is why we chose them.

Dr R. Marks (Physician, Cardiff): The main factor determining whether or not the skin looks young is the age of the eyes that behold the skin! There are a number of factors that determine the age of the skin, such as the general turgor and resilience of the skin when tested by indentation. This is a function, usually, of the amount of water in the connective tissue, which as has been shown on a number of occasions, rises *pari passu* with the amount of hyaluronic acid present. One cannot shrug off all the effects on appearance of decreased epidermo-poiesis, or skin thinning. Undoubtedly in old age the stratum corneum binds together less well, the skin becomes much more flaky and the whole skin surface tends to be a greyer, less lovely thing.

The large doses of estrogen in our culture pots were primarily due to the fact that estrone is a wretchedly insoluble matarial, and those are the amounts that we calculated were present, although as to the actual tissue dose, we cannot tell you. I do not think that any *in vitro* experiment can really tell the effective tissue dose of estrogen from what is put into the culture pots.

Mr I. L. Craft: Would Mr Gordon like to reply to Professor Lauritzen's comments on the reliability of the vaginal smear in assessing steroid status.

Mr H. Gordon (Gynaecologist, London): This was a gross over-simplification, and it is just not true. Certainly changing hormonal status can be followed, for example in a normal menstrual cycle with smears. The secondary estrogen peak in the second half of the cycle can even be identified in the absence of infection. I will agree that the intermediate cell pattern, as distinct from the well-estrogenized pattern on the one hand, and the total atrophy pattern on the other, is difficult to interpret, and is associated with a variety of different conditions, as wildly different as androgen-secreting tumours, pregnancy and the second half of the menstrual cycle. But if the two extremes are taken, it is possible to identify on the one hand an epithelium with a high karyopyknotic index which can only occur as a result of an estrogen effect, and on the other a very high percentage of para-basal cells which indicates a negligible hormonal effect associated with atrophy.

What we have been able to show is that it is quite wrong to consider a menopausal population as something homogeneous. Some women are producing a lot of hormones from somewhere well into old age; some others do not appear to have that ability, and from a very early stage show evidence of vaginal atrophy. It is quite an improper generalization to say that there is no correlation between estrogen status and vaginal cytology.

Dr T. Pyörälä (Gynaecologist, Jyräskylä): I have a comment which is relevant to Professor Lauritzen's observation. I have done a small trial to investigate the haemodynamic effects of estriol valerate on post-menopausal patients. The illustration shows (Figure 1) that in post-menopausal patients the estradiol valerate treatment caused an increase in blood volume, an increase in cardiac output, an increase in stroke volume, and a decrease in heart rate. It is possible that the peripheral circulation, especially skin circulation, can be increased, but we do not know how.

Dr D. W. Sturdee (Gynaecologist, Birmingham): For the treatment of atrophic vaginitis, local estrogen cream is advocated, particularly in women in whom oral estrogen therapy seems to be contraindicated. But a recent study has shown that estrone and conjugated estrogen cream have been absorbed in considerable amounts through the vagina. I wonder, therefore, if there is any particular advantage of local estrogen cream over oral therapy, and whether any studies have been done on the differences of the effects of these two routes of administration.

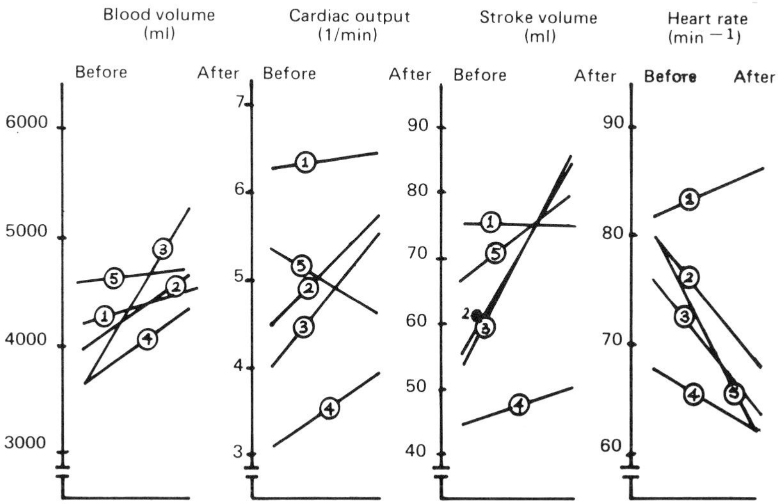

Figure 1 The effect of 20 days estradiol valerate treatment on blood volume, cardiac output, stroke volume and heart rate

Mr H. Gordon: I would agree that a lot of local estrogen is absorbed, but probably to a lesser extent, and less predictably than oral estrogen. Personally I do not think that it has much advantage. Perhaps its only advantage is that it is more acceptable for some patients who come with vaginal symptoms, and who in general are a bit reluctant to take tablets, but seem to see the point in applying the medication to the area causing the complaint. From that point of view only it is more acceptable to some women.

Section G

URINARY TRACT

Chairman: J. MALVERN

24

Post-menopausal changes in micturition habits and in urine flow and urethral pressure studies

J. L. Osborne

As beauty is in the eye of the beholder so the normality or otherwise of the micturition pattern of any subject relies upon the observers concept of normality. This concept of normality is inevitably influenced by the assessors own micturition habit, based upon the assumption that 'I am normal but I am not so sure about anyone else'.

It is therefore important that any observations should be objective, as far as is possible, and based upon the study of 'normal' subjects; not upon the study of patients attending a hospital outpatient department who may not be typical of the population at large.

To assess any changes in micturition with age and changing hormonal climate a longitudinal study of subjects over a number of years would be required; as this was not possible, a parallel study of a group of 600 women between the ages of 35 and 60 years working for a well known store, all considered to be fit for employment and drawn from different parts of the British Isles was carried out.

Each subject was asked to complete a questionnaire about their general health, past history and micturition habit. From the information obtained the following figures have been extracted.

The need for objective assessment is demonstrated by the first slide (Figure 24.1) which contrasts the number of hours between voiding of a group of women who complained of frequency with a larger group not admitting to this symptom.

It can be seen that although the mean of the time interval between voiding has been shifted 1 hour to the left in the group complaining of frequency that there is a considerable overlap between the groups.

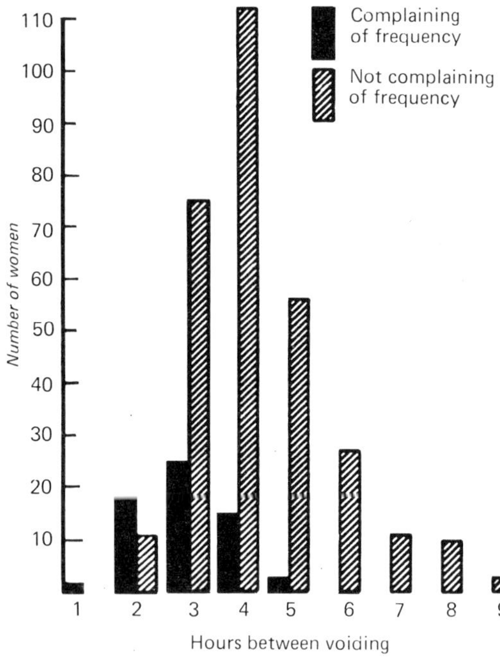

Figure 24.1 Comparison of the number of hours between voiding for women who complain of frequency and a larger group who do not

When the distribution of the frequency of voiding is plotted for each five year age group from 35 years to 55 years (Figure 24.2) it can be seen that there is no significant difference in the distribution of frequency of micturition with age and the menopause.

The next symptom to be studied is nocturia; the subjects were asked if they were awakened at night to pass urine and how often this occurred. Only those subjects who admitted to nocturia at least once every night were classed as having nocturia for the purposes of this study. Plotting the incidence of nocturia as a percentage of the patients in each age group there appears to be an increase in incidence over the age of 50 years (Figure 24.3). When the subjects are divided into those that are pre-menopausal and those that are post-menopausal the incidence of the symptom is 16% and 25% respectively. These results give a χ^2 of 6·4 with one degree of freedom and a

Fisher P of 0·011. This difference is therefore significant at the 5% level but not at the 1% level.

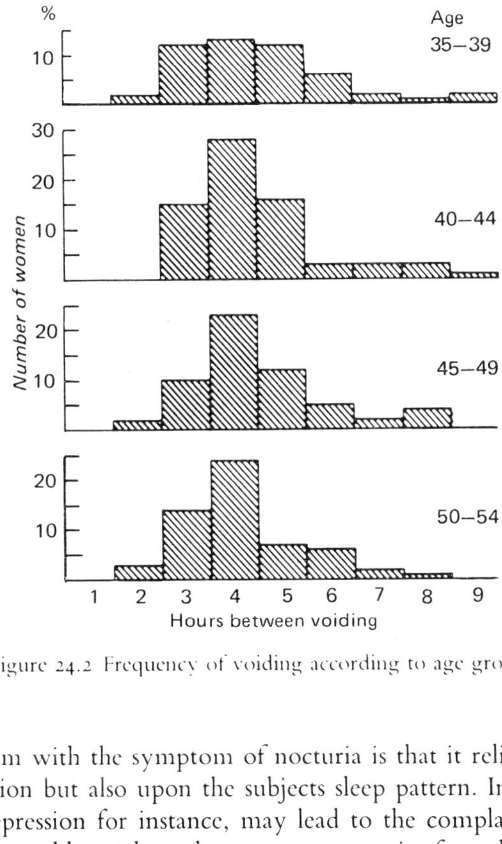

Figure 24.2 Frequency of voiding according to age group

The problem with the symptom of nocturia is that it relies not only on bladder function but also upon the subjects sleep pattern. Insomnia due to any cause, depression for instance, may lead to the complaint of nocturia because being unable to sleep the woman may arise from her bed to pass urine for the sake of something to do. This distinction is difficult to make from questionnaire answers although at interview it is not difficult.

As with frequency, the symptoms of urgency which occurred in 10% of the group, urge micturition (5%) and dysuria (16%) showed no significant change with age. In fact the highest incidence of dysuria occurred in the 35 to 39 year group.

It was somewhat surprising to find that the incidence of clinically significant stress incontinence (26% overall) did not change significantly (Figure 24.4); the 35 to 39 year group may not be typical because it contained a disproportionately large number of nulliparous women. The figure of 26%

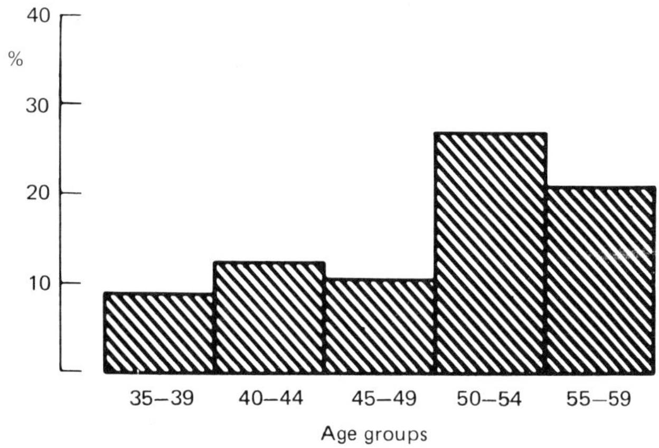

Figure 24.3 Frequency of nocturia according to age group

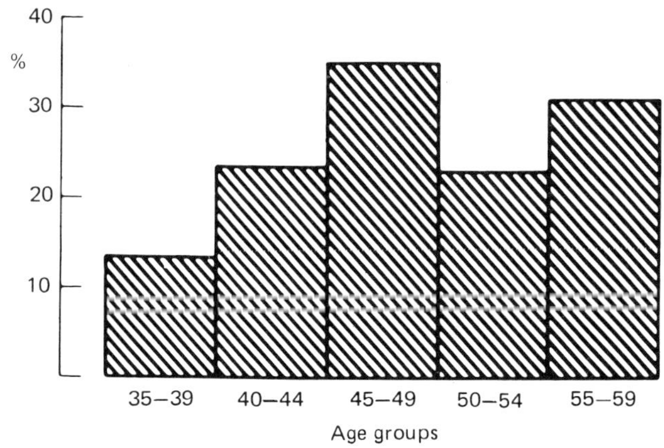

Figure 24.4 Frequency of stress incontinence according to age group

quoted here is only half that found by Wolin *et al.*[1] and Nemir and Middleton[2] but they assessed whether their subject ever leaked whereas we were only assessing the number of women in whom it was a troublesome symptom.

It has been shown by Edwards and Malvern[3] that the amplitude of the urethral pressure profile decreases with age, it would be reasonable to assume that this decrease is due, at least in part, to the decreasing vascularity of the peri-urethral tissues associated with falling estrogen levels and that this process would therefore be reversible with estrogen therapy.

The failure of this survey to demonstrate a change in the incidence of clinically significant stress incontinence may well be because only those women with a bladder neck which is not cough proof and strain proof are at risk as far as stress incontinence is concerned and that this percentage of the population does not change with the advent of the menopause although the degree of leakage may increase if the urethral resistance falls; quantitative assessment of stress incontinence may be possible to assess accurately in the future with electric nappy devices but at present is rationally inaccurate.

In conclusion little change in micturition patterns has been found with advancing age in this survey of fit women except in the symptom of nocturia. This survey may not be typical of the population as a whole but it does provide a counterbalance to those figures produced from the study of women attending hospital who are also not typical.

References

1. Wolin, L. H. (1969). Stress incontinence in young healthy nulliparous female subjects. *J. Urol.*, **101**, 545
2. Nemir, A. and Middleton, R. P. (1954). Stress incontinence in young nulliparous women. *Am. J. Obstet. Gynecol.*, **68**, 1166
3. Edwards, L. and Malvern, J. (1974). The urethral pressure profile: theoretical considerations and clinical application. *Br. J. Urol.*, **46**, 325

25

The effect of estrogens on bladder function in the female

P. J. B. Smith

Bladder function in a woman consists of the regular storage and intermittent voiding of urine. In both capacities the bladder function is closely related to that of the urethra. As yet there is no evidence of any direct effect of estrogen on the bladder itself but there is clear evidence of estrogen activity affecting the urethra and more particularly its distal segment. This paper summarizes this evidence and indicates how estrogen activity in the distal urethra may affect bladder function, particularly in the post-menopausal woman.

By far the commonest bladder dysfunction in women consists of attacks of frequency and painful micturition somewhat loosely defined as the urethral syndrome. Women with this symptom constitute a large part of a urologist's work load. In a study of nearly 3000 new patients seen over a 2-year period, 928 were female, and of these 719 presented with symptoms of the urethral syndrome (Table 25.1). Taking the age at which these women first experienced their symptoms and expressing this as the sexual or physiological age (Table 25.2) it can be seen that 292 women were first afflicted with the condition after their menopause.

Table 25.1 Incidence of urethral syndrome

Total patients seen over 2-year period	2895
Total females seen over 2-year period	928
Total patients with urethral syndrome	719

Estrogen activity in the female undergoes a gradual decline after the menopause but this can vary, some women maintaining adequate estrogen levels in the absence of a menstrual cycle for many years[1].

Table 25.2 Sexual age at onset of urethral syndrome

Sexual age	*Number of patients with urethral syndrome*
Pre-puberty	22
Reproductive	405
Post-menopausal	292

In other cases the decline in estrogen activity may be so severe as to result in senile vaginitis, a condition rapidly responding to estrogen therapy[2].

Clinical evidence of senile vaginitis was noted in many of the 292 post-menopausal women presenting with the urethral syndrome. This association has been noted previously[3] as also has been the concomitant relief of urinary symptoms after estrogen therapy in these patients[4, 5].

As well as this pathological correlation, both vagina and distal urethra are closely similar in their anatomy particularly in the squamous epithelium lining both their surfaces. They also have, in part, a common origin from the urogenital sinus of the embryo[6].

This close relationship between development and structure of vagina and urethra was first commented on by Parkes and Zuckerman[7] and in later animal experiments extra-genital estrogen sensitivity, manifested by macturation of squamous epithelium, was demonstrated in tissues derived from the urogenital sinus and in particular the distal urethra[8].

A cytohormonal study based on the method of Papanicolou[9] and using the macturating index as described by Frost[10] was carried out on 402 females embracing all three stages of sexual life (Table 25.3)[11]. The smear or cellular pattern thus obtained reflected the underlying tissue pattern and biological response of the urethral and vaginal tissues to estrogen activity.

This showed that the human female urethra was sensitive to estrogen as shown by the cytology of its squamous epithelium and that the cytological changes in the urethra were paralleled by similar changes in the vagina. Both showed similar reactions to the physiological variations (even those within the menstrual cycle) in estrogen activity that occur throughout a woman's life.

The distribution of smears in the 123 post-menopausal women (Table 25.4) indicated varying levels of estrogen activity. This is in accord with

Table 25.3 Cytohormonal analysis

	Sexual age by history of all cases
Pre-pubertal	18
Reproductive	261
Post-menopausal	123

Table 25.4 Cytohormonal analysis. Age distribution in post-menopausal urethral smears

Type of smear	*Age* 40–50	50–60	60–70	70–80
Cyclic	12	3	0	0
Crowded	3	43	39	0
Atrophic	0	2	13	8

the much larger cytohormonal studies of Stoll[12] and Meisel[1] thus confirming that abrupt atrophic changes in the urethra or vagina do not necessarily follow at the menopause. In 85 the smears had a 'crowded menopausal' appearance with intermediate and para-basal cells indicating a decline in estrogen activity (Figure 25.1). Fifteen had smears showing normal cyclic activity indicating full estrogen activity, (Figure 25.2). In only 23 was there a true atrophic smear consisting of parabasal cells indicating the absence of estrogen activity (Figure 25.3). There is however, a progressive decline in estrogen activity with advancing age.

It is clear, therefore, that estrogen deprivation in the post-menopausal woman may result in atrophic distal urethritis. The segment of urethra becomes rigid, inelastic and has a thin inflamed and occasionally ulcerating epithelium. This interferes with bladder function firstly by producing bladder outflow obstruction and raised residual urine due to distal urethral stenosis. Secondly, the urethritis combined with inadequate flow rate and abnormal flow pattern may result in the inability to prevent the ascent of introital organisms. These organisms produce local urethral discomfort and in many

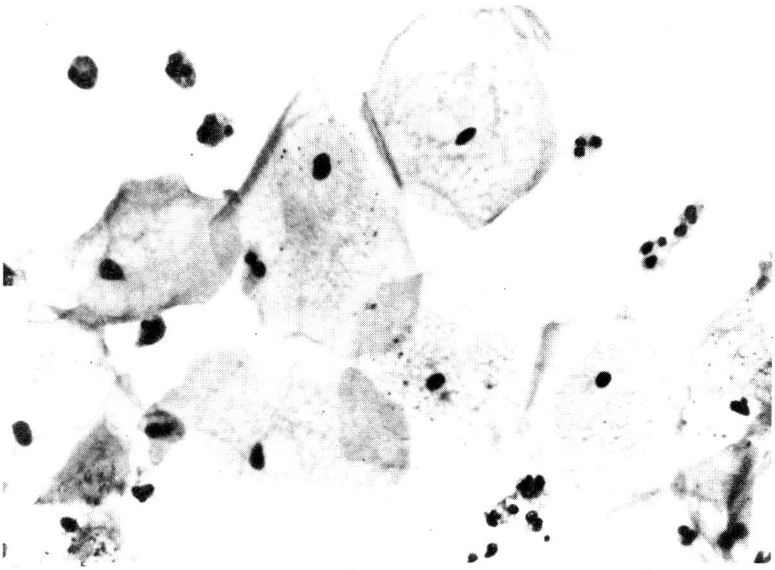

Figure 25.1 Parabasal cells in urethral smear

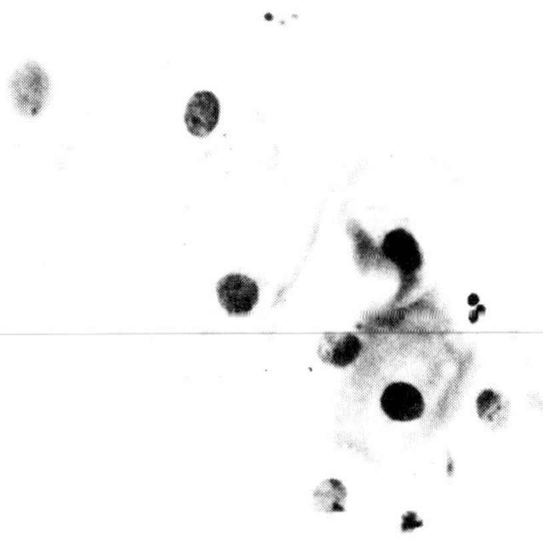

Figure 25.2 Intermediate cells in urethral smear

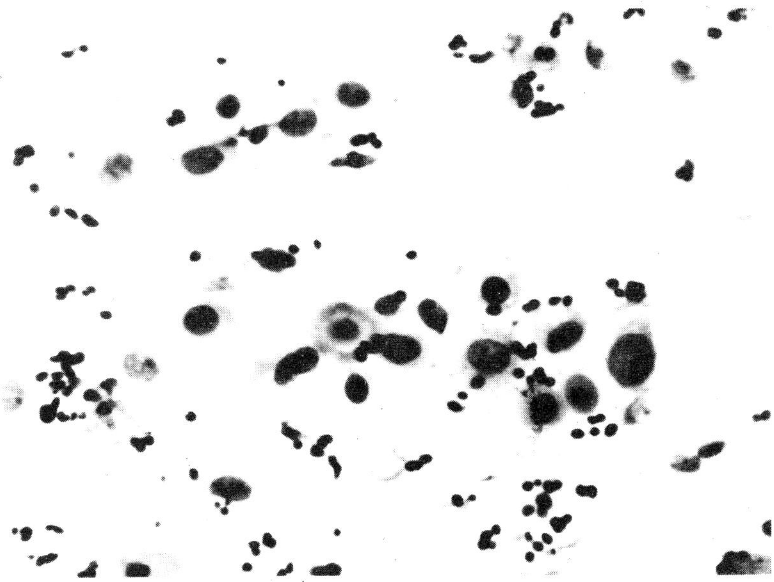

Figure 25.3 Superficial cells in urethral smear

cases a secondary bacteiuria due to bladder involvement. Both conditions will result in a urethral syndrome with frequency, urgency and dysuria, and hence interference with the normal storage pattern of urine. The obstructive and inflammatory elements are usually combined and treatment is aimed at both, consisting of urethral dilatation or urethrotomy (both up to 30 Ch.) plus supportive estrogen therapy. This therapy usually takes the form of conjugated estrogen (Premarin) either as tablets 1·25 mg daily or vaginal cream, 4 g. This treatment is given for 3 out of 4 weeks for a total of 3 months.

Table 25.5 Urethral syndrome and trabeculation

Total number of patients	500
With trabeculated bladder	92
With trabeculated bladder post-menopausal	42

In the first series a study was made of 500 women with the urethral syndrome[13] (Table 25.5). Obstruction, as shown by the presence of bladder trabeculation, was present in 92 women and of these 42 were post-menopausal. The initial treatment was by dilatation alone but this was insufficient in just under half. However, the use of estrogen markedly improved this 'failure' group (Table 25.6).

Table 25.6 Urethral syndrome and trabeculation. Results of treatment—post-menopausal group

Total patients	42
Improved with dilatation	35
No improvement with dilatation	7
Relapse after initial improvement with dilatation	13
Prolonged remission with estrogens	11

With this encouragement a further study was made of 292 post-menopausal women with the urethral syndrome. This time, cytohormonal studies were used to diagnose the estrogen deficiency and consequent atrophic urethritis. The results of combined estrogen therapy and dilatation are shown in Table 25.7 and are obviously a considerable improvement.

Table 25.7 Urethral syndrome and cytohormonal analysis

Total number of patients seen over 2-year period	719
Total number of cases in post-menopausal group	292
Total number of cases with senile urethritis	68
Treated satisfactorily with estrogen + dilatation	64
Treated unsatisfactorily with estrogen + dilatation	4

Whilst urethral stenosis is usually associated with ascending infection recent evidence using urodynamic techniques has revealed an association between obstruction and detrusor instability. Whilst this is more obvious in the male, a study of 557 women of all ages (Figure 25.4) shows an increasing incidence of bladder instability with age and suggests a possible association with estrogen deficient urethritis and stenosis.

Furthermore, in a study of obstruction in the female measured by urodynamic techniques with the formula:

$$\frac{\text{Peak flow pressure}}{\text{Max. flow rate}^2}\left(\frac{P}{F^2}\right) > 0{\cdot}3$$

the same tendency to an increase in obstruction with age is seen (Figure 25.5). When instability and obstruction are compared 21 of the 53 obstructed cases were unstable, i.e. 40% as opposed to only 27% instability in the much larger unobstructed group.

Estrogen therapy does not affect instability and if symptoms are sufficiently severe bladder distension may be required.

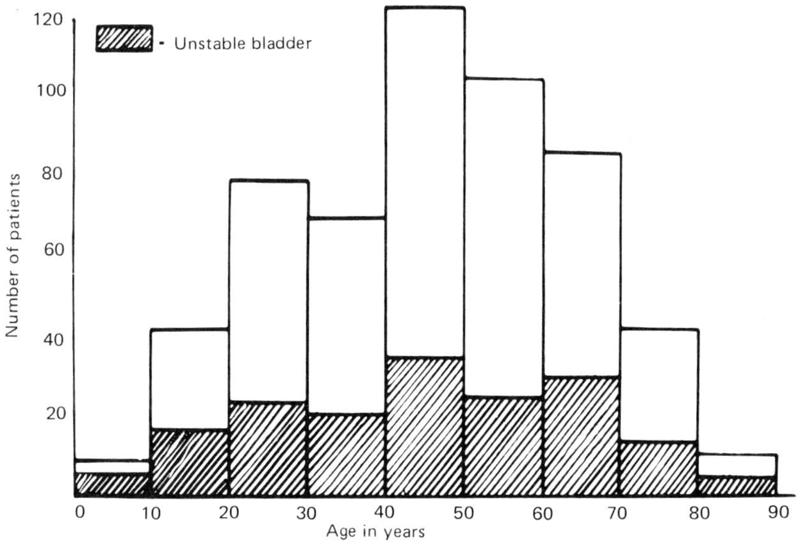

Figure 25.4 Incidence of bladder instability in 557 women

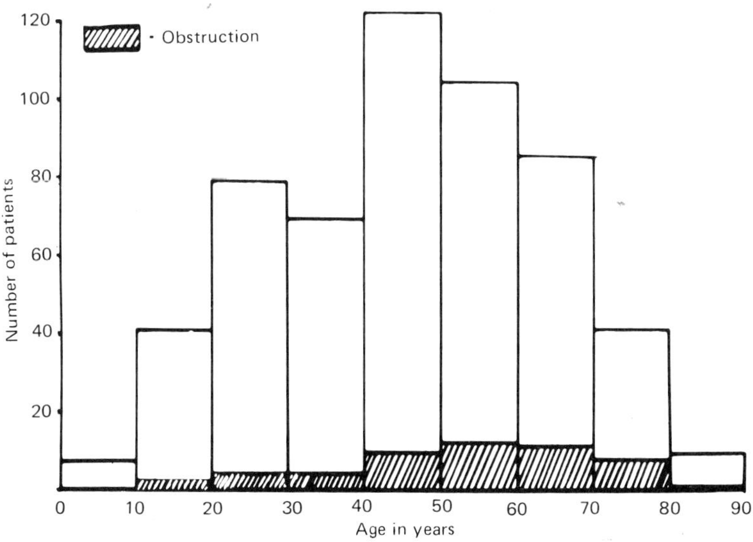

Figure 25.5 Incidence of obstruction in 557 women

Summary

The distal urethra of the human female is sensitive to physiological variations in estrogen activity. In some post-menopausal women the estrogen deficiency may be such as to result in atrophic distal-urethritis and stricture formation. This will in turn affect bladder function by producing obstruction, raised residual urine and ascending infection with symptoms of frequency and dysuria. This state of affairs responds best to urethral dilatation or urethrotomy plus 3 months low dose conjugated estrogen. The occasional finding of detrusor instability in these women may be associated with the obstructive effect of the atrophic urethritis but this condition itself does not respond to estrogen therapy.

References

1. Meisel, A. (1966). The menopause. A cytohormonal study. *Acta Cytol.*, **10,** 49
2. Midwinter, A. (1969). The management of the menopause. *Practitioner*, **202,** 372
3. Everett, H. S. (1941). Urology in the female. *Am. J. Surg.*, **52,** 521
4. Salmon, U. J., Walter, R. and Geist, S. H. (1941). The use of oestrogens in the treatment of dysuria and incontinence in post-menopausal women. *Am. J. Obstet. Gynecol.*, **42,** 845
5. Youngblood, V. H., Tomlin, E. M., Williams, J. O. and Kimmelsteil, P. (1958). Exfoliative cytology of the senile female urethra. *J. Urol.*, **79,** 110
6. Langman, J. (1963). *Human Enbryology*, 1st Edn. (Baltimore: Williams & Wilkins Co.)
7. Parkes, A. S. and Zuckerman, S. (1931). The menstrual cycle of the primates. II. Some effects of oestrin on baboons and macaques. *J. Anat.*, **65,** 272
8. Zuckerman, S. (1940). Histogenesis of tissue sensitive to oestrogens. *Biol. Rev. Cambridge Philosoph. Soc.*, **15,** 231
9. Papanicolau, G. N. (1933). The sexual cycle in the human female as revealed by vaginal smears. *Am. J. Anat.*, **51,** Suppl.
10. Frost, J. K. (1962). Quoted from Novak and Woodruff 1962. *Gynaecological and Obstetric Pathology*. (Philadelphia and London: W. B. Saunders Co.)
11. Smith, P. (1972). Age changes in the female urethra. *Br. J. Urol.*, **44,** 667
12. Stoll, P. (1960). Vaginal smears in the menopause. *Acta Cytol.*, **4,** 148
13. Roberts, M. and Smith, P. (1968). Non-malignant obstruction of the female urethra. *Br. J. Urol.*, **40,** 694

26

Urethral profile studies on menopausal women and the effects of estrogen treatment

R. F. Harrison

Continence in the female depends on maintenance of a level of pressure in the outflow tract urethra that is greater than intravesical pressure.

This ability is a function of the periurethral tissues and external sphincteric mechanism and their control and is often imperfect. Up to 50% of healthy young girls have been known to have involuntary loss of urine in times of sudden stress and as age increases, frequency, urgency and incontinence become more common.

In the menopausal female, whose pelvic floor musculature may have already been disadvantaged by childbirth or excessive abdominal pressure, and whose whole ambience of life has already been altered by other menopausal symptoms, the exacerbation of urinary tract symptoms such as frequency, urgency and incontinence could possibly be a result of periurethral tissue weakening induced directly or indirectly by estrogen deprivation. The alleviation of such symptoms which have been noted to be a sequel to menopausal therapy (as reported elsewhere and here today) may possibly be due to the rejuvenation of pelvic tissue following re-introduction of estrogen replacement therapy.

To test the validity of such a premise a comparative series of urethral pressure studies were performed on patients before and 6 months after commencement of hormone replacement therapy. Under control conditions, the maximum urethral pressure depends on the pressure exerted on the urethra at its mid point by the surrounding supports, and any alteration in the pressure readings following therapy may, therefore, be considered to be a measure of the effect that hormone replacement therapy has had on the periurethral tissue tonus in the patient.

Methodology

Patient selection

Patients attending the Menopause Clinic at Chelsea Hospital for Women for the first time were asked to take part in the study. They were unselected apart from having first been diagnosed as menopausal by another doctor on clinical criteria. 18 patients embarked on the study aged between 45 and 58, parity 0–4. Of the 18, 8 were not considered in the final analysis. Two stopped therapy due to severe mental disease, and two considered they did not need treatment. Two left the country and one left the clinic after the first visit never to return. Data on one patient were not available in time to be included. Results of urethral pressure profile studies on the remaining 10 are thus presented.

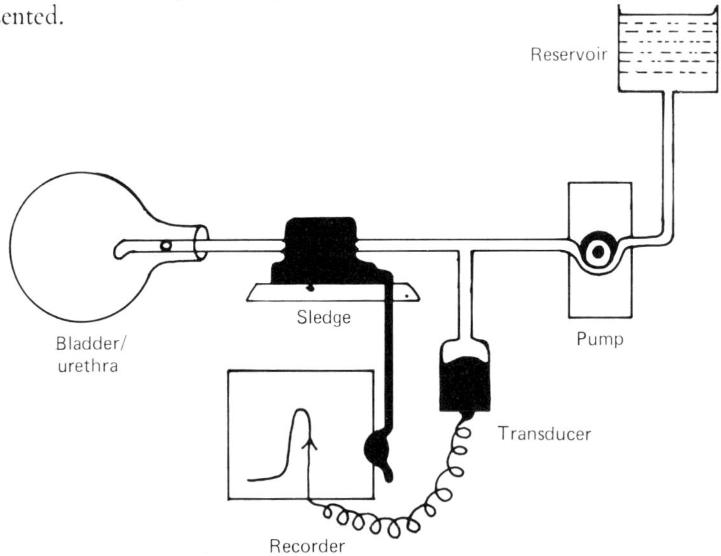

Figure 26.1 Diagram of the urethral pressure profile apparatus

Pressure profile

The simple technique of urethral pressure estimation described by Malvern and Edwards[1], was used by the author. This method is relatively free from sources of error and complication (Figure 26.1). Normal saline at body temperature is infused through the profile catheter at 2 ml/min. This continuous column of fluid is also connected via a side arm to a pressure transducer which connects with a single channel recorder so that the pressure obtained at the side holes on the catheter is transmitted and recorded on a trace. The catheter is withdrawn from the bladder to atmosphere via the urethra, hence providing readings at consecutive points opposite the side holes along the whole length of its journey. As the mechanical drive method of catheter withdrawal is linked to the spindle driving the chart paper at a constant speed, comparative traces can be obtained (Figure 26.2). From this trace the maximum urethral pressure is measured in centimetres of water by subtracting the resting bladder pressure from the total pressure obtained.

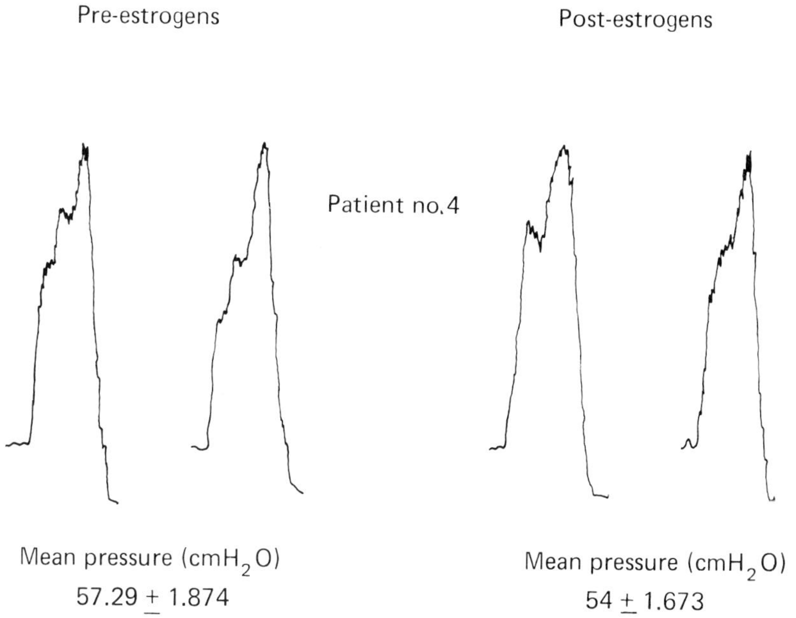

Figure 26.2 Comparison of comparable weekly urethral pressure studies, pre- and post-therapy

Results

Two studies were carried out on each patient a week apart prior to start of treatment and two further studies were performed a week apart after 6 months' estrogen hormone replacement therapy. At least three comparable measurements were made at each study; hence the patients acted as their own controls. Patients were also questioned and a note made of any urinary symptoms at each visit.

Mean maximal urethral pressure comparison, pre- and post-therapy (Table 26.1)

Mean and standard error of mean of maximal urethral pressure was computed for each patient before and after treatment and a comparison between the figures obtained was made using Student's '*t*' test. Four patients showed a significant difference of at least 5% after therapy. However, closer perusal

Table 26.1 Maximum urethral pressure comparison pre- and post-estrogen therapy

Patient	*Pre-* (*Mean* ± *S.E.M.*)	*Post-* (*Mean* ± *S.E.M.*)	*t*	*P* (5%)
1	103·167 ± 2·587	97·25 ± 5·949	0·912	NS
2	83·714 ± 3·63	79·37 ± 2·57	0·976	NS
3	12·333 ± 0·615	68·5 + 2·487	21·928	< 0·001
4	57·285 ± 1·874	54 ± 1·673	1·308	NS
5	65·625 ± 1·164	60·333 ± 0·919	3·568	< 0·01
6	45·429 ± 0·922	42·475 ± 1·887	1·275	NS
7	85·6 ± 0·927	67 ± 2	8·437	< 0·001
8	52·5 ± 1·628	48·2 ± 1·158	2·153	NS
9	67·25 ± 1·887	68·2 ± 3·68	0·230	NS
10	60·167 ± 2·971	51 ± 2·47	2·370	< 0·05

of results shows that in only one of these was there an increase in the mean pressure (case 3). In the other three there actually (5, 7 and 10) was a significant fall in pressure after 6 months' therapy. This finding is a little harder to explain than finding no significant difference after therapy in the other six patients. All cases, except patient 3 (Figure 26.3) who showed a significant increase in maximal urethral pressure after treatment, had normal pre-treatment urethral pressure amplitudes when values were corrected for age by the formula devised by Edwards and Malvern[2] (Normal amplitude (cmH_2O) = 92-pt. age in years). It is thus perhaps difficult to record a significant increase in urethral pressure when that pressure is already normal. Even when there was a significant fall, pressure still remained within normal limits (Figure 26.4) after therapy.

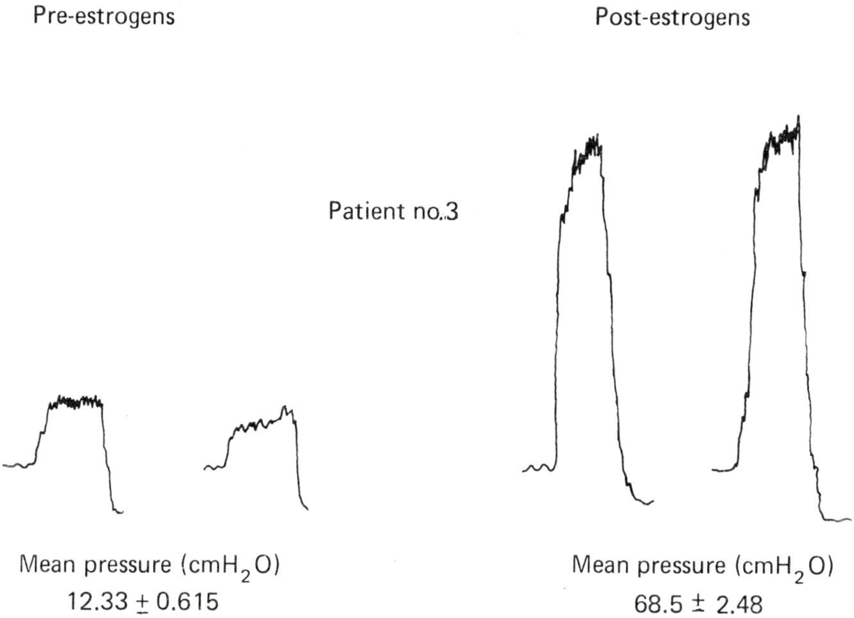

Figure 26.3 Comparison of urethral pressure studies: significant increase after therapy

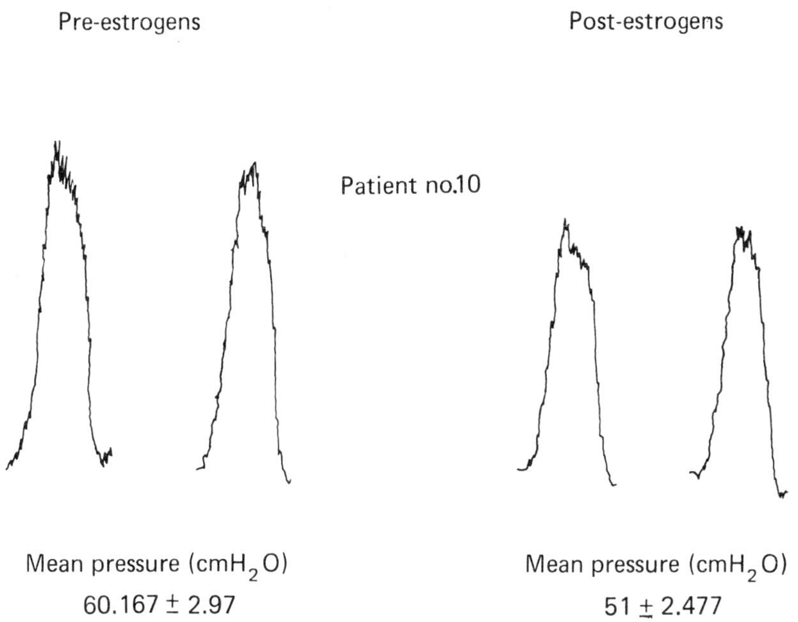

Figure 26.4 Comparison of urethral pressure studies: significant decrease after therapy

Table 26.2 Menopausal patients urinary symptoms comparison pre- and post-estrogen therapy

Patient		Symptom			
		Frequency (Time mins)	*Nocturia (Times)*	*Urgency (Severity)*	*S. Incontinence (Incidence)*
1	Pre-	Nil	Nil	Nil	Nil
	Post-				
2	Pre-	10 mins	2	+ + +	+ +
	Post-	Nil	Nil	±	Nil
3	Pre-	30 mins	Nil	+ + +	Nil
	Post-	Nil		Nil	
4	Pre-	30 mins	4–5	+ + +	+ +
	Post-	Nil	2	Nil	± (week of tablets)
5	Pre-	Nil	Nil	Nil	Nil
	Post-				
6	Pre-	Nil	0–1	+ +	Nil
	Post-		Nil	+	
7	Pre-	Nil	2	+ + +	+ +
	Post		2	+ + +	+ +
8	Pre-	Nil	Nil	+ +	Nil
	Post-			+ +	
9	Pre-	Nil	2–3	+ + +	Nil
	Post-		0–1	Nil	Nil
10	Pre-	60	2	±	Nil
	Post-	60	2	±	

Comparison of urinary symptoms pre- and post-therapy (Table 26.2)

Eight of the 10 patients gave a significant history of urinary tract symptoms before treatment. They fell into four categories: frequency (more often than 3-hourly), nocturia, urgency and stress incontinence. Following 6 months' therapy, five of these eight (2, 3, 4, 6, 9) had significant alleviation of all of whatever mixture of symptoms they had previously complained of. The other three were no worse than before and two had no symptoms in the first place (1, 5).

Comparison of significant difference 'P' in urethral pressure with alteration of urinary symptoms following therapy (Table 26.3)

Although five patients' symptoms improved, only in patient No. 3 was there exhibited a significant increase in maximal urethral pressure after treatment. Where the profile decreased significantly symptoms either stayed the same (7, 10) and the other case had no symptoms in the first place.

Table 26.3 Significance of change in maximal urethral pressure compared with change in urinary symptoms after estrogen therapy

Patient	*P*	*Change Ur. Symptoms*
1	NS	—
2	NS	Improved
3	< 0·001	Improved
4	NS	Improved
5	< 0·01	—
6	NS	Improved
7	< 0·001	Same
8	NS	Same
9	NS	Improved
10	< 0·05	Same

— = No symptoms to change

Conclusion

This small pilot study shows that although urinary symptoms appear to be alleviated in some patients on hormone replacement therapy the effect appears to be other than an effect on periurethral tissue as measured by urethral pressure studies.

It may be that the profile does not measure what it is claimed to do or that, as some of the symptoms relieved are not necessarily dependent on periurethral tissue, the necessary improvement might have been achieved in other areas of the lower urinary tract. A placebo effect of therapy *per se*, or an indirect effect following alleviation of other menopausal symptoms by estrogens, might also explain these results.

Acknowledgments

To Mrs. Minardi for helping to organize the patients and to Sister Secluna for her help with the profile studies.

References

1. Malvern, J. and Edwards, L. (1972). International Continence Society Meeting, Paris
2. Edwards, L. and Malvern, J. (1974). The urethral pressure profile: theoretical considerations and clinical applications. *Br. J. Urol.*, **46**, 325

Discussion on Section G:

Urinary Tract

Chairman: *Mr J. Malvern*

Mr J. Malvern (Chairman): Each of the speakers has approached his topic slightly differently. Mr Osborne has taken a group of people who have not gone to hospital, but have been working quite healthily in a store, and determined the incidence of the symptoms in the various age groups. Mr Smith selected his patients from those attending his hospital, while Mr Harrison has analyzed urethral pressure measurements in a small group of well motivated patients attending a menopause clinic.

Dr C. B. Hammond (Gynaecologist, Duke University): I too was surprised that with progressing age through the menopause, there was not an increase in the symptoms of stress incontinence. Mr Osborne mentioned low parity in the 35–40 year old group. Does he have figures on parity for the older group? I should be surprised if they did not have relatively low parity.

Mr J. Osborne (Gynaecologist, London): I do not have figures with me, but we did look at it, and there was no significant difference in the parity of the older age groups as compared with the normal population.

Dr C. B. Hammond: Were they all of low parity, relatively speaking?

Mr J. Osborne: No, they were not all of low parity. They encompassed quite a wide range of parity. Most of them were from socio-economic groups 3 and 4, of both high and low parities with no significant bias.

Dr C. B. Hammond: After the course of treatment which included the urethrotomy, the Premarin therapy for 3 months, and then its cessation, what was the eventual outcome? Did the symptoms recur, and if so, how quickly?

Mr P. J. B. Smith (Urologist, Bath): I cannot answer that question with accuracy. What we considered a success was that 3 months after completion of treatment, the patient was fit and well. That is a fairly crude clinical estimate. We followed these women up for a total of 6 months. The trial is still in progress, and my impression is that some of those women—and I stress that it is only an impression, because we do not have enough figures, are now beginning to come back after 18 months to 2 years. I agree that we are only treating an episode, and the condition probably does recur. I hasten to add that because someone has atrophic urethritis, it does not mean that she will have symptoms of the urethral syndrome. It is important to realize that we are treating women both with symptoms and atrophic urethritis.

Professor C. Lauritzen (Gynaecologist, Ulm): From my studies of the literature on the effect of estrogens on the bladder and the urethra, I recollect reading that estrogens may increase the tone of the detrusor of the bladder, and androgens may increase the tone of the so-called sphincter. That has been shown for the human in Langreder's monograph*, and I recollect some papers on small rodents where it has been shown that if they are given nortestosterone or testosterone, a retention of urine can be produced because of hyperplasia and hypertrophy of the so-called sphincter. Secondly, in my own experience, and in the experience of many others, ectropion of the urethra, that is the protrusion of the dorsal wall of the outer urethra, can be cured completely within a few weeks by giving estrogens.

Mr P. J. B. Smith: I agree with Professor Lauritzen's last statement. I think what happens is that the distal urethra is almost vaginal tissue, and with post-menopausal atrophy, there is regression of the anterior wall of the vagina. This is pulled back with the anterior vaginal wall, due to its own natural retraction. By giving estrogens the distal urethra regrows and this can be corrected, virtually within days. If with many so-called caruncles, which are fulgurated, one only gave the woman a tube of Premarin, or some similar vaginal estrogen cream, just as good result would probably be achieved.

But with regard to the question of the direct influence of estrogens and androgens on bladder tone, I did not realize that there was any effect.

Mr J. Osborne: I am not too sure of Professor Lauritzen's references, but I think that the evidence is that estrogens may have a mild alpha-adenergic receptor stimulating effect. Under those circumstances, one would not expect the effect on the dome of the bladder, the trigone and the urethra to be the same, because the dome of the bladder has a large number of beta-adenergic receptors, whereas there are a greater number of alpha-adenergic receptors in the trigone and in the urethra. As El-Badawi and Schenk† using histochemical techniques have shown that these receptors in different parts of the bladder can be differentiated, one would not expect a uniform effect of estrogens on the whole of the bladder, and the urethra. If the estrogens have any effect at all, they would tend to increase the activity of the trigone and the urethra, but have no effect on the dome of the bladder.

Mr R. F. Harrison (Gynaeaologist, London): The effect of estrogens may not just be on the musculature of the bladder and the urethra but may also influence the tone of the surrounding tissues. This concept of increasing vascular support is well illustrated by the penis whose tone increases if the vascularity to it is increased. This may be a factor in the female as well.

* Langreder, W. (1961). *Gynaekologische Urologie*. (Stuttgart: Thieme)

† El-Badawi, A. and Schenk, E. A. (1968). *J. Urol.*, **99,** 585

Dr Muriel G. Yates (General Practitioner, Liverpool): Is there any place for estrogen therapy in the treatment of elderly post-menopausal incontinent women where urinary infection has been excluded and where no senile confusion state or dementia exists? If the estrogen does increase muslce tone, is there any place for it?

Mr J. Malvern: One of the essentials in discussing the subject of the urinary tract is to clearly define the disorder which is requiring treatment. One group of patients can be suffering from incontinence caused by urethral sphincter mechanism incompetence and another group of patients may be suffering from urgency, frequency and such symptoms which have a very different aetiology. The use of estrogens in patients with urethral sphincter mechanism weakness is probably small, but as was shown, by Mr Smith, the administration of estrogens to patients who have an irritable bladder, or urgency and frequency, secondary to some urethral syndrome, may well be of considerable benefit.

Mr P. J. B. Smith: I would agree. I do not think that any work that we have done has ever demonstrated significant improvement in true incontinence, but I hasten to add that it is worth checking some of these elderly women for bladder instability, most of whom will respond to distension therapy, a simple enough treatment and well worth doing. The important thing to stress is that I am not talking about true urethral stricture but atrophic narrowing. Hinman* described it very nicely by saying that what it does is to alter the flow pattern down the urethra. If you and I look at our urethral stream, we hopefully show a good '404 bore' type flow, a good spiral flow. If the outlet is narrowed, the urine flows in an eddy formation, with urine actually reaching the external meatus, then eddying back up into the bladder. The flow pattern alters, rather than the flow rate.

Having said that, in a lot of the women mentioned by Dr Yates it is the outflow part of the bladder, the proximal urethra, that is at fault, and that can be caused by a variety of factors. I do not think that estrogen has any specific effect in that area, and although people keep reporting an improvement in urinary symptoms. If one reads the papers carefully, particularly one by Heber† from Australia, all that they are saying is that they are a bit better. In other words, they are not so wet. That is very little consolation, and I think that it is a mistake to throw the estrogens around these women. One must find evidence of atrophic urethritis, which one can find by doing a vaginal smear—because a vaginal smear equals a urethral smear—and one must have evidence of distal urethral narrowing, which is obtained by looking at it. When these co-exist, then urethrotomy and estrogens do help, but it is only a small group, and I regret to say that as yet the estrogens are unlikely to help the large majority of the patients mentioned.

Mr J. Malvern: So often, when some interest is shown in a patient's urinary problem, there will be an initial symptomatic improvement. Unfortunately the long term outcome is less satisfacory.

* Hinman, F. Jnr. (1968). *J. Urol.*, **99,** 811

† Heber, K. R. (1970). *J. R. Austral. Coll. GPs*, **15,** 81

Section H

RISKS OF ESTROGEN THERAPY

PART 1: *THROMBOEMBOLISM*

Chairman: S. CAMPBELL

27

A double blind cross-over study with conjugated equine estrogens on blood clotting

L. Poller

The present report describes blood clotting studies performed during the study initiated by Dr. Coope on the clinical and laboratory effects of the administration of natural estrogens for menopausal symptoms. Synthetic estrogens are known to carry a thrombosis risk and in our studies which have extended over a number of years since the early 1960s we have shown that all oral contraceptive preparations monitored which contained synthetic estrogens produced acceleration of blood clotting tests and increased platelet aggregation[1–6].

An outline of the blood coagulation mechanism is given in Figure 27.1. When it is shed from a vessel, blood coagulates. In the absence of trauma to tissue, this clotting usually takes several minutes. The clotting delay depends on the time taken for the blood to generate its own 'intrinsic' thromboplastin. In the presence of injuries, tissue juices are liberated which activate clotting by a different mechanism; tissue juices are liberated and the 'extrinsic' clotting system is activated. Both the 'extrinsic' and 'intrinsic' systems operate concomitantly in promoting normal haemostasis.

Different laboratory tests which have been designed to measure these two systems of blood clotting. The broad spectrum screening test for 'extrinsic' clotting is the prothrombin time and for 'intrinsic' clotting, the cephalin time test (PTT). In addition to these screening tests, we have individual clotting factor assays designed to measure the levels of these specific clotting components. The specific assays tend to be more sensitive to changes than the broad spectrum screening tests, although less useful in the assessment of the overall effects on blood coagulation.

The changes we have observed during conventional estrogen/progestogen administration have not been detected during progestogen only administration. These changes may be responsible in part or whole for the increased risk of thromboembolism associated with 'pill' administration. Claims have, however, been made by the manufacturers that the so-called 'natural' conjugated estrogens derived from equine urine (Premarin), do not cause

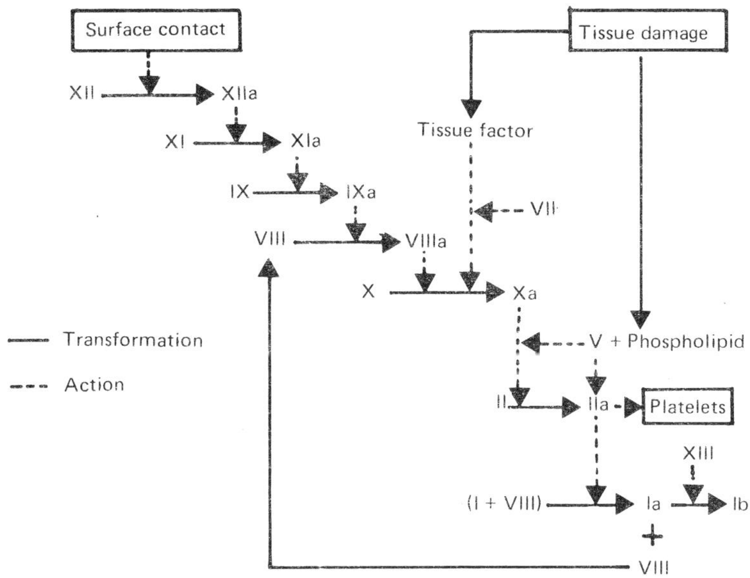

Figure 27.1 Blood coagulation mechanism

acceleration of blood clotting. These important claims required confirmation by laboratory study. Particular importance arose from the long-term use of these so-called 'natural' estrogens in women of the older age groups where the incidence of thromboembolism is greater.

The present, double-blind cross-over study in patients from a single group practice given natural estrogens and placebo alternately was designed to discover first whether menopausal symptoms respond to estrogens and whether there were adverse effects on blood clotting. Blood clotting tests and platelet aggregation studies were performed before starting and during the period of the double-blind study.

This presentation is confined to the coagulation and platelet results, the other results being discussed by Dr. Coope.

Method of study

The women came from a single, mixed rural and industrial practice composed of 6500 patients. They presented at the surgery with a variety of symptoms which were considered to be due to the menopause.

30 women participated in the study with ages ranging from 40 to 61, the mean being 52.

All patients came to the haematology laboratory at Withington Hospital, Manchester for their blood tests.

The trial was conducted on a double-blind cross-over basis. Cases were randomly allocated to two groups each consisting of 15 patients.

One group received natural conjugated equine estrogens (Premarin 1·25 mg) daily for 21 days, for three courses, with a break of 7 days in between each course. This group was then given placebo tablets containing lactose with the same coating as the Premarin, in the same dosage for a similar period. The other group received placebo first and the natural conjugated estrogens subsequently.

The patients were informed that they would be given a 3 months' course of hormone and 3 months of an inert preparation. The patients, the medical and the coagulation laboratory staff were not informed of the order of the treatment.

Blood clotting and platelet studies

The following tests were performed before starting and during the final week of both estrogen and placebo administration: prothrombin time; kaolin-activated partial thromboplastin (cephalin) time; factor VII assay, factor X assay.

The following were also performed on each occasion: thrombelastography; (r); (*k* value) and (ma value); platelet aggregation time (Chandler's tube technique); haemoglobin and platelet count.

Results

Full clinical and laboratory results have been described elsewhere[7].

PROTHROMBIN TIME

Figure 27.2 shows there was a significant difference between the base-line results and the treated group at the 3-month stage and between the treated group and the placebo series after a similar time interval. There was, however, no significant difference between the placebo group and their base-line prothrombin time.

PARTIAL THROMBOPLASTIN (CEPHALIN) TIME

There was no significant change in either group during the period of study.

FACTOR VII ASSAY

The results are illustrated in Figure 27.3. There was a significant difference between the base-line factor VII assay and the results in the same women after 3 months' estrogens. The placebo group also gave a result which just reached the significance level but when the group was sub-divided further into those who had received estrogen first and those who had placebo first, only the former were significantly increased, i.e. the significant increase in factor VII was only found in the women who had received a 3 months' course of the estrogen and there was a carry-over of the raised VII levels for a further 3 months.

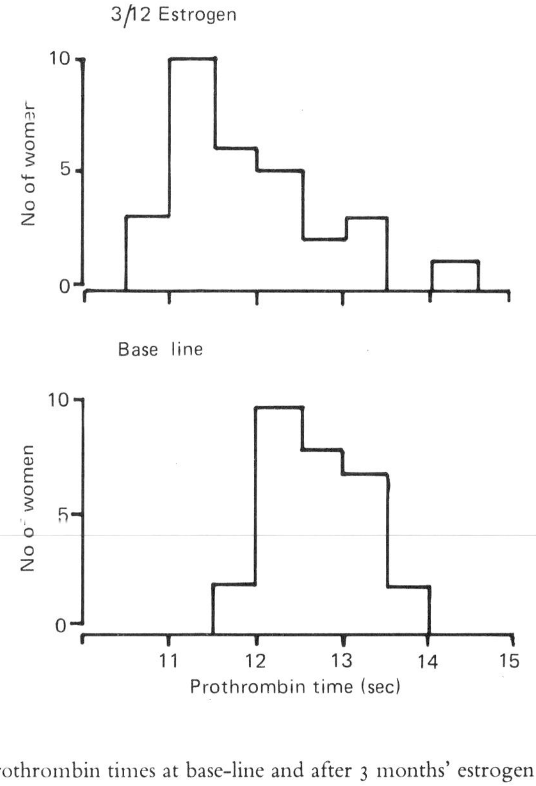

Figure 27.2 Prothrombin times at base-line and after 3 months' estrogen administration

FACTOR X ASSAY

Results are given in Figure 27.4. The factor X assays showed a significant difference between the estrogen group and the base-line readings, but again no significant difference was observed between the natural estrogen group and the placebo. Half of the latter group had of course received 3 months of estrogen replacement prior to placebo and there was thus again evidence of an effect 3 months after withdrawal.

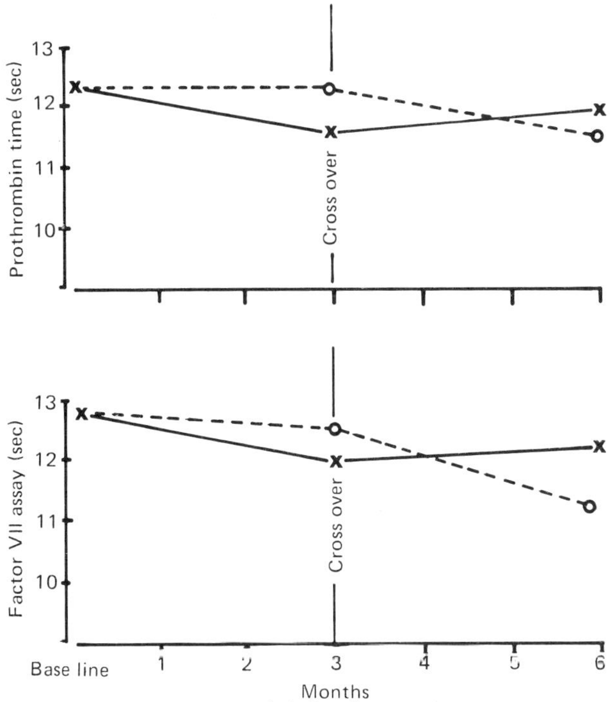

Figure 27.3 Prothrombin times and factor VII levels during the trial. X—X estrogen first, O - - - - O placebo first

THROMBELASTROGRAPHY

There was no significant change in either group in the three parameters measured during the period of study.

PLATELET AGGREGATION STUDIES (CHANDLER'S TUBE TECHNIQUE)

There was no significant difference between the base-line results and the estrogen and placebo groups during the respective 3-months' administration.

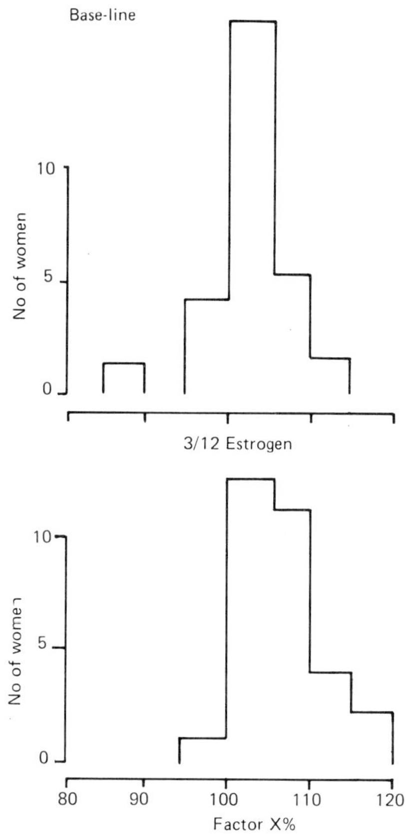

Figure 27.4 Factor X levels

HAEMOGLOBIN AND PLATELET COUNT
There was no significant alteration in the above, in either group.

Comments

This investigation of the effects of natural estrogen replacement in menopausal women has produced interesting findings both from the clinical standpoint and also from the study of blood clotting.

The clinical changes were complicated and masked by the placebo response. Unequivocal results, however, arose from the effects of natural estrogens on blood coagulation. It has been widely claimed, without adequate laboratory data, that natural estrogens had little or no effect on coagulation in contrast to synthetic estrogens which raise levels of certain clotting factors.

The findings of our present study are therefore disturbing. After only 3 months' natural estrogen there was a marked acceleration of extrinsic clotting shown by the prothrombin times and factor VII assays. Factor X, which is involved in both extrinsic and intrinsic clotting was also significantly increased. The adverse effects on clotting are substantially similar to those we have previously described after the identical period of synthetic estrogen–progestogen oral contraceptive administration[2] (Figure 27.5) and contrast unfavourably with the lack of acceleration of blood clotting previously found by us with the progestogen-only contraceptives, chlormadinone and norethisterone at the same stage[7].

In our earlier studies changes following administration of conventional oral contraceptives became progressively more marked after 3 months and

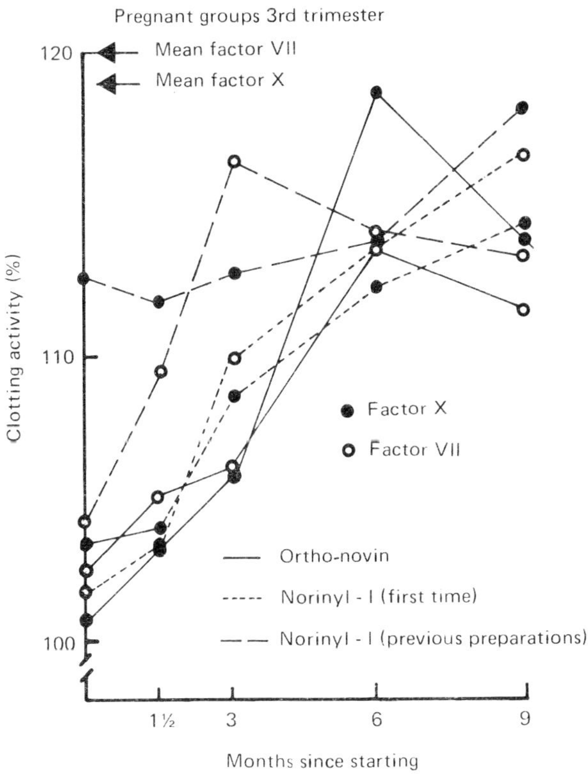

Figure 27.5 Factor VII and factor X levels following combined estrogen/progestogen administration in a related study

involved a wider spectrum of tests and platelet function[2]. Further studies are in progress to determine whether the adverse effects of natural estrogens on blood clotting show a similar progression.

The incidence of thromboembolism increases with age, and in menopausal women who are a substantially older group than women on oral contraceptives the acceleration of clotting during estrogen therapy must give rise to concern although they are not necessarily synonymous with a thrombotic tendency. In these older women, moreover, there is no compensatory reduction in mortality and morbidity from the thromboembolism associated with pregnancy, such as is the case with younger women taking oral contraceptives. There was, in fact, an appreciable incidence of superficial venous thrombosis in this study. Four cases occurred in the 30 women during the 6 months' period although there was no obvious bias to either placebo or estrogen groups. The numbers are of course too small to draw any conclusions on the danger of thrombosis from natural estrogens and this can only be derived from larger, long-term epidemiological studies which appear to be urgently required.

Finally, it must be emphasized that the results of this double-blind study only monitor changes for a 3-month period of estrogen administration. Most of the patients are now receiving long-term replacement and are being followed up. The incidence of thromboembolism with long-term therapy requires adequate assessment. It is also necessary to determine whether more marked changes in blood clotting and platelet function will result from longer periods of estrogen administration.

References

1. Poller, L. (1973). Oral contraception and blood clotting. In *Recent Advances in Thrombosis* (Edinburgh: Churchill-Livingstone)
2. Poller, L. and Thomson, Jean M. (1972). The partial thromboplastin time test. *J. Clin. Pathol.*, **25,** 1038
3. Poller, L., Thomson, Jean M. and Sear, C. H. J. (1971). The identification of a congenital defect of factor VII in beagle dogs. *J. Clin. Pathol.*, **24,** 626
4. Poller, L., Thomson, Jean M., Tabiowo, A. and Priest, Celia N. (1969). Progesterone oral contraception and blood coagulation. *Br. Med. J.*, **1,** 554
5. Poller, L., Thomson, Jean M. and Thomas, P. W. (1972). Effects of progestogen oral contraception with Norethisterone on blood clotting and platelets. *Br. Med. J.*, **4,** 391
6. Coope, Jean, Thomson, Jean M. and Poller, L. (1965). The effects of natural oestrogen replacement therapy on menopausal symptoms and blood clotting. *Br. Med. J.*, **4,** 155
7. Thomson, Jean M. and Poller, L. (1965). Oral contraceptive hormones and blood coagulability. *Br. Med. J.*, **2,** 231

28

Effects of synthetic and natural estrogens on the coagulation system in post-menopausal women

J. Bonnar

The effects of hormones on the blood clotting system can be studied in two different ways. The first involves detailed laboratory studies of hormones in small groups of women to define any consistent effects on the proteins concerned with blood coagulation. The second involves epidemiological studies in a large population to determine the incidence of thrombosis in women taking hormones compared with a matched population of women not using such therapy. The controlled studies carried out by the Royal College of General Practitioners in the United Kingdom and by Sartwell and his co-workers in the United States indicate that during the reproductive years the risk of developing deep vein thrombosis and pulmonary embolism is increased at least five-fold by the use of oral contraceptives[1]. The epidemiological data on the thromboembolic complications associated with oral contraception did not become available until almost 15 years after the introduction of oral contraception. If, as seems likely, estrogen replacement therapy after the menopause is to be used on a scale as great as oral contraception, it is important that the effects of this therapy on the clotting system in post-menopausal women should be carefully investigated, as this may assist in the development of formulations which do not increase the risk of thrombosis. In this way, we may avoid exposing millions of women to the risk of thromboembolism. We have investigated three formulations of estrogen therapy, which are used in post-menopausal women to determine their effects on certain coagulation factors and inhibitors.

Patients and methods

Three groups of women with menopausal complaints were investigated. The characteristic presenting symptoms of all the patients were hot flushes, sweats and palpitations, together with a variety of other symptoms, which included forgetfulness, vertigo, headache, insomnia, fatigue, nervousness, depression and joint aches. The patients were asked to take no other medication for the duration of the study and anyone receiving cortico-steroids, psychotropic drugs or antibiotics was excluded. Patients with organic gynaecological disorders or breast disease, cardiovascular disease, blood dyscrasias, liver dysfunction, renal disease and previous thromboembolic disorders were also excluded. Three hormonal formulations were investigated as follows:

1. *Sequential mestranol (Menophase)*

This sequential preparation which contains both mestranol and norethisterone was given in 28-day packs. Venous blood samples were taken for measurement of coagulation factors and inhibitors and plasma levels of luteinizing hormone (LH) and follicle stimulating hormone (FSH). The plasma LH and FSH were measured by double antibody radioimmunoassay; the standards used in the hormone assays have been described elsewhere[2]. Coagulation factors II, V, VIII, IX, X, VII and X complex, and coagulation inhibitors antithrombin III and anti factor Xa were assayed by methods described by Biggs[3]. 15 women received treatment with Menophase for a period of 6 months and the hormone and coagulation factor assays were carried out as follows: Before treatment, after 1, 2, 4 and 6 months of treatment, and two months after the hormone therapy was discontinued. The mean age of the women was 55 years (S.D. = 6).

2. *Estradiol valerate (Progynova 2 mg) and*
3. *Conjugated estrogens (Premarin 1·25 mg)*

The effect of these preparations was investigated over a 14-week period with coagulation factor assays before treatment, after 6, 10 and 14 weeks of treatment and 6–8 weeks after the hormone therapy had been discontinued. Coagulation factors II, V, VIII, VII and X complex, factor X and the coagulation inhibitor antithrombin III were measured. 16 women taking Progynova were studied (mean age 51 years, S.D. = 3·5) and 17 women taking Premarin (mean age 49 years, S.D. = 5).

Statistical analysis of results

Wilcoxon's signed Rank's test and Student's t test were used to determine the statistical significance of changes in the clotting factors.

Results

1. *Sequential mestranol (menophase)*

Out of the 15 patients admitted to this study, four were excluded in the final analysis as two of these patients were found to have low levels of LH and FSH and enquiry revealed that they were both taking other hormonal preparations (Mixogen). A further two patients did not complete the study. Figure 28.1 shows the mean levels of the gonadotrophin hormones in the women who were treated with Menophase. The elevated levels of LH and FSH decreased during the first 2 months of treatment to the pre-menopausal range and 2 months after treatment was discontinued, the levels had returned to the pre-treatment value. Figure 28.2 shows the serial changes of coagulation factors X, VII and X complex and factor IX. The pre-treatment levels

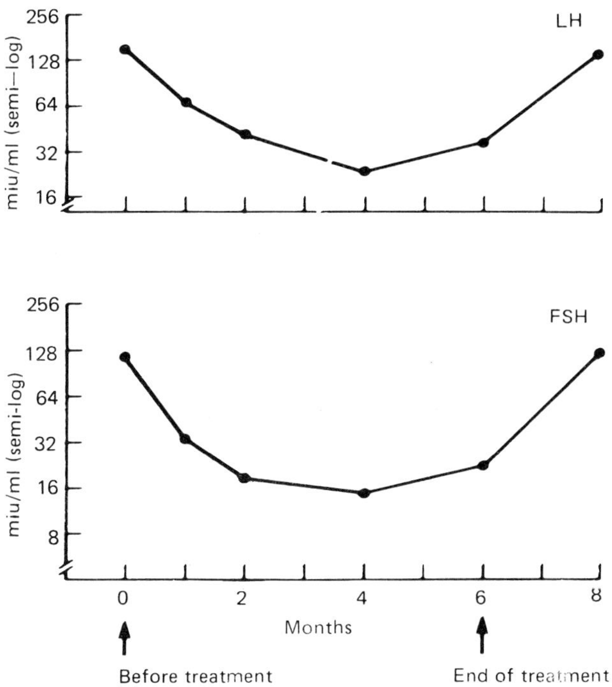

Figure 28.1 Effect of sequential mestranol/norethisterone on plasma levels of luteinizing hormone (LH) and follicle stimulating hormone (FSH)

of the coagulation factors for each patient were expressed as 100% and the subsequent percentage changes calculated on this basis. Factor X showed a sharp increase and after 2 months' therapy had risen to mean value of 162% ($p < 0{\cdot}02$). The levels of factor X subsequently showed a significant decrease and after 6 months therapy the mean value was 122%. Factor IX also increased, but not as rapidly as factor X and the highest mean value of 138% was found after 6 months of treatment. Factor VII and X complex increased during the first 4 months of treatment, but after 6 months had returned to the pre-treatment range. 2 months after discontinuing the

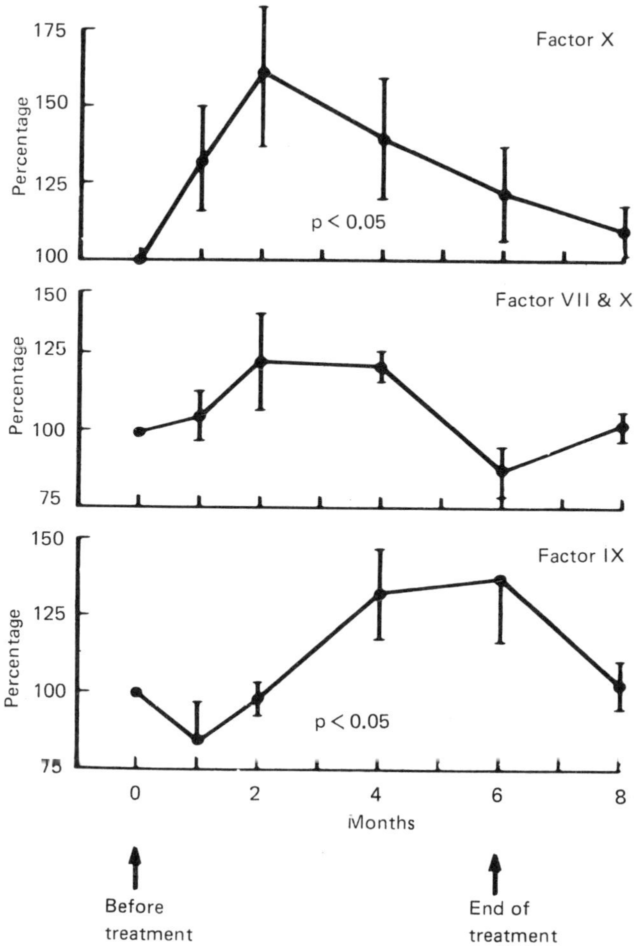

Figure 28.2 Effect of mestranol/norethisterone on vitamin K dependent factors in post-menopausal women

hormone therapy, the coagulation factors had returned to their pre-treatment values. Figure 28.3 shows the levels of factor V and factor VIII; no significant change was detected with factor V and with factor VIII a significant decrease was detected after 2 months' treatment but not at any other time.

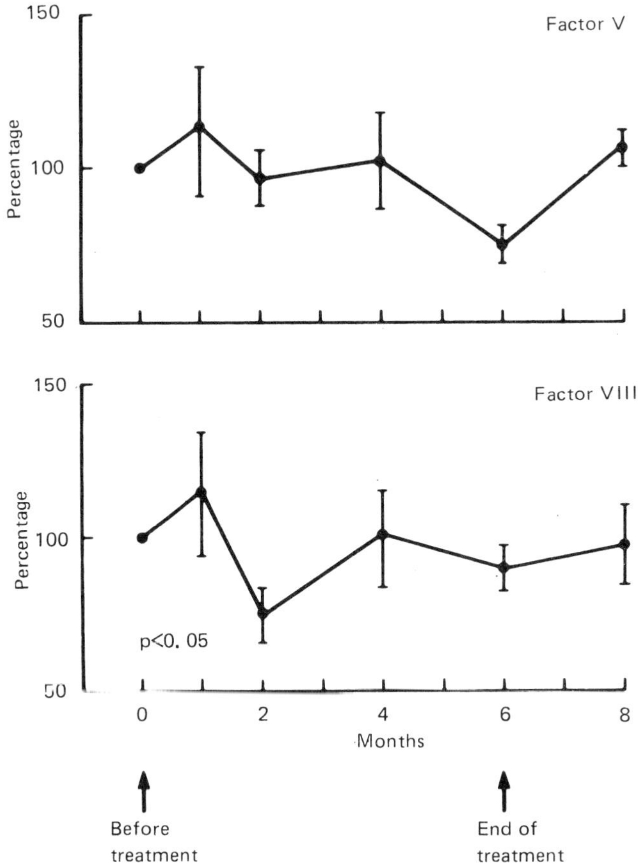

Figure 28.3 Effect of mestranol/norethisterone on coagulation factors V and VIII in post-menopausal women.

Figure 28.4 shows the serial changes of the coagulation inhibitors anti-factor Xa and anti-thrombin III; as shown the levels of both these inhibitors decreased during the months of treatment and this was most marked with anti-factor Xa, the mean value decreasing to 82% after 1 month of treatment.

The lowest value of anti-thrombin III detected was 89% after 2 months' treatment. The levels of anti-factor Xa had returned to the normal pre-treatment values two months after the therapy was discontinued.

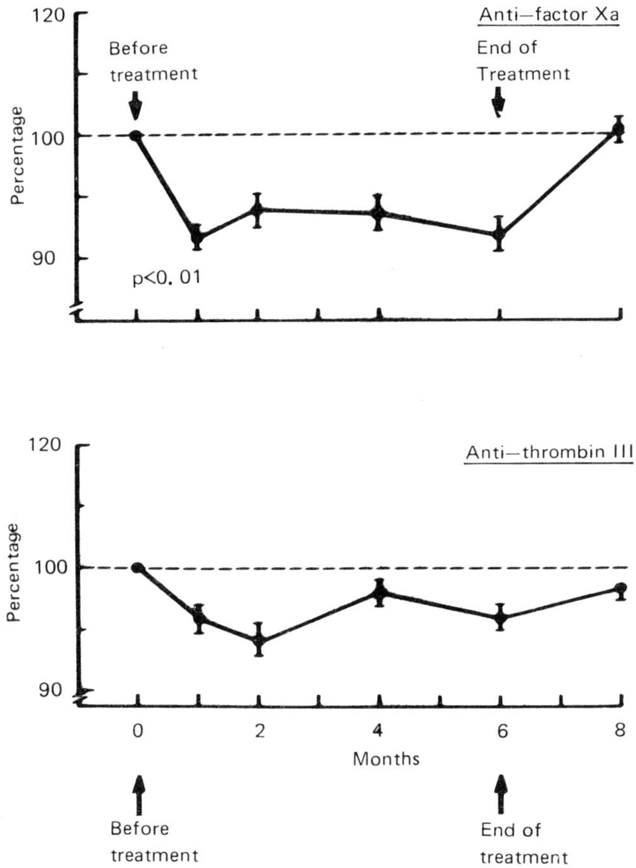

Figure 28.4 Effect of mestranol/norethisterone on coagulation inhibitors in post-menopausal women

2. *Estradiol valerate* (*Progynova 2 mg*) and

3. *Conjugated estrogens* (*Premarin*)

Figure 28.5 shows the serial levels of factor II, factor X and VII and X complex. A rise of factor II and factor X was found during treatment with estradiol valerate and the values were still elevated 6–8 weeks after treatment. No increase was found with factor II and factor X during treatment with conjugated estrogens, but a rise of the VII and X complex was found with both preparations and this was highly significant in the women receiving estradiol valerate. As shown in Figure 28.6 no evidence of depression of anti-thrombin III was found in the women receiving estradiol valerate and conjugated estrogens.

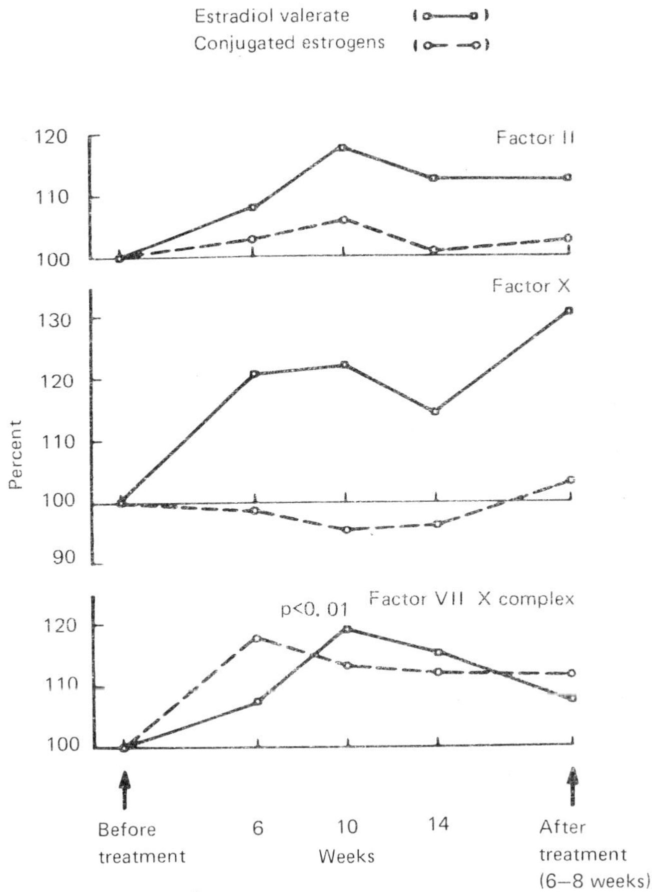

Figure 28.5 Effect of estradiol valerate (2 mg) and conjugated estrogens (1·25 mg) on coagulation factors II, X, and VII and X complex.

Discussion and conclusion

Estrogen preparations present considerable problems in terms of comparing the potency of the various formulations. The women who received treatment with Menophase had up to 50 μg of mestranol B.P. and norethisterone up to 1 mg, the dosage of these hormones being varied to mimic the levels of estrogen and progesterone which occur in the normal menstrual cycle.

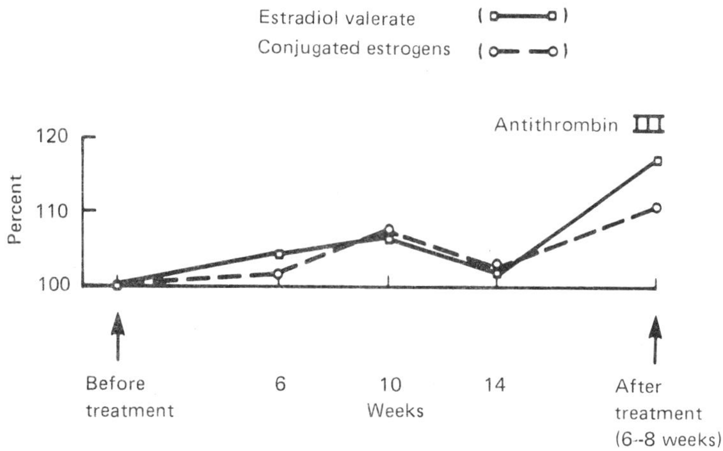

Figure 28.6 Effect of estradiol valerate (2 mg) and conjugated estrogens on levels of antithrombin III

The women receiving Progynova had estradiol valerate 2 mg which would be equivalent to 50 μg of ethinyl estradiol. The patients on conjugated estrogens (Premarin 1·25 mg) were receiving estrogen which would have approximately half the potency of the other preparations, at around 25 μg of ethinyl estradiol.

Of the three preparations studied the formulation containing mestranol had the most marked effect on the coagulation system, with a sharp increase of vitamin K dependent factors, particularly factor X and a significant decrease of the coagulation inhibitors anti-thrombin III and anti-Xa. The changes induced with estradiol valerate and conjugated estrogens were less apparent. Both hormones appeared to produce a rise of factor VII and X complex and in the patients receiving estradiol valerate a rise of factor X but neither of these two preparations was shown to have any effect on the levels of anti-thrombin III.

A state of homeostatic balance appears to exist in the plasma between the clot promoting potential and the inhibitors of clotting. If this balance is deviated towards an increase of the clotting potential and a decrease of the inhibitors, then it is reasonable to deduce that such a change will predispose to thrombosis, given a trigger stimulus to activate the coagulation system. The basic assumption in this type of study is that the increase of coagulation factors and reduction of anti-thrombotic activity in the blood may be equated with the hyper-coaguable state or a thrombotic tendency. Definite clotting changes develop in women taking estrogen containing preparations for oral contraception and epidemiological evidence has shown that such medication carried a proven thrombotic risk. Hormones or combinations which from clotting studies, do not produce these untoward changes, may therefore be less thrombogenic in clinical usage.

The findings of the present study give every reason to suspect that the use of synthetic estrogen preparations will carry a thrombogenic hazard and our own results would suggest that mestranol may be more hazardous than estradiol valerate.

Apart from a slight rise of the VII and X complex we were not able to detect other changes with conjugated estrogens. The women studied during treatment with coagulated estrogens, however, were receiving approximately half of the amount of estrogen to those taking mestranol and estradiol valerate. In a higher dosage, a different effect might well be found with conjugated estrogens. In the control and safety of drug and hormonal formulations for post-menopausal women, it would seem that some attention should be paid to their thrombogenic potential before these preparations are made available for widespread use. If we are to learn anything from the experience with oral contraception there is an overwhelming case for setting up forthwith a controlled prospective study and a register of all post-menopausal women in the British Isles, receiving estrogen therapy to carefully document both the beneficial effects and any adverse effects such as thromboembolic disease and vascular complications. The Royal College of General Practitioners and Royal College of Gynaecologists would seem the appropriate bodies with the expertise for this important study.

Acknowledgment

This work was supported by research grants from Syntex Pharmaceuticals Ltd. and by Schering Chemicals Ltd.

References

1. Vessey, M. P. (1973). The epidemiology of venous thromboembolism. In: *Recent Advances in Thrombosis*. Editor, L. Poller (London, Churchill-Livingstone)
2. Bonnar, J., Franklin, M., Nott, P. N. and McNeilly, A. S. (1975). Effect of breast feeding on pituitary ovarian function after childbirth. *Br. Med. J.*, **4**, 82
3. Biggs, R. (1972). *Human Blood Coagulation, Haemostasis and Thrombosis*. (Oxford: Blackwell Scientific Publications), p. 602–647

Discussion on Section H:

Risks of Estrogen Therapy (Part 1) Thromboembolism

Chairman: *Mr S. Campbell*

Mr J. Maddison (Community Medicine, Twickenham): I have been working on HRT for almost 18 years and I have treated between 3000 and 4000 women, nearly all of them with Premarin, and I have never had a single case of thrombosis in all that time.

Mr S. Campbell (Chairman): And have detailed follow-up studies been carried out on all those patients?

Mr J. Maddison: Yes. Many of them have been on the therapy for 15 or 16 years and some of them are well into their seventies, and even approaching 80.

Mr S. Campbell (Chairman): That would be well worth publishing.

Mr E. S. Saunders (Gynaecologist, London): Any kind of estrogen that is swallowed goes to the liver, where it is split up into different fractions. Which of those fractions is responsible for the coagulopathy, we do not know. We have tried to bypass this by treating patients with implants, parenterally. We would be most interested to hear of a comparative study of the effects on coagulation by oral application and by means of parenteral treatment.

Dr L. Poller (Haematologist, Manchester): Dr Coope will confirm that there were four cases of superficial thrombophlebitis in our 30 patients: something not to be lightly disregarded.

Secondly, parenteral estrogens have been used as haemostatics for a considerable time. There is no doubt that parenteral administration of estrogen has an effect on blood coagulation.

Professor J. Bonnar (Gynaecologist, Dublin): I am interested that someone has treated 3000 to 4000 patients for a substantial number of years, and I hope that he has records, because that is what we need.

I would be the first to say that if the epidemiological studies show that the natural estrogens are free of thromboembolic hazards, then they may well be a major advance in therapy for women. Nonetheless, in 3000–4000 women, some of them approaching 70, one would have expected two or three instances of thromboembolic complications, even without estrogen therapy. Suffice to say that we cannot draw conclusions from the small studies. We need large population studies.

Parenteral estrogens are interesting. We have studied estradiol implants, but the study was complicated by the fact that the implants were put in at hysterectomy, and the operation of hysterectomy induces fairly extensive coagulation changes. The estradiol implant appeared to have less effect on coagulation, and that could reflect its very slow rate of release.

When I talk about clotting, I am not really referring to short-term courses treating women with severe symptoms. We all know that they need treatment. I am referring to the blanket, prolonged, 10–20 years therapy which to my mind has a big question mark opposite it.

Mr S. Campbell: Dr Poller mentioned cases of superficial thrombophlebitis. Mr McQueen has some information from our study at Chelsea Hospital for Women.

Mr J. McQueen (Gynaecologist, London): It is postulated that estrogen treatment is associated with an increased risk of venous thrombosis. Leg scanning employing fibrinogen labelled with iodine-125 has been shown to be a reliable means of detecting subclinical calf vein thrombosis (Negus, D., Pinto, D. J., Le Quesne, L. P., Brown, N. and Chapman, M. (1968). *Br. J. Surg.*, **55**, 835) and in our hospital we have considerable experience at detecting subclinical postoperative thromboses employing this sensitive test (McCarthy, T. G., McQueen, J., Johnstone, F. D., Weston, J. and Campbell, S. (1974). *J. Obstet. Gynaecol. Br. Commonwlth.*, **81**, 486).

During our double-blind cross-over trial using conjugated estrogens, 1·25 mg cyclically, versus a placebo, we performed the test three times on each patient, that is on admission to the trial, and within the last 2 weeks of each 6-month period of treatment.

Iodone-125 labelled fibrinogen was given intravenously, and the scanning was performed after 3 days. This would detect any forming thrombus. In 124 scans, on 50 patients, we found no evidence of leg vein thrombosis, and at no stage in the trial did any of our patients develop clinical evidence of deep or superficial vein thrombosis. Since we have finished the trial, we have had three patients who complained of calf tenderness and pain. We performed a scan within 48 hours of the pain, and detected no evidence of deep vein thrombosis.

Professor J. Bonnar: Were these patients subject to surgery?

Mr S. Campbell: No.

Dr P. Bye (Schering Chemicals, Sussex): Professor Bonnar has pointed out that he—and no doubt everybody else—is not concerned solely with the effects in the short term on the coagulation factors, but they want to know what the long-term epidemiological consequences will be.

No one has today mentioned one very important aspect of this. Professor Oliver talked about the differences in the incidence of coronary disease between men and women, and how the graphs converged in old age. It is clear that we cannot blame this convergence on estrogens since estrogen levels are declining in the older age group. What other factor then is coming into this? If we bear in mind the evidence of Elkeles, who in 1967 studied X-rays of the abdominal aorta in women, and found that in the 50–60 age group the incidence of calcification was 25% in males, and 13% in females, but that after the age of 60 the incidence was 70% in females and 41% in males, then we can see that atherosclerosis is, as we have long been taught, the dominant factor in causing vascular complications in old age. Therefore, it may well be that with HRT even if we are losing something in the short term on the swings of coagulation problems, we are gaining more on the roundabouts of atherosclerosis prevention in the long term.

Professor J. Bonnar: The only worry about that is that estrogens made no difference to the incidence in men; all they did was to give the men thrombosis, and thromboembolism.

Mr S. Campbell: These were synthetic estrogens.

Dr P. A. van Keep (Gynaecologist, Geneva): There are some major series of patients, such as those of Burch and Byrd who studied 11 000 women-years treated with conjugated estrogens in the post-menopause. The study recorded cause of death and the occurrence of all kinds of phenomena, but has not specifically recorded thromboembolic phenomena, and has observed them only extremely rarely.

Might there perhaps be a difference between what is seen in the United Kingdom and abroad? My colleagues, when I discussed this before, all agreed that thromboembolic episodes in women in the post-menopause, treated with estrogen, are extremely rare. The question has been asked at various similar meetings, and no one could recall such a case. Might there be some different effect as between the United Kingdom and other countries.

Mr S. Campbell: I do not thank that there is any data from this country on the incidence of thromboembolism with HRT, but would the panel comment.

Professor J. Bonnar: I would go back to the contraceptive pill. It was the United Kingdom which, against tremendous denials and condemnations from across the Atlantic, put out the data, which eventually proved to be correct. This is an island, and people are well followed up in Britain. If people die, we know about it. In many countries of the world, this is not so. I would honestly respect the epidemiological work in Britain as of a scientific calibre that is probably second to none. Not only that, I would add that such work is often carried out in university departments and is not out to prove anything. It is hard work, often involving general practitioners, and only by doing such studies can we get the facts.

With the pill and with post-menopausal estrogens we are speaking in terms of millions of women; we are not talking about a couple of hundred here, and a couple of hundred there. When we put such a therapy as HRT out for widespread use, for prolonged use, we must have pause for thought and reappraisal. That is the point I would wish to make on the basis of the laboratory data so far produced.

Dr L. Poller: When questions were raised about the pill, it was not until specific studies were made with particular reference to pill administration that the truth emerged. Although there was a vast amount of banked data which one would have thought might have answered these questions, it was just not reliable. It did not reflect the true incidence of venous thromboembolism in the population.

Dr P. A. van Keep: Professor Bonnar has not been completely fair. On the Continent too, good research is done and I should remind you that it was clincians who first drew our attention to the risk of thromboembolism during oral contraception and that it was epidemiologists who confirmed this, and not haematologists.

Mr B. Eton (Gynaecologist, Hastings): With the pill we have learned that the risks of thromboembolism are dose-related. Professor Bonnar has said that the effect of 1·25 mg Premarin corresponds roughly in its thrombogenic effects to about 25 μg ethinyl estradiol.

Professor J. Bonnar: I did not say thrombogenic effect; I said estrogen potency.

Mr B. Eton: In that case, 0·625 mg Premarin, for instance, must correspond in potency to only 12·5 μg ethinyl estradiol, which is a very small dose compared to the common contents of the contraceptive pill, and we can assume, therefore, that the effect on the coagulation factors must also be very much reduced.

Professor J. Bonnar: That is a difficult one to answer. I do not know if it would be an effective therapeutic dose. When the pill came in, we were using potencies of hormones vastly in excess of what was required. Almost every 3 months we get a new pill with less and less in it, and this has been happening for 3 or 4 years. Most of the pills introduced originally have now been withdrawn. I am worried that we shall make the same mistake with the post-menopausal estrogens. Could we get the work done now to look at the effects, and identify the hormones and dosages which appear to provide minimum disturbance of areas such as coagulation and perhaps use those? Hopefully we should find an effective dose that does not have a thrombogenic potential.

Dr R. C. Greenberg (Community Psychiatrist, London): I can summarize the last MRC Report on coronary thrombosis in two sentences. As far as I understand it, it says: 'If an apple a day does not keep the doctor away, an aspirin a day keeps the second coronary away'. What is the view about the use of aspirin as an interim prophylactic measure where pills of this kind are being used?

Dr L. Poller: I reserve judgement on the value of aspirin. It is very effective compared with conventional anticoagulants, which themselves tend to be of limited value in the prevention of arterial thrombosis. I am not at all happy about the role of aspirin. It is a very dangerous drug!

Mr E. van Hall (University of Leiden): When we talk about the frequency of thromboembolic processes, we nearly always think only about leg vein thrombosis I would point out another possibility. There are neurologists who have the impression that an increased frequency of small cerebral accidents can occur which are not clinically obvious, but which can have very important social consequences. When people report on studies to the effect that they have never seen a case of thromboembolism, such a possibility should perhaps be kept in mind.

Professor J. Bonnar: I agree. I hope that we shall move away one day from learning at the expense of patients. We should pay some attention to history, and the day is over when we can say: 'I have treated so many and I have had no problems'. Maternal deaths in this country are few and far between, but they still occur. Very few doctors ever see any, but that does not mean to say that they do not exist.

Surgeon Lt. Cdr. P. R. Brinsden (Gynaecologist, Royal Navy): Our colleagues in the United States have been using these drugs for 10 to 15 years or more and I cannot believe that they have been doing so without making some epidemiological studies. Can the panel, or any members of the audience, quote any figures, to help us to put this into perspective, since we only seem to be starting in this field.

Professor J. Bonnar: The only long-term studies in the States on estrogens have been on oral contraception. Sartwell and his colleagues (Sartwell, P. E. and Anello, C. (1969). In: *The Second Report on the Oral Contraceptives by the Advisory Committee on Obstetrics and Gynecology*. U.S. Department of Health, Education and Welfare, Food and Drug Admin. Washington, D.C.) have figures similar to those from Oxford namely a fivefold increase in thromboembolic complications.

The epidemiological studies on post-menopausal estrogens have not yet been completed and there are very few of them in existence. Keep in mind that the patients on which these drugs are being used—largely in the private sector in the United States—are not usually the subject of such studies.

Mr S. Campbell: There is the well-known Boston Collaborative Survey of patients who were mainly on Premarin, which did not show a significant increase in thrombo-embolic disease, but there are criticisms of this study, and Dr Oliver mentioned them this morning.

Dr Jean Coope (General Practitioner, Bollington): I should like to comment on the study by Burch, J. C., Byrd B. F. and Vaughn, W. K. (1974). The effects of long-term estrogen on hysterectomized women. *Am. J. Obstet. Gynecol.*, **118,** 778 which con-concerns a great number of post-hysterectomy cases who were treated with estrogens over a very long time. In that study there was no comparison of data from that group with data from a comparable control group. The mortality rates were compared with those in the general population: The patients involved were probably social class 1, very wealthy private patients, and the mortality rate from carcinoma, or from any other pathology cannot be compared with the rate in the general population in a country like the U.S.A.

Dr Gahwyler (Ayerst Laboratories, New York): A question has been raised about some studies done in the United States, and I should like to refer to a study published recently by the Kaiser Foundation and Health Service in California. The study was a prospective study on 4000 healthy women of reproductive age and a similar number of women in an age group 40–45 and upwards with 2500 controls, about 1300 on oral contraceptives and about 400 on oral estrogens for replacement therapy. They studied only one criterion, that is thromboembolism in all these women, prospectively, over a period of 3 years. They found that there was a statistically significant difference between the control group and the group on the O.Cs, but the estrogen replacement therapy group, which admittedly was small, did not show any difference in the incidence of thromboembolism. It is the first published study that I have seen, but I know of several large institutions that are trying to do such epidemiological studies now.

Mr S. Campbell: We must repeat the call for long-term epidemiological studies. As a doctor running his own menopause clinic, I should like to stress that we should not regard all post-menopausal women as a homogenous population, and that we should assess them for risk factors such as hypertension and history of thromboembolism and also for endogenous estrogen production if vasomotor symptoms are not present.

Secondly we should warn all patients about possible thromboembolic complications. I personally do that in my clinic, and not one single patient has opted not to go on the treatment, despite my warnings. Maybe I do not warn them as sternly as Professor Bonnar would like me to, but I think that we should do it, and that we should always use the smallest doses of estrogen consistent with the elimination of symptoms.

Section H

RISKS OF ESTROGEN THERAPY

PART 2: *CANCER*

Chairman: R. B. K. RICKFORD

29

The effects of estrogen replacement therapy on the risk of cancer during the post-menopausal years

C. J. Dewhurst

The two organs which it has been suggested have a raised cancer risk as a result of estrogen therapy given to post-menopausal women are the uterus and breast. In this paper I will concentrate more on the former than on the latter since the breast is the subject of the paper which follows this one.

I am going to suggest that we do not know whether prolonged estrogen therapy *alone*, and I stress the word 'alone', after the menopause predisposes to uterine cancer. One reason why we do not know is that a number of the papers customarily quoted when this matter is considered do not concern estrogen therapy alone but cyclical estrogen and progestogen therapy. Progestogens are known to have a destructive effect upon endometrial carcinoma[1–3] even though the carcinoma may be in an advanced stage; moreover, so far as I am aware, cyclic estrogen and progesterone therapy has been linked with the causation of endometrial cancer on only one occasion[4]. It is important, therefore, to ensure that any papers which are being considered as to the safety or otherwise of estrogen therapy are those which concern estrogen therapy alone.

Let us first consider some background information. It has been maintained by a number of authors over the years that estrogen therapy, if unopposed, may lead to endometrial hyperplasia and ultimately to carcinoma[5–10]. It has also been shown that in young women who suffer for several years from dysfunctional uterine bleeding in which unopposed estrogen stimulation is almost certainly a feature, have developed adenocarcinoma of the uterine body; four women with such adolescent dysfunctional bleeding reported by Southam and Richert[11] developed adenocarcinoma of the uterine body at the ages 23, 29, 30 and 33. Other examples of adenocarcinoma of the uterine body in relatively young patients with gonadal dysgenesis treated by unopposed estrogen therapy have also been reported[12–16]. The average age at which the cancer developed in these latter patients with gonadal dysgenesis was only some 30 years which is many years earlier than the average age of corpus cancer in other circumstances. Although most of such cases have received large doses of estrogens for long periods of time a more recent report[17] indicates that much smaller doses such as ethinyl estradiol 0·02 mg daily can produce cystic glandular hyperplasia after only 3 or 4 years' treatment. A further point to be considered is that adenocarcinoma of the uterus has been associated with the presence of estrogen-producing tumours of the ovary in some 15–27% of post -menopausal women with this type of feminizing tumour[18].

With this general background it is perhaps surprising that papers which have been devoted to the supposed cancer risk in patients receiving prolonged estrogen therapy do not appear to show a raised risk of uterine carcinoma. Let us look at some of the reasons why this might be so.

I would like to consider in certain detail five papers devoted to the incidence of uterine cancer in post-menopausal patients treated with estrogens[19–24].

The paper by Schleyer-Saunders[24] gives only the most sketchy details of the dosage and duration of estrogen treatment among 500 patients. The paper states that no patient developed cancer 'that could be attributed to estrogens'. The same author in a later paper[25] reports that uterine cancer developed in two patients in the first 150 treated patients and two others in a second group of 470 patients. The period of time considered in the second paper is longer than in the first and it is possible that the two cases of uterine cancer in the second group of 470 were not included in the first paper which dealt with 500; however, the two cases of uterine cancer which occurred in the first group of 150 must have been included in the first paper by Schleyer-Saunders. It is not easy, therefore, to understand the original comment made that 'no patient developed cancer that could be attributed to estrogens' except by assuming that the two cancers which did occur were not thought to be related to the estrogen therapy and no attempt is made to justify this view. A further point of criticism of these papers is that close scrutiny does not provide reassurance that there was detailed follow-up nor objective scientific assessment of the patients and a large question mark must hang over these results.

The second paper frequently considered is that by Geist *et al.*[23] who reviewed 206 women who received estrogen injections for from 6 months to

$5\frac{1}{2}$ years. There was no case of cancer in the group. Details are few and the frequency of injections is not given and dosages varied. It will be noted here that although some patients were treated for 5 years or more many must have been treated for far shorter periods of time, perhaps 6 months only. Within such a relatively short period of time it is perhaps not surprising that no case of cancer developed and it is not reassuring to read the author's comments that the continued administration of estrogens usually resulted in an appearance of cystic endometrial glands resembling the swiss-cheese pattern. As the precise duration of treatment in these patients is unknown and in many must have been short, very little reassurance can be gained from this paper. This is especially the case when we remember that the patients with gonadal dysgenesis who developed endometrial carcinoma in association with estrogen therapy had been treated for an average time of 10 years.

A third frequently quoted series is that by Gordan[21, 22]. 220 patients were treated with estrogens for a total of 1545 patient years (average 7 years) with one case of carcinoma of the endometrium developing. Further scrutiny of this paper, however, reveals that when patients were not troubled, or were troubled to only a very small extent by vaginal bleeding estrogens were given alone; if a patient was troubled more seriously by bleeding, however, a progestogen was given as well during the last period of estrogen therapy. Some, at least, of these patients, therefore, must be excluded and in this exclusion it must be assumed were those patients who were probably most affected by previous endometrial proliferation and who might have been most at risk of cancer had a progestogen not been introduced into treatment as well.

A fourth paper frequently quoted is that by Wallach and Henneman[19]. These authors reported on their use of estrogens in 292 patients for a mean period of 5·1 years. Four patients developed endometrial carcinoma, one after 2 years of cyclic therapy with stilboestrol alone and three after parenteral depot or pellet estrogen treatment for 6–15 years. Again we appear to see the influence of the duration of treatment since three patients developing cancer after treatment for 6–15 years in a group whose mean period of treatment was merely 5·1 years indicates that many of the 292 patients must have been treated for only a very few years.

A fifth paper frequently quoted is that by Wilson[20] which concerns only estrogen and progestogen cyclic therapy and cannot therefore be considered by us here as at all reassuring for patients receiving estrogen treatment alone.

The very closest scrutiny of these papers which appear to show that estrogen therapy does not significantly increase the risk of uterine cancer appears to me to question the validity of any such assumption. Two papers from one author[24, 25] give very few details and there are obvious inaccuracies of reporting. A second author[23] treated only *some* of his patients for a maximum period of 5½ years and many for a far shorter time. The third series[19] concerns a longer average period of treatment of 5·1 years but shows three cancers developing in those patients treated for well above the average period of time, namely 6–15 years. In the fourth series[21, 22] it seemed evident that those patients most at risk received progestogens as well as estrogens and therefore these patients must be excluded from our consideration. Similarly, the fifth series[20] concerned estrogen and progestogen therapy and gives no reassurance whatever about the safety of unopposed estrogens for many years.

I believe that the evidence I have reviewed here indicates clearly that adequate evidence has not yet been presented that unopposed estrogen therapy is safe so far as uterine cancer is concerned. It would seem that greater claims may have been made than are justified. This latter point seems to me to be highlighted by a further uncritical and inaccurate assessment of the papers I have just reviewed by Defares[26]. This author excludes the series[19] with its four cases of endometrial cancer on the grounds that some of these occurred when estrogens were given by injection yet he includes the series[24, 25] which employed estrogen implants; he further claims that the duration of therapy in Wilson's series[20] was 17 years whereas, in fact, it was for an average time of 7·8 years; he states that Geist's[23] patients were treated for 5½ years whereas we have seen that this was the longest period of time any patient was treated, the span of treatment varying from 6 months to 5½ years.

May I now briefly turn to a consideration of breast cancer. Here may I say that I have found no figures to support a significant increase in the incidence of breast cancer as a result of estrogen therapy. Comparisons are difficult because of the general absence of comparable groups of untreated patients and estimated incidence rates have to be used instead. However, Gray and Barnes[27] found an incidence rate of approximately 0·25 per 100 patients per year with breast cancer and Burch *et al.*[28] an incidence rate of approximately 0·2 per 100 patients per year; these figures are compared with a predicted rate of 0·17 per 100 patients per year by Feinleib and Garrison[29] and a rate of 0·16 per 100 patients per year estimated by Burch[28]. It has also been commented by others that national statistics do not support either an increased incidence or death rate as a result of the widespread introduction of estrogen therapy into the United States in the last 25 years[29, 30].

References

1. Bergsjö, P. (1965). Progesterone—progestational compounds in the treatment of advanced endometrial carcinoma. *Acta Endocrinol.*, **49,** 412
2. Hustin, J. (1970). Endometrial carcinoma and synthetic progestogens; results of intra-uterine treatment. *J. Obst. Gynaecol. Brit. Cmnwlth.*, **77,** 915
3. John, A. H., Cornes, J. S., Jackson, W. D. and Bye, P. (1974). Effect of a systemically administered progestogen on histopathology of endometrial carcinoma. *J. Obst. Gynaecol. Br. Cmnwlth.*, **81,** 786
4. McCarroll, A. M., Montgomery, D. A. D., Harley, J. G., McKeown, E. F. and MacHenry, J. C. (1975). Endometrial carcinoma of the cyclical oestrogen–progestogen therapy for Turner's Syndrome. *Brit. J. Obst. Gynaecol.*, **82,** 421
5. Gusberg, S. B. (1947). Precursors of corpus carcinoma: estrogens and adenomatous hyperplasia. *Am. J. Obstet. Gynecol.*, **54,** 905
6. Gusberg, S. B., Moore, D. B. and Martin, F. (1900). Precursors of corpus cancer: II. Clinical and pathological study of adenomatous hyperplasia. *Am. J. Obstet. Gynecol.*, **68,** 1472
7. Hertig, A. T. and Sommers, S. C. (1949). Genesis of endometrial carcinoma: I. Study of prior biopsies. *Cancer*, **2,** 946
8. Hertig, A. T., Sommers, S. C. and Bengloff, H. (1949). Genesis of endometrial carcinoma: III. Carcinoma in situ. *Cancer*, **2,** 964
9. Meissner, W. A., Sommers, S. C. and Serham, G. (1957). Endometrial hyperplasia, endometrial carcinoma and endometriosis produced experimentally by estrogen. *Cancer*, **10,** 500
10. Gusberg, S. B. and Hall, R. E. (1961). Precursors of corpus cancer: III. The appearance of cancer of the endometrium in estrogenically conditioned patients. *Obstet. Gynecol.*, **17,** 397
11. Southam, A. L. and Richert, R. M. (1966). Prognosis for adolescents with menstrual abnormalities. *Am. J. Obstet. Gynecol.*, **94,** 637
12. Dowsett, J. W. (1963). Corpus carcinoma developing in a patient with Turner's syndrome treated with estrogen. *Am. J. Obstet. Gynecol.*, **86,** 622
13. Carlorbe, P., Chartier, M. and Vink, le Tan. (1967). Cancer de l'uterus probable apres traitement prolonge d'un syndrome de Turner par les oestrogenes. *Sem. Hop. Paris*, **43,** 1083
14. Scott, T. (1967). Turner's syndrome and vermiform phlebectasia of the bowel. *Trans. Am. Clin. Climatol. Ass.*, **79,** 45
15. Cutler, B. S., Forbes, A. P., Ingersol, F. M. and Scully, R. E. (1972). Endometrial carcinoma after stilbestrol therapy in gonadal dysgenesis. *N. Engl. J. Med.* **287,** 628
16. Wilkinson, E. J., Friedrich, J. R., Mattingly, R. F., Regali, J. A. and Garancis, J. C. (1973). Turner's syndrome with endometrial adenocarcinoma and stilbesterol therapy. *Obstet. Gynecol.*, **42,** 193
17. Dewhurst, C. J., de Koos, E. B. and Haines, M. (1975). Oestrogen therapy in gonadal dysgenesis. *Br. J. Obstet. Gynaecol.* (in press)
18. Novak, E. R. and Woodruff, J. D. (1962). *Novak's Gynecologic and Obstetric Pathology with Clinical and Endocrine Relations*
19. Wallach, S. and Henneman, P. H. (1959). Prolonged estrogen therapy in postmenopausal women. *J. Am. Med. Ass.*, **171,** 1637
20. Wilson, R. A. (1962). The roles of estrogen and progesterone in breast and genital cancer. *J. Am. Med. Ass.*, **182,** 327

21. Gordan, G. S. (1962). Round Table Conference. The Menopause and the roles of estrogens. *Excerpta Medica Foundation, May*
22. Gordan, G. S. (1970). Postmenopausal osteoporosis: Problems of diagnosis and therapy. *The Female Climacteric,* **1,** no. 3
23. Geist, S. H. Walter, R. I. and Salmon, U. J. (1941). Are oestrogens carcinogenic in the human female? *Am. J. Obst. Gynecol.*, **42,** 242
24. Schleyer-Saunders, E. (1960). The management of the menopause. *Med. Press,* **244,** 337
25. Schleyer-Saunders, E. (1971). Results of hormone implants in the treatment of the climacteric. *J. Am. Geriat. Soc.*, **19,** 114
26. Defares, J. G. (1971). Cancer preventible? *Lancet,* **i,** January 16
27. Gray, L. A. and Barnes, M. L. (1971). Effects of estrogenic therapy on the breast. *Southern Med. J.*, **64,** 835
28. Burch, J. C., Byrd, Jr., B. F. and Vaughn, W. K. (1974). The effects of long-term oestrogen on hysterectomized women. *Am. J. Obstet. Gynecol.*, March 15, 778
29. Feinleib, M. and Garrison, R. J. (1969). Interpretation of the vital statistics of breast cancer. *Cancer,* **24,** 1109
30. Shimkin, M. B. (1963). Cancer of the breast. *J. Am. Med. Ass.*, **183,** 146

30

Estrogens and breast cancer

R. A. Sellwood

Introduction

It seems clear that there is a relationship between the ovarian hormones and cancer of the breast but in spite of very extensive clinical and laboratory research the nature of this relationship remains unexplained.

In small rodents ovarian hormones are an important factor in the development of cancer of the breast. Female mice which normally have a high incidence of mammary cancer are protected by bilateral oophorectomy before the age of 3 months and in male mice tumours may be induced by ovarian grafts or administration of estrogens.

In women bilateral oophorectomy or irradiation of the ovaries causes dramatic remission of advanced cancer of the breast in approximately 30% of patients. Primary tumours may diminish dramatically in size, fungating ulcers shrink and heal, lytic lesions of bone recalcify and remodel and leucoerythroblastic blood pictures return to normal. Cancer of the breast is relatively rare in women whose ovaries are removed early in life and in those with a short menstrual history due to a late menarche or early menopause. In women castrated before the age of 35 the incidence of breast cancer is only one third of that observed in normal women.

Several studies of urinary estrogen excretion in patients with cancer of the breast have been reported but the results are conflicting and confusing. Some workers have claimed that women with cancer excrete more estrogens than normal, but others have found that they excrete less and in one study the output of estrogen was normal. Measurement of urinary estrogens has proved an unsatisfactory method of study for several reasons. Estrogen production varies according to the stage of the menstrual cycle and there are practical difficulties in acquiring the multiple complete 24-hour specimens needed to represent the whole cycle. Most estrogen is metabolized in the liver and does not appear in the urine and that proportion which does may bear little relationship to that present in the body fluids. For these reasons it seems likely that assays of estrogens in blood will be of more value than those in urine.

It is now possible by means of radioimmunoassay to measure simply, accurately and relatively cheaply the concentrations of ovarian hormones in small quantities of serum.

In this study we have measured the concentration of estradiol 17β, one of the most powerful of the estrogens, progesterone and the pituitary hormone prolactin in serum from normal women and compared these findings with those in women with benign or malignant disease of the breast.

Method

Subjects

Samples of blood were taken daily or as often as possible during at least one menstrual cycle as follows:

(a) 32 normal women with no history of breast cancer. Eleven subjects were aged 20 to 29 years, ten 30 to 39 and eleven 40 to 49.
(b) 32 women with benign disease of the breast. 19 had painful lumpy breasts and were considered on clinical grounds to have generalized fibro-adenosis. Six were aged 20 to 29 years, eight 30 to 39 and five 40 to 49.

The remaining 13 had had one or more cysts aspirated from one or both breasts. Of these five were aged 30 to 39 years and eight aged 40 to 49 years.
(c) Ten women with cancer of the breast aged 40 to 49 years.

All samples were taken approximately 3 months after mastectomy. None of the subjects had a history of gynaecological disease or was taking any hormonal preparation.

Collection of blood samples

Peripheral venous blood (approx 10 ml) was collected daily between 9 a.m. and 12 noon. The blood was allowed to clot, centrifuged and the serum removed and stored at −20 °C.

Measurement of serum estradiol-17β, progesterone and prolactin

Radioimmunoassay of estradiol-17β was carried out by the method described by Cameron and Jones[1], that for progesterone by the method described by Farr[2] and that for prolactin by Cole and Boyns[3].

Expression of results

The lengths of the cycles varied greatly so that a reference point other than the first day of the cycle needed for comparative purposes. The day of the mid cycle peak of estradiol-17β was used as the reference point and designated as Day 0. Preceding days were given negative numbers and the days following positive numbers. Due to the difference in profiles of the three hormones Day −11 to Day −4 was referred to as the follicular phase and Day +4 to Day +12 as the luteal phase for estradiol −17β; but Day −12 to Day 0 was referred to as the follicular phase and Day +2 to Day +16 as the luteal phase for progesterone; and Day −12 to Day −4 was referred to as the follicular phase, Day −3 to Day +3 as the ovulatory phase and Day +4 to Day +16 as the luteal phase for prolactin.

The results for estradiol and progesterone were compared in each group by the statistical method of paired comparison. The results for prolactin in each phase were calculated and comparisons carried out with the Student's '*t*' statistical test.

Results

Normal women

(a) ESTRADIOL-17β

During the follicular phase of the cycle the concentrations of estradiol-17β were low (mean 35·3±4·39 SE mean pg/ml), rose to a peak at the time of ovulation (mean 192·9±12·7 SE mean pg/ml) and during the luteal phase (Day +4 to Day +12) to a plateau (mean 67·3±1·47 SE mean pg/ml). In the luteal phase of the cycle the mean concentrations of estradiol-17β in women in the fourth decade were significantly higher than those of women in the fifth ($p < 0·001$) and the third decades ($p < 0·01$).

(b) PROGESTERONE

During the follicular phase of the cycle the concentrations of progesterone were low (mean 0·7+0·04 SE mean ng/ml). In the luteal phase they rose to a maximum on about Day +6 to Day +8 (mean 13·4±1·3 SE mean ng/ml) and fell again before menstruation (mean 1·4±0·27 SE mean ng/ml).

In the luteal phase of the cycle the mean concentration of progesterone in women in the fifth decade was significantly lower than that in those in the third ($p < 0·02$) or fourth decade ($p < 0·001$).

(c) PROLACTIN

The mean concentration of prolactin in the follicular phase was 0·11± 0·009 SE mean mU/ml. During the ovulatory phase the concentrations rose to a peak on Day 0 (0·21±0·05 SE mean mU/ml). During the luteal phase there was considerable individual variation as revealed by the large increase of the standard error of the mean. There was a peak on Day +7 and from Day + 10 to the time of menstruation the concentrations rose sharply to a maximum of 0·26±0·12 SE mean mU/ml.

When age was taken into account it was found that women in the fourth decade of life had concentrations greater than either older or younger women. This difference was significant when older women were considered ($p < 0·02$).

Benign breast disease

In women with fibroadenosis the concentrations of estradiol-17β and progesterone were normal but the concentration of prolactin in women over 30 was significantly higher than normal. In women in the fourth decade of life this difference was significant during the follicular phase ($p < 0·001$) and in the fifth decade in both follicular and luteal phases ($p < 0·001$).

In women with cysts in the fifth decade of life the concentration of estradiol-17β in the luteal phase and the concentration of prolactin throughout the cycle was significantly higher than normal ($p < 0·001$). In younger women there was no difference in any of the three hormones.

Cancer of the breast

In both the follicular phase and luteal phase of the cycle the concentration of estradiol-17β in patients with cancer of the breast was slightly but significantly greater than in normal women ($p < 0·05$). However, the main feature was one of great individual variation.

In the luteal phase, the concentration of progesterone was significantly higher than normal, although the difference was very small. The concentration of prolactin did not differ significantly from normal.

Discussion

The pattern of secretion of the two hormones estradiol-17β and progesterone throughout the normal menstrual cycle has been well established by other workers. The results from the previous studies and from this one indicate that the concentrations of estradiol are low during the follicular phase of the menstrual cycle, that there is a well defined peak at the time of ovulation and a second rise to a fairly high plateau during the luteal phase. The concentrations of progesterone are very low during the follicular phase, but after ovulation they rise over a period of days to a plateau before falling before menstruation.

The results for prolactin differed from those for estradiol and progesterone in that very consistent patterns of secretion were not found. The concentrations of prolactin varied widely from day to day with peaks at variable times within the individual cycles studied. This may have resulted from the circadian periodicity in the serum concentrations of prolactin now known to exist in man. When the results for the total group of normal women were studied however certain generalizations could be made. Concentrations of prolactin were lower during the follicular than the luteal phase of the cycle; there was a low peak at the time of ovulation; and during the luteal phase the concentrations rose again exhibiting a biphasic pattern with a peak on Day +6 and a further one on Day +14. One group of workers has reported a similar pattern.

It is difficult to explain why women in the fourth decade of life had higher concentrations of estradiol and prolactin than younger or older women or why women in the fifth decade of life had significantly lower concentrations of progesterone than younger women. There is no doubt that in this type of study age is an important consideration.

The symptoms and signs of fibroadenosis are usually most marked before menstruation when estradiol and progesterone are present in high concentrations for several days. It has seemed reasonable to assume that one or both of these hormones has an aetiological role. These data provide no evidence that either hormone is involved in any way. In older women with fibroadenosis (fourth and fifth decades) concentrations of prolactin were significantly greater than normal throughout the menstrual cycle. It is known that prolactin may amplify or affect in other ways the activity of other hormones and its potentiating effect on aldosterone and antidiuretic hormone are well recognized. The possibility of a similar relationship to estradiol and/or progesterone requires investigation.

In women with cystic disease the endocrine profiles were quite different. In women in the fifth decade of life concentrations of estradiol and prolactin were strikingly greater than normal. Prolactin was raised throughout the menstrual cycle but the increase of estradiol was confined to the luteal phase. Unlike women with fibroadenosis these patients provided clear evidence of an endocrine abnormality but this does not imply that the abnormality was necessarily the cause of the breast condition. The occurrence of cysts in post-menopausal women treated with estrogens however does suggest that the high concentrations of estradiol may have been an aetiological factor.

In women with cancer of the breast the most striking feature was the marked variation in the results particularly those for estradiol. The variation took place on either side of the mean normal profile. Although the mean concentrations of estradiol and progesterone were slightly but significantly greater than normal, it was extremely difficult to apply statistical methods in a meaningful way. Greater numbers must be studied before conclusions can be drawn.

Acknowledgements

This work was supported by grants from the Cancer Research Campaign, the Medical Research Council and the Management Committee of the University Hospital of South Manchester.

We wish to thank Professor K. Griffiths and Dr E. N. Cole for kindly carrying out the estimations of prolactin.

References

1. Cameron, E. D. H. and Jones, D. A. (1972). Some observations on the measurement of estradiol-17β in human plasma by radioimmunoassay. *Steroids*, **20**, 737
2. Furr, B. J. (1973). Radioimmunoassay of progesterone in peripheral plasma of the domestic fowl in various physiological states and in follicular venous plasma. *Acta Endocrinol.*, **72**, 89
3. Cole, E. N. and Boyns, A. R. (1973). Radioimmunoassay for human pituitary prolactin, using antiserum against an extract of human amniotic fluid. *Hormone Res.*, **4**, 261

Discussion on Section H:

Risks of Estrogen Therapy (Part 2) Cancer

Chairman: *Mr R. B. K. Rickford*

Mr R. B. K. Rickford (Chairman): Professor Sellwood gave estrogens to his male rats and they developed carcinoma. Did he ever think of giving them estrogens and progestogens.

I also hoped that he might explain to me, as a mere gynaecologist, why we are sometimes asked to take ovaries out of patients with carcinoma of the breast, and why some patients with carcinoma of the breast are given massive doses of estrogens.

Professor R. A. Sellwood (Surgeon, Manchester): I shall take the second question first. We have the concept of estrogen-dependence. Someone coined the term a long time ago, to explain the dramatic remission of the disease that occurs in about 30% of pre-menopausal women following removal of the ovaries. I cannot explain why in post-menopausal women, or at least in women who are 5 or 6 years beyond the menopause, an equally dramatic remission can be obtained by giving estrogens. Perhaps we are wrong to talk about estrogen dependence. Perhaps we should simply say that anything we do which drastically alters the sex hormone environment alters the responsiveness of the tumour. The estrogens that we give are synthetic and generally speaking they are either stilbestrol or ethinyl estradiol. One could postulate that their effect is to block the receptors on the tumour cells on which the endogenous estrogens normally work and produce their effect, but I have no evidence that this is so.

The work on rats was not mine. It is American work and I do not think that anyone has studied the effects of estrogen and progestogen together in the male rat.

Mr E. S. Saunders (Gynaecologist, London): Professor Dewhurst has been kind enough to mention my work. My statistics published in 1960 concerned 500 cases which were treated with hormone implants. The duration was 15 years, and not 5 years. The expected number of cancers, according to the general population, would have been about 30; there were no cancers in my treated patients.

Professor Dewhurst referred to another group where two cases of cancer of the uterus were found. Those two cases are very interesting, from every point of view. One case came to see me because of severe flushes and palpitations, and also osteoporosis. I gave her the usual implant. Ten days later that woman came back complaining of bleeding. A thorough examination was done, and a curettage showed a polyp which was examined by the pathologist who reported malignant changes on the tip of the polyp. We cannot claim than an implant done 10 days earlier provoked a cancer of the endometrium. The second case of cancer was also interesting. The patient was aged about 49 or 50, with a history of irregular periods, a slight loss every few weeks, and because of her severe menopausal symptoms—she showed no signs of malignancy—I gave her an implant. Three weeks later she came with bleeding. A curettage showed carcinoma of the endometrium. From the point of view of statistics, I have to put those cases in, although I am convinced that they have nothing to do with the implant.

A second statistic of mine has not been mentioned. The material was presented at a Congress in Vienna. There were 600 cases, selected menopausal women, about the same age group. They were divided into two groups. Three hundred were given a placebo but the other three hundred were treated with implants. Ten years later a follow up of most of the cases showed that the women who had received implants had $2\frac{1}{2}$ times less cancer than the others.

To conclude: Professor Dewhurst has said that there is no evidence that estrogen might not produce a cancer, but there is no evidence either that estrogen has produced cancers.

Mr S. Campbell (Gynaecologist, London): In our 6-month crossover placebo trial which we described earlier, the patients had an outpatient (Vabra) curettage on admission to the study and again after 6 months Premarin and 6 months placebo. Twenty-six of the 39 patients who had intact uteri had withdrawal bleeding on Premarin 1·25 mg, an incidence of 67% which is very much higher than the 10–20% which is quoted in the literature. A total of 6 patients (9%) had cystic glandular hyperplasia while on Premarin 1·25 mg but did not have it on placebo. That is a very high incidence and although I quite accept that this may not be a pre-cancerous lesion, it worries me considerably.

We have had one case of cancer of the endometrium in a patient who before she came to our clinic, had been one year on continuous Premarin. We put her on a cyclical dosage but discovered cancer of the endometrium a few months later when we performed Vabra curettage.

The conclusion I would draw is that we cannot be complacent about the risks of cancer of the endometrium. We must use the minimum dosage to control symptoms, and for any patient with regular withdrawal bleeding I would recommend a 6-monthly Vabra curettage or preferably the addition of a progestogen to the therapy. More and more I am using a regime of continuous estrogen, and for the first week of every calendar month prescribing norethisterone, 5 mg daily. Since adopting this regime we have had no cases of hyperstimulation of the endometrium and I feel very much happier when I see that situation.

Professor C. J. Dewhurst (Gynaecologist, London): I share Mr Campbell's concern about cystic glandular hyperplasia. The fact that millions of women on the Pill which contains estrogen and progestogen, do not develop cancer, is irrelevant as to whether estrogens alone do. That is one of my points. I do not think that these facts are clearly stated in many of the papers, and my purpose here is to suggest that we should still look, and go on looking critically at the evidence that estrogens alone over long periods of time are free from risk.

Ms. Tove Wisborg (Copenhagen): In the past 10 years we have seen five cases of estrogen-produced ovarian cancer and one case of breast cancer. We thought that there might be a connection with a continuous high level of estrogen in the body, compared with normal cyclic variations. Perhaps it might be advisable not to use continuous estrogen in post-menopausal women, but to use intermittent therapy.

Professor R. A. Sellwood: I would be most interested in the data. The information is new to me.

Professor C. J. Dewhurst: For other reasons, I would always approve intermittent therapy, but that is hardly relevant to the question.

Mr E. V. van Hall (Leiden): Did Professor Selwood do the same studies in post-menopausal breast cancer patients? They are the more interesting group. Also it would be interesting to look at estrone, and perhaps androgens.

Professor R. A. Sellwood: We have done this in post-menopausal women. We have got a group of about 30 or 40 post-menopausal women with cancer of the breast, and 30 or 40 normal women. The estradiol 17-β is so low in the post-menopausal women that it is at the lower limit of sensitivity of our assay, and I can make no comment about it. We have not yet measured the prolactin in those women. It should be more interesting.

Of course Mr Van Hall is right. What we really want to measure is estrone, but as yet we cannot produce an antibody.

Professor C. Lauritzen (Gynaecologist, Ulm): I have some comments on estrogens and mammary carcinoma.

We have discussed estrogens, carcinoma of the breast, and of the endometrium, but we would be very short-sighted, or even blind, to look only at estrogens. I cannot let the discussion go without mentioning that genetic factors in the human are of great importance in mammary carcinoma, and the risk factor if a mother has a carcinoma of the breast, for the daughter, is about 5, and for disturbances of the cycle, such as anovulation, it is 2. This is a great difference*†.

Professor R. A. Sellwood: It is even greater when a sister has cancer of the breast.

Professor C. Lauritzen (Ulm): There is also growing evidence that mammary carcinoma may also be virus-induced.‡

I refer to the study of McMahon and co-workers*, which has not been mentioned. The risk for mammary carcinoma increases fourfold if the first pregnancy is later than 25 years. The prolactin levels are much higher at night than by day, so prolactin levels

* MacMahon and Cole (1969). *Cancer*, **24,** 1146

† Zippin and Petrallis (1971). *Cancer*, **28,** 1381

‡ Moore *et al.* (1971). *Nature (London)*, **229,** 611

should be studied at night*. If Professor Sellwood has some plasma left, he should use it to determine androgens too.

Mr R. B. K. Rickford (Chairman): Could an American surgeon give his views on the length of time that post-menopausal women should take estrogens? To the grave? To 80, to 70, or how long?

Dr C. B. Hammond (Gynaecologist, Duke University): It is nice to be asked an easy question! I plan to touch on this tomorrow in my paper and I can only give my own personal opinion. I think that there is a group of patients in whom estrogen therapy, or hormonal therapy, is beneficial. It should be carried out for the treatment of the symptoms that they have. I am not a member of the school which advocates estrogen for all women for all time, and I should like to leave it at that until I can present the data.

Dr P. Bye (Schering Chemicals, Sussex): On the question of mammary carcinoma, it may be germane to quote from a publication that has just come out—a WHO monograph on carcinogenic risks of various types of drugs. The latest volume deals with the sex hormones. They reviewed all the data on long-term studies, those that Professor Dewhurst mentioned, and others. They made the same methodological criticisms that he made, but they came to the conclusion that despite the methodological shortcomings, they could go so far as to say that whereas it had not been proved that the risk of mammary carcinoma was reduced by the use of estrogens, at least it could be said that there was no indication of any increased risk.

Dr N. G. Mussalli (Gynaecologist, Welwyn Garden City): Professor Sellwood has described clinical investigations and hormone assays in patients with breast cancer, with cystic disease of the breast and in normal controls. Extensive work has been done, especially by veterinary colleagues, on the physiology of the breast in relation to lactation. This involved tissue cultures using hormones. Could the responsiveness of the target organ be helpful in investigating this disease?

Professor R. A. Sellwood: The questioner I believe suggests that if we set up cultures of mammary tumours against a battery of either hormonal or cytotoxic agents, rather in the same way that we set up cultures of a bacterium against antibiotics, we might find a sensitivity, so to speak. We might be able to pick out the tumour that will respond to estrogen, and the one that will respond to androgen. Quite a lot of tissue culture work has been done and I have done some myself. Overall I would say that the results are very disappointing. This is because it is so very difficult to culture cancer of the breast. Almost every other cancer can be cultured by fairly straightforward methods but cancer of the breast is so often nearly all fibrous tissue and very few tumour cells. All of us who have worked in the field have had the most terrible difficulty in getting reliable standard cultures of the type that would be needed to do this. One or two people claim to have done so, and there have been suggestions that it might be possible, but I cannot go further than that.

Dr Muriel G. Yates (General Practitioner, Liverpool): Could Premarin be given to a patient with severe menopausal symptoms who has had a radical mastectomy?

Professor R. A. Sellwood: I know of no reason why not except for a patient with

* Nokin *et al.* (1972). *Br. Med. J.*, **3**, 561

advanced cancer of the breast who was being treated by bilateral oophorectomy. That would imply that she was a pre-menopausal woman, and most unlikely to be undergoing menopausal symptoms. If the symptoms were produced by doing the oophorectomy, I would not then give the hormone; having done the operation to remove estrogens, and I would not put them back.

Miss G. S. Agerbak (Copenhagen): On the basis of the data we have heard today, does the panel consider it possibly advantageous to advocate a sequential therapy, that is estrogen plus progestogen at the end of the cycle for post-menopausal women?

Professor C. J. Dewhurst: The problem would be one of patient acceptability. I should have thought that many patients would not want to go on menstruating, which by and large they would do for a period of time. However, from the point of view of cancer risk, combined estrogen/progestogen therapy would be preferable to estrogens alone. I believe that it would be preferable to use a progestogen occasionally, two or three times a year, to strip the endometrium effectively, so that probably the hyperplasia about which I am concerned would not then occur.

Mr S. Campbell: Professor Dewhurst is absolutely right. Post-menopausal women do not like to have regular periods, but on the other hand, if they are given a choice between suffering menopausal symptoms or having regular withdrawal bleeding, they opt for regular withdrawal bleeding any day; they are very willing to accept this small inconvenience.

Mr R. B. K. Rickford: To sum up. Estrogens are possibly dangerous, depending perhaps on dosage, and also perhaps on the length of time that they are given to post-menopausal women. There may be a lot to be said for giving a progestogen with them.

Section I

THERAPEUTIC PROBLEMS

Chairman: J. C. McCLURE BROWNE

31

The premature menopause

H. S. Jacobs and M. A. F. Murray

It is not possible to provide a completely satisfactory definition of the premature menopause. Ideally the definition should be based on accurate epidemiological studies so that its timing could be stated, in years, as two standard deviations less than the (appropriate) population's mean age at the final cessation of menstruation. Unfortunately the data required for such a definition are not available. A clinician treating patients complaining of infertility is faced with another problem—how can he know whether the individual patient's amenorrhea represents the final cessation of menstruation? Finally, it is an important feature of the condition that the fundamental cause is primary ovarian failure rather than any other cause of permanent amenorrhea. These three factors—the uncertainties of timing and of permanence, and the implicit ovarian component—explain the different definitions offered by various authorities. In this review, the concept of finality is sacrificed because it is impractical. The term premature menopause is taken to mean primary ovarian failure occurring before the age of 45. Since ovarian failure may occur with or without menstruation having become established, we consider the term should include pre-pubertal ovarian failure.

The endocrine profile of the premature menopause differs in no way from that of the normal menopause. The diagnostic criteria are therefore the same but occur in a younger age group. However the implications are more serious; they include the patient's disappointment over her sterility and the grave problem of precocious estrogen deficiency. As we shall show, there are other causes of severe estrogen deficiency and infertility which are common and can be readily reversed by appropriate therapy. An accurate diagnosis is therefore essential.

The symptoms and signs of the premature menopause are essentially those of estrogen deficiency. Atrophic changes in the genital tract account for distressing symptoms during coitus and indubitably contribute to impaired libido. Changes in the skin are often obvious; those in the bones may be covert but they are sinister and herald early and severe osteoporosis if the patient is left untreated. Vasomotor instability is common but seems to be a feature of post-pubertal estrogen deficiency. We have been impressed by a number of patients who reported a general sense of well-being during estrogen replacement which they had not previously realized was absent.

Table 31.1 Primary ovarian failure

Chromosomal	—e.g.	Turner's Syndrome
Enzyme defect	—e.g.	17α Hydroxylase deficiency
Iatrogenic	—e.g.	Cytoxic drugs Pelvic irradiation Ovariectomy
Autoimmune	—e.g.	Associated with Addison's Disease and anti steroid-producing cell antibodies
Idiopathic	—e.g.	Premature menopause

The causes of premature ovarian failure are given in Table 31.1. The list is not exhaustive but is intended to indicate common conditions or to draw attention to disorders whose existence represents particularly interesting experiments of nature. The rarest of all is a deficiency of the 17α-hydroxylase enzyme in the steroid producing cells of both the adrenals and the ovaries. The result is estrogen deficiency leading to a failure of sexual maturation, and hypertension resulting from an excess of the mineralocorticoids which are precursors of aldosterone. Chromosomal lesions are familiar and well documented. Here it is only necessary to recall that mosaic and isochromosomal forms may lead to difficulty in diagnosis if only the buccal smear is relied upon: karyotype analysis is therefore obligatory for correct diagnosis. It is important to exclude other congenital lesions and to be aware of the increased incidence of thyroid disorders both in the patient and in her mother.

A form of ovarian failure that is occurring with increasing frequency is that caused by anti-cancer chemotherapy and/or inadvertent ovarian irradiation in patients with various lymphoreticular disorders. The improved prognosis for patients with these diseases has prompted several studies of gonadal function in treated patients. In a retrospective analysis of 22 patients with Hodgkin's disease, Thomas *et al.*[1] found a close relationship between the development of ovarian failure and the ovarian dose of irradiation. Doses above 500 rads were commonly associated with ovarian failure and frequently occurred with an inverted Y irradiation field, despite prior elective oophoropexy—which by itself was without effect on either ovarian function or transport of gametes. The development of amenorrhea, estrogen deficiency and high serum gonadotrophins in one patient was followed 2 years later by resumption of ovulation cycles and pregnancy, so in this condition the prognosis of the reproductive state may be difficult to establish, despite the presence of the usual diagnostic criteria of ovarian failure (see below).

Immunological studies of patients with primary ovarian failure have defined a small but important group of patients. Autoimmune oophoritis is common in patients with autoimmune Addison's disease of the adrenal and is usually associated with circulating anti steroid-producing cell antibodies, which are apparently active *in vitro*[2]. In one patient a pharmacological dose of glucocorticoids lead to resumption of menstrual cycles, presumably by suppressing the immunological process[2]. Moraes Ruehsen *et al.*[3] found a high incidence of associated autoimmune diseases in patients with autoimmune oophoritis and Addison's disease. As with patients with chromosomal causes of ovarian failure, thyroid disease occurred with an increased frequency but these patients also had a greatly enhanced incidence of parathyroid failure, of diabetes mellitus and of pernicious anaemia.

When the above conditions have been excluded it must be admitted that the cause of premature primary ovarian failure is usually unknown. Some cases no doubt represent one end of the extremes of the normal survival of a sufficient complement of ovarian follicles, but a better understanding of the normal factors determining persistence of ovarian function will be required before any of the many hypotheses to explain the premature menopause can be excluded.

The endocrine profile of primary ovarian failure is of low concentrations of serum estradiol-17β associated with elevated levels of both gonadotrophins. In establishing the diagnosis it is essential that production of both gonadal and trophic hormones is assessed. Serum luteinizing hormone (LH) and follicle stimulating hormone (FSH) concentrations can be readily measured by radioimmunoassay and these measurements have been made available throughout the United Kingdom by the Supra Regional Assay Service. Although patients with primary ovarian failure have elevated concentrations of serum LH, there may be considerable overlap with the levels found in patients with other forms of amenorrhea and serum FSH concentrations offer easier discrimination[4]. Estrogen production may be assessed by examination of the lower genital tract; a simple biological index is provided by the progestogen withdrawal test, since withdrawal bleeding is very rare when estradiol concentrations are below 50 pg/ml[5]. It is emphasized that an accurate diagnosis of ovarian failure requires assessment of both estrogen and gonadotrophin production. Figure 31.1 shows serum estradiol-17β concentrations in a group of patients with the premature menopause, in patients with hyperprolactinaemic amenorrhea and in patients with amenorrhea and a partially recovered form of anorexia nervosa. The lowest estradiol concentrations occurred in patients with hyperprolactinaemic amenorrhea.

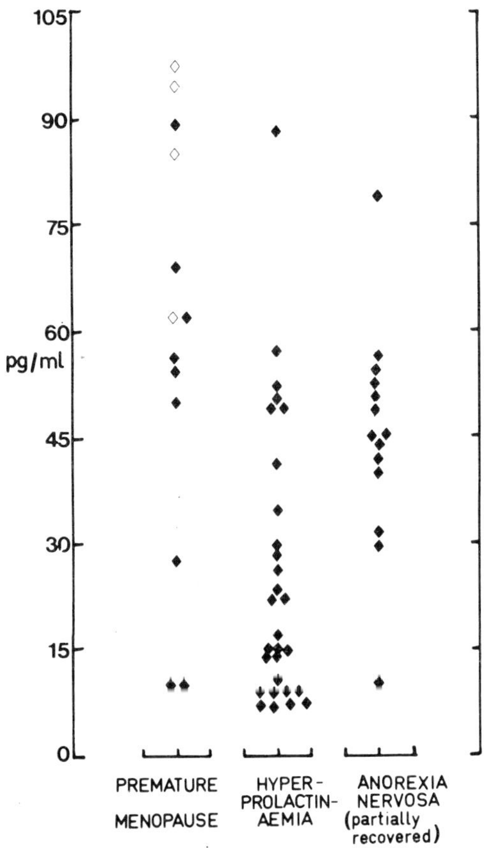

Figure 31.1 Serum estradiol-17β concentrations in patients with premature menopause, hyperprolactinaemia or partially recovered anorexia nervosa. The open symbols indicate those patients who had positive progestogen withdrawal tests.

Very low levels were also seen in patients with partially recovered anorexia nervosa. The latter two groups of patients, which together accounted for about 50% of 75 consecutive cases of amenorrhea seen in our Gynaecological Endocrine Clinic[6], could readily be mistaken for patients with primary ovarian failure if only the estrogen status were assessed. Little help in reaching the diagnosis is obtained from the history, because galactorrhea only rarely accompanies hyperprolactinaemia[7] and the age of presentation (Figure 31.2)

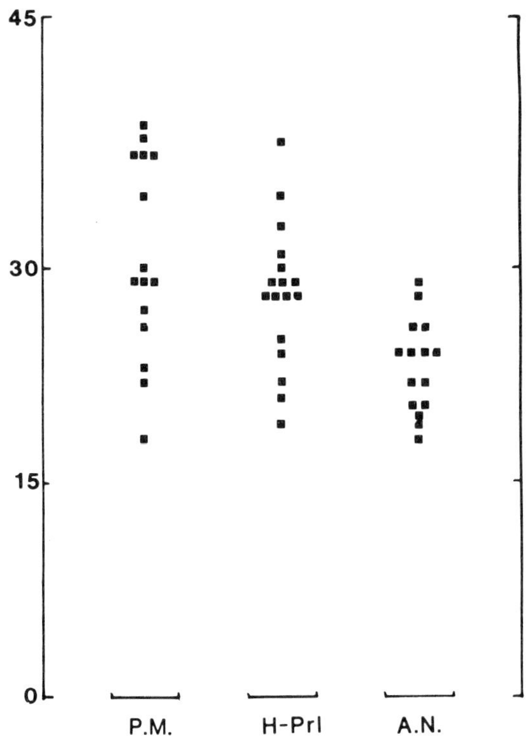

Figure 31.2 The age at presentation of patients with premature menopause (P.M.) hyperprolactinaemic amenorrhea (H-Prl) and partially recovered anorexia nervosa (A.N.)

and duration of amenorrhea (Figure 31.3) are very similar in the three groups. Moreover mis-diagnosis is encouraged by the typical failure of patients with all of these conditions to respond to clomiphene, and in many cases, to ovulate in response to gonadotrophin therapy.

Serum gonadotrophin concentrations in these patients are shown in Figures 31.4 and 31.5 and from these data it appears that ovarian failure can easily be identified, since all the patients diagnosed as having the premature menopause had FSH concentrations of at least three times the upper limit

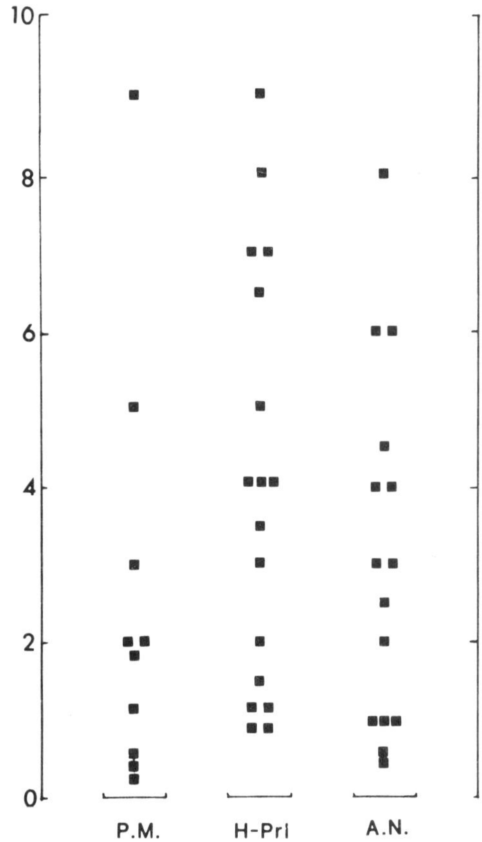

Figure 31.3 Duration of amenorrhea (in years) in patients with premature menopause (P.M.), hyperprolactinaemic amenorrhea (H-Prl) and partially recovered anorexia nervosa. The shortest history was obtained from patients with the premature menopause.

of normal. However four patients (indicated in Figure 31.1 by the open symbols) had positive progestogen withdrawal tests and estrogen levels over 60 pg/ml, despite elevated LH and FSH concentrations. Two of these patients have so far undergone laparotomy: one had large pale ovaries with a histological appearance similar to that described in the resistant ovary syndrome[8], and one patient had bilaterally atrophic ovaries associated with a small tumour on one side. Removal of this tumour, which was thought to be a thecoma, lead to a fall of estradiol concentrations and the development of symptoms and signs of estrogen deficiency. One other patient, aged 38, with gross elevation of both gonadotrophins (and an exaggerated response of LH and FSH to gonadotrophin releasing hormone) made an

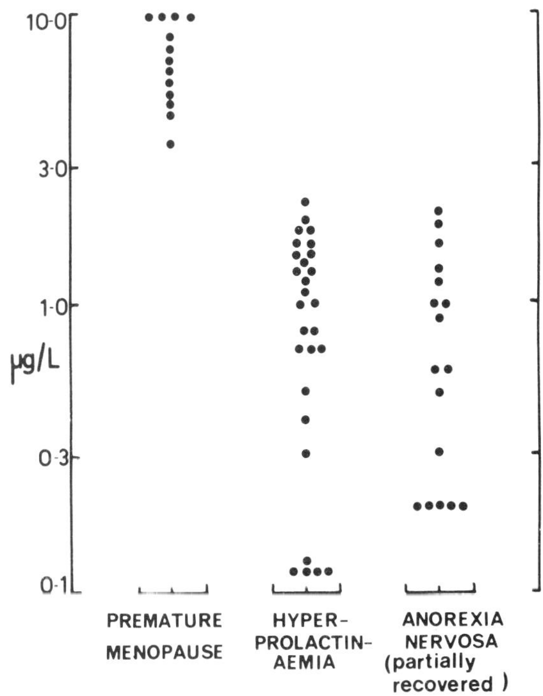

Figure 31.4 Serum LH concentrations in patients with premature menopause, hyperprolactinaemia or partially recovered anorexia nervosa.

unequivocal ovulatory response to clomiphene. The serum progesterone concentration 12 days after completing the clomiphene (50 mg a day for 5 days) was 8·8 ng/ml and the LH and FSH concentrations in that sample had fallen to within the normal range. This patient presumably represents an example of the 'premature perimenopause', since her results are similar to those observed in spontaneous perimenopausal cycles by Sherman and

Korenman[9]. Ovarian visualization has not yet been achieved in the fourth patient with a positive progestogen test, but these cases are described in detail to emphasize the importance of combined assessment of both gonadotrophin and estrogen production in young women with apparent primary ovarian failure.

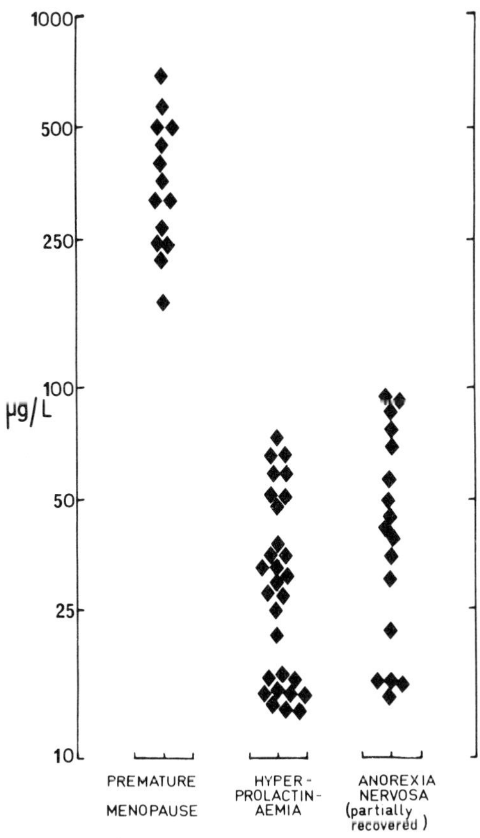

Figure 31.5 Serum FSH concentrations in patients with premature menopause, hyperprolactinaemia or partially recovered anorexia nervosa.

The management of patients with a premature menopause is essentially the differential diagnosis and treatment of estrogen deficiency. Anorexia nervosa, both in the phase of weight loss and when partially recovered, gonadotrophin deficiency and hyperprolactinaemia must be identified because there are now precise and specific treatments available[6]. The association of high gonadotrophin concentrations with estrogen levels more appropriate to the women with intact menstrual cycles indicates the need for ovarian visualization, at least in women complaining of infertility. The need for a biopsy representative of the whole ovary means that laparotomy rather than laparoscopy is usually required. Chromosomal lesions should be sought because their presence indicates the need for the exclusion of associated and often serious congenital abnormalities. The clinician must be aware of the rare but important association with Addison's disease. Other autoimmune disorders should be excluded: the most common—and often the most difficult one to be certain about—is hypothyroidism. The symptoms may be mild and masked by those of estrogen deficiency. Moreover blood tests can be confusing because total thyroxine concentrations may be low, due to the low thyroxine binding globulin concentrations consequent upon estrogen deficiency. Moreover TSH measurements, if not made with care, can be spuriously high because of cross reactions from the gonadotrophins[10].

When the diagnosis of primary ovarian failure is established, it is essential to inform the patient of the diagnosis and its implications for her fertility and for hormone replacement. The latter should be administered cyclically. As yet no strong arguments have been advanced for either sequential or combined estrogen plus progestogen therapy. Our own preference is for the latter since it allows greater flexibility in the choice of cycle length.

Acknowledgments

We thank Dr W. D. Odell for the antisera used for the gonadotrophin measurements. The reference preparations were provided by the Medical Research Council of the United Kingdom. We thank Mr E. J. Fox for expert technical assistance.

We thank the physicians and gynaecologists of St Mary's Hospital for permission to investigate patients under their care.

References

1. Thomas, P. R. M., Winstanley, D., Peckham, M. J., Austin, D. E., Murray, M. A. F. and Jacobs, H. S. (1976). Reproductive and endocrine function in patients with Hodgkin's disease: effects of oophoropexy and irradiation. *Br. J. Cancer* (in press)
2. Irvine, W. J. (1974). Autoimmunity in endocrine disease. *Proc. R. Soc. Med.*, **67,** 548
3. Moraes Ruehsen, M., Blizzard, R. M., Garcia-Bunuel, R. and Seegar Jones, G. (1972). Autoimmunity and ovarian failure. *Am. J. Obstet. Gynecol.*, **112,** 693

4. Jacobs, H. S. (1975). Endocrine aspects of anovulation. *Postgraduate Med. J.*, **51,** 209
5. Hull, M. G. R., Franks, S., McNeilly, A. S., Murray, M. A. F. and Jacobs, H. S. (1975). The progestogen test in the investigation of Amenorrhea. *J. Endocrinol.*, **67,** 17
6. Jacobs, H. S., Hull, M. G. R., Murray, M. A. F. and Franks, S. (1976). Therapy orientated diagnosis of secondary amenorrhea. *Horm. Res.* (in press)
7. Franks, S., Murray, M. A. F., Jequier, A. M., Steele, S. J., Nabarro, J. D. N. and Jacobs, H. S. (1975). Incidence and significance of hyperprolactinaemia in women with amenorrhea. *Clin. Endocrinol.*, **4,** 597
8. Van Campenhout, J., Vauclair, R. and Maraghi, K. (1972). Gonadotropin-resistant ovaries in primary amenorrhoea. *Obstet. Gynecol.*, **40,** 6
9. Sherman, B. M. and Korenman, S. G. (1975). Hormonal characteristics of the human menstrual cycle throughout reproductive life. *J. Clin. Invest.*, **55,** 699
10. Jacobs, H. S. and Lawton, N. F. (1974). Pituitary and placental glycopeptide hormones. *Br. Med. Bull.*, **30,** 55

32

The rationale of operative removal of the ovaries at hysterectomy

T. L. T. Lewis

Hysterectomy is one of the more common operative procedures carried out by the gynaecologist. I am excluding from my considerations in this paper operations for ovarian disease where hysterectomy may also be carried out, such as endometriosis, oophoritis, ovarian carcinoma and benign cysts, in which it is necessary to remove ovaries in order to eradicate disease; and hysterectomy for carcinoma of the uterine cervix or body when the ovaries are routinely removed in case they contain metastases, or to obtain a better clearance. I want instead to concentrate on the problem with which the gynaecologist is frequently faced when he is performing an abdominal hysterectomy for menorrhagia due to ovarian dysfunction or to benign lesions such as fibroids. If either ovary is diseased the gynaecologist will have to remove the abnormal part of the ovary or, more probably, the whole ovary on that side. But what should he do when both ovaries appear quite normal? In this context the patient is usually over the age of 35 or 40 years and is still menstruating.

The advantages to the patient of conserving her ovaries are:

1. She will not be precipitated immediately into a premature menopause.
2. The menopause will occur naturally at a later date, probably some years after the hysterectomy.
3. Menopausal symptoms, if they occur, are likely to be less severe because the rate of hormonal withdrawal is less rapid.

4. The ovaries *may* continue to function after the menopause.
5. The risks of coronary artery disease and osteoporosis in later life *may* be lessened.

The advantages to the patient of removing her ovaries are:

1. She is protected from subsequent malignancy arising in the ovaries.
2. She will not suffer from benign ovarian cysts.
3. She cannot experience pain in her ovaries, nor can they be in the way of intercourse, giving rise to deep dyspareunia.

I wish to discuss first the advantages of removing the ovaries.

The risk of subsequent ovarian malignant disease if the ovaries are conserved

There is no reason to believe on theoretical grounds that carcinoma of the ovary is either more or less common after hysterectomy. We may as well suppose therefore, that the risk of malignancy after hysterectomy is the same as it is in the female population as a whole.

Figure 32.1 shows the death rates from cancer of the breast, uterus and ovary per 100 000 female population in the United States from 1930 to 1967. In 37 years it appears that the risk of death in one year from cancer of the ovary has doubled in the U.S.A. from 4 per 100 000 to 8 per 100 000.

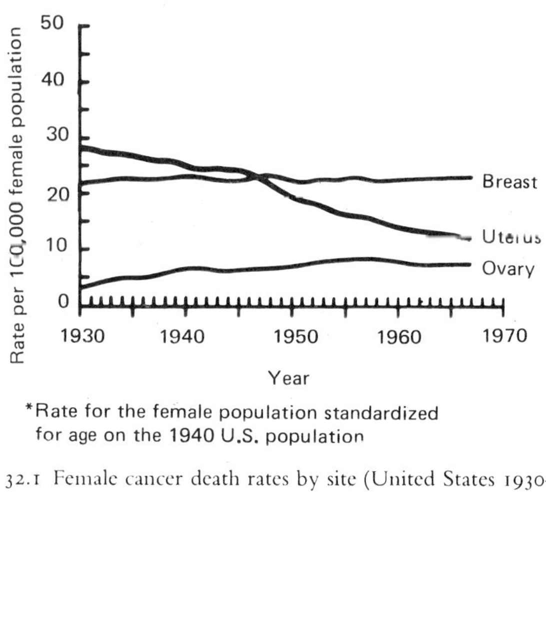

Figure 32.1 Female cancer death rates by site (United States 1930–1967)

Because the survival rate in carcinoma of the ovary is so poor the death rate approximates to the incidence.

From 1960 to 1972 the total number of deaths from malignant disease of the ovary in England and Wales rose from 2927 to 3623 (Figure 32.2). In 1972 the number of deaths from carcinoma of the breast was 11 149, from carcinoma of the cervix 2218 and carcinoma of the body of the uterus 1139. Since the number of deaths from cancer of the lung in women in 1972 was 5897 it would be more reasonable to persuade them not to smoke than either to remove their ovaries or to take cervical smears.

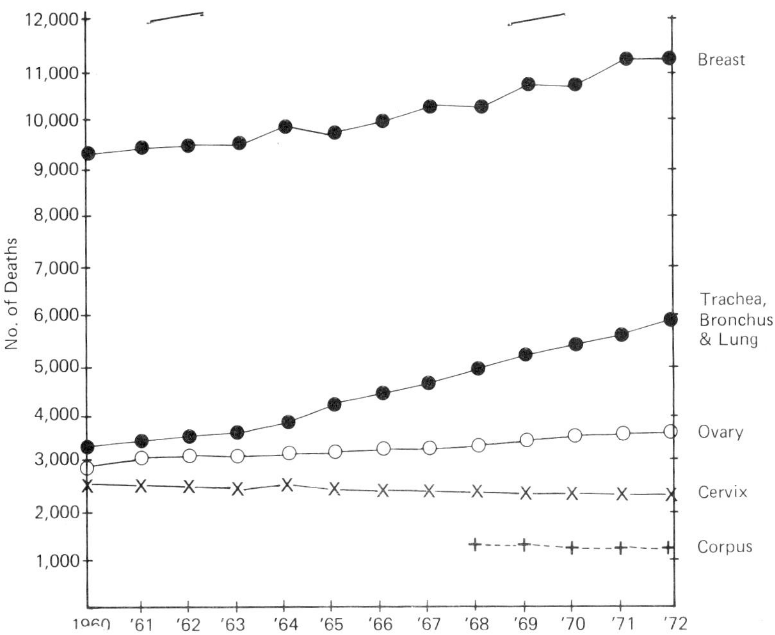

Figure 32.2 Total deaths by cause in England and Wales (Registrar General's Statistical Review)

In 1954 Randall and Gerhardt[1] worked out from figures of the incidence of disease in the State of New York the chance of a woman developing cancer of the ovary as about 1 in 100 during most of her life, although it becomes less as she grows older (Table 32.1).

There are two ways of trying to decide what is the risk of ovarian carcinoma occurring after hysterectomy. One way is to find out how many patients with ovarian cancer have had a hysterectomy. In the series of cases in Table 32.2 the proportion of women having had a hysterectomy varies from 4·2% to 26%.

Table 32.1 Probable risk of cancer after stated age in percentages

Age	*All sites*	*Breast*	*Cervix*	*Endometrium*	*Ovary*
20	23·8	5·4	2·3	1·6	1·0
30	23·7	5·4	2·3	1·6	1·0
40	23·1	5·2	2·0	1·5	0·9
50	24·5	4·6	1·6	1·4	0·8
60	18·7	3·9	1·1	1·1	0·6
70	14·9	3·0	0·7	0·7	0·4

Table 32.2 Incidence of previous hysterectomy in patients with ovarian cancer

Author	*No. of patients*	*Previous hysterectomy*
Speert (1949)[2]	260	26%
Golub (1953)[3]	211	4·2%
Counseller *et al.* (1955)[4]	1500	4·5%
Fagan (1956)[5]	172	7·5%
Bloom (1962)[6]	141	10·6%

The authors of the papers from which these figures are taken all advised the removal of ovaries when doing a hysterectomy in a woman over the age of 45 years. But these figures do not include the number of hysterectomies performed with conservation of ovaries which were *not* followed by malignancy. A more realistic way therefore, of determining the risk after hysterectomy is to follow-up cases operated on to see how many develop malignant disease of the ovary (Table 32.3).

Although it is not clear for how many years these cases were followed up the incidence of ovarian carcinoma after hysterectomy is so low, well below the expected incidence in the population at large in fact, that one is tempted to suggest that perhaps hysterectomy has a protective effect. Jeffcoate[7] said that he thought the risk of ovarian cancer after hysterectomy was less than it was for all women. He stated that he had not had the experience of treating a patient for cancer of an ovary which he himself had previously conserved. I would like to side with Jeffcoate and, being a gynaecologist, suggest that when the ovaries are carefully inspected and palpated at operation and pronounced normal the risk of subsequent cancer in them is, in fact, reduced.

Table 32.3 Incidence of ovarian cancer in patients who had hysterectomy and conservation of ovaries

Author	*No. of patients*	*Ovarian cancer*
Reycroft (1955)[8]	4500	0·2%
Funk-Brentano (1958)[9]	580	0·17%
Whitelaw (1959)[10]	1215	0
Gevaerts (1962)[11]	303	0

The risk of ovarian cysts or pelvic pain if the ovaries are conserved

Several series have been published in which is given the number of patients in whom a subsequent laparotomy was performed for reasons other than malignancy following hysterectomy and conservation of ovarian tissue (Table 32.4).

It has to be remembered that if the ovaries are conserved and pelvic pain is complained of a laparotomy is more likely to be done than in patients from whom the ovaries have been removed. For instance, in the above

Table 32.4 Risk of non-malignant pathology in ovaries conserved at hysterectomy

Author	*No. of patients*	*Subsequent laparotomy*
Grogan and Duncan (1955)[12]	391	19 (4·9%)
Whitelaw (1959)[10]	1215	4 (0·3%)
Schabort (1960)[13]	169	15 (8·9%)
Gevaerts (1962)[11]	303	6 (2%)

series, Gevaerts[11] reported six laparotomies, five of which were for adhesions. Jeffcoate said that the only ovaries that are painful after hysterectomy are those in which the operation was done for pelvic inflammatory disease. In other cases pelvic pain is usually due to causes not in the ovary, as for example, spastic colon. Whitelaw[10] showed that it is possible to do a large number of hysterectomies and to conserve the ovaries with very little risk of subsequent disease in them.

I wish now to turn to the other side of the coin and to consider what are the advantages of conserving the ovaries. There are two questions which have to be answered.

Do the ovaries continue to function after hysterectomy?

There are numerous studies to show that the ovaries continue to function after hysterectomy until the patient reaches the age of the normal menopause. As long ago as 1951 Richards[14] followed up 332 patients at the Chelsea Hospital for Women who had had a hysterectomy before the age of 45 years. He found that if both ovaries were conserved 27% had hot flushes within 2 years of operation; that if one ovary was removed 52% had hot flushes; and that if both ovaries were removed 98% had hot flushes. He suggested that one in four patients with both ovaries conserved got hot flushes because of tension put on the slender ovarian pedicle by the surgeon which brought about thrombosis of the ovarian blood vessels. Bancroft-Livingstone[4] found continuing ovarian activity for up to 3 years after operation in 95% of patients treated by hysterectomy and conservation of the ovaries. In 1958 in West Fife, Whitelaw[16] found by vaginal smears and gonadotrophin estimation that the estrogenic activity of ovaries conserved at hysterectomy persists for years; and there was, moreover, no indication that the onset of the menopause was hastened by hysterectomy. By basal temperature charts and measurement of urinary pregnanediol Whitelaw demonstrated continuing ovulation in nine out of 24 patients who had had their uteruses removed. Leverton[17] found that in 80% of cases bilaterally conserved ovaries functioned adequately for about 7 years. And then in 1969 in Melbourne, Australia, Beavis *et. al.*[18] studied ovarian function in 69 patients subjected to hysterectomy between the ages of 25 and 48 years. The ovaries were completely conserved in 48 patients and partially conserved in 21. Ovarian function was monitored for up to 2½ years by weekly urinary estrogen and pregnanediol estimations. In the group with both ovaries conserved function continued completely normally up to the expected time of the menopause. 73% of the cycles were ovulatory and the cycle duration was 28 days. In the group with ovarian tissue partially conserved the incidence of anovulatory cycles was higher.

There is, in my opinion, good evidence to support the theory of a protective effect by the ovaries against coronary artery disease and osteoporosis in later life. This has been considered in this Symposium by Dr M. F. Oliver and Dr J. M. Aitken. The protective effect after hysterectomy clearly depends on the continuing function until the menopause of conserved ovaries.

In 1964 Randall *et al.*[19] reported on 6767 pre-menopausal women of a median age of 42 years complaining of menorrhagia who were followed after treatment for more than 20 years. One third had a hysterectomy with both ovaries conserved, one third had their ovaries removed or irradiated and one third had one ovary removed or were given a small dose of irradiation. They found that in the women who had had their ovaries removed or irradiated there were nearly three times the number of deaths from cerebrovascular accidents.

Do the ovaries continue to function after the menopause?

The concensus of modern opinion seems to be that the production of steroids by the post-menopausal ovary is negligible. Longcope[20], for instance, found that there was a constant low concentration in the blood of estradiol which did not alter with injections of human chorionic gonadotrophin. The concentration in the blood of estrone varied with the daily secretion of estrone and androstenedione by the adrenal gland. Androstenedione seems to be the main source of post-menopausal estrone as the result of peripheral conversion[21]. A contrary view on the function of ovaries after the menopause has been given in this symposium by Professor I. D. Cooke.

Conclusion

What then should be the surgeon's policy at hysterectomy for benign uterine conditions, assuming that the ovaries look and feel normal? I believe that the ovaries continue to function after hysterectomy until the natural menopause; and that the advantages to the patient of their continuing function far outweigh the relatively small risks of malignancy or subsequent benign disease of the ovaries. I think therefore that they ought to be conserved whenever possible in the pre-menopausal woman. After the menopause the problem is different. If the ovaries no longer function there is little point in conserving them. *If* their continuing function after the menopause can be established the advantages of conservation again outweigh the risks.

References

1. Randall, C. L. and Gerhardt, P. R. (1954). *Amer. J. Obstet. Gynec.*, **68,** 1378
2. Speert, H. (1949). *Ann. Surg.*, **129,** 468
3. Golub, L. J. (1953). *Amer. J. Obstet. Gynec.*, **66,** 169
4. Counseller, V. S., Hunt, W. and Haigler, F. H., Jr. (1955). *Amer. J. Obstet. Gynec.*, **69,** 538
5. Fagan, G. E., Allen, E. D. and Klawans, A. H. (1956). *Obstet. Gynecol.*, **7,** 418
6. Bloom, M. L. (1962). *S. Afr. med. J.*, **36,** 714
7. Jeffcoate, T. N. A. (1967). *Principles of Gynaecology*, 3rd Edition. (London: Butterworths), p. 932
8. Reycraft, J. L. (1955). *Amer. J. Obstet. Gynec.*, **69,** 543
9. Funk-Brentano, P. (1958). *Rev. Franç. Gynécol.*, **53,** 217
10. Whitelaw, R. G. (1959). *J. Obstet. Gynaec. Brit. Emp.*, **66,** 413.
11. Gevaerts, P. O. H. (1963). Abdominale totale uterus extirpatie o sapravaginale uterus amputatie? Thesis, Leiden, Holland
12. Grogan, R. H. and Duncan, C. J. (1955). *Amer. J. Obstet. Gynec.*, **70,** 1277
13. Schabort, J. W. (1960). *Trans. Coll. Physns S. Afr.*, **4,** 11
14. Richards, N. A. (1951). *Proc. R. Soc. Med.*, **44,** 496
15. Bancroft-Livingston, G. (1954). *J. Obstet. Gynaec. Brit. Emp.*, **61,** 628
16. Whitelaw, R. G. (1958). *J. Obstet. Gynaec. Brit. Emp.*, **65,** 917
17. Leverton, J. C. S. (1958). *J. Obstet. Gynaec. Brit. Emp.* **65,** 839
18. Beavis, E. L. G., Brown, J. B. and Smith, M. A. (1969). *Obstet. Gynaec. Brit. Cwlth*, **76,** 969
19. Randall, C. L., Paloucek, F. P., Graham, J. B. and Graham, S. (1964). *Amer. J. Obstet. Gynec.*, **88,** 880
20. Longcope, C. (1974). *The Menopausal Syndrome*, Edited by R. B. Greenblatt, V. B. Manesh, and P. G. McDonough, Medcorn Press
21. Grodin, J. M., Siitteri, P. K. and MacDonald, P. C. (1973). *J. Clin. Endocrinol.*, **36,** 207

33

Contraindications to estrogen therapy and management of the menopausal syndrome in these cases

Audrey Midwinter

The only contraindication to estrogen therapy is the presence of an estrogen-dependent malignancy. This is the view expressed by those who would abolish the menopause. The ultra cautious would support the statement expressed in the British Medical Journal namely that 'long term studies of the clinical incidence of thromboembolic and other sequelae are needed before large scale replacement therapy can be recommended'[1].

The first, and I think important, contraindication to therapy is the woman with sufficient endogenous estrogen, but the question is what is sufficient and how many women do not require therapy. Providing agreement can be reached about symptoms to include, and the weighting to be placed on frequency and severity of a complaint, epidemiological surveys[2] will give estimates of those women who feel less than healthy but have not consulted a doctor. Experiment has shown that women with plasma estrogens below 40 pg/ml are symptomatic[3]. However it is not feasible on a population basis to measure plasma estrogens serially, blood lipids or bone densities to detect women who will never need supplementary estrogen. Cytological studies, easier to perform may be altered by infection or drug administration. Caution must therefore be exercised when a woman without symptoms asks for replacement therapy as a result of reading a magazine article. It would be unreasonable to accept even a low incidence of serious side effect from a drug if that drug was not needed.

The absolute contraindications, namely estrogen dependent malignancies will not be elaborated, except to emphasize that not all carcinomas of the breast are estrogen dependent. Non-malignant breast conditions such as chronic mastitis are often more painful after exhibition of estrogen, and their presence is a relative contraindication to therapy[4, 5]. Although the Boston Collaborative Drug Surveillance[6] programme found only 3 out of 6300 women using estrogen for 5 years or more had benign breast tumours, women with such conditions may have been denied treatment.

Carcinoma of the cervix is not estrogen dependent and many women have now had estrogen therapy following Wertheims hysterectomy. Myomata and endometriosis are non-malignant conditions affected by estrogen levels. Although with the smaller substitution doses of estrogen it is unlikely that fibroids enlarge and degenerate as they sometimes do with oral contraception, it is noted that breakthrough bleeding is more common if fibroids are present[7]. Surgical cure of endometriosis includes removal of ovaries[8] and these often younger patients complain bitterly of menopausal symptoms. Estrogen substitution which is started within a few weeks of hysterectomy has not provoked endometriotic symptoms, probably because doses are usually low enough not to stimulate endometrium.

An association between administered estrogen and thrombosis in the younger women has been established[9, 10] with an incidence of 1 : 2000 for estrogen and 1 : 1500 for those on oral contraceptives. The dosage and type of estrogen are not necessarily the same as those used in menopausal substitution therapy. Gow[11] using mestranol in post-menopausal women reported four of 25 patients developed a deep venous thrombosis. The Boston programme[10] reported no cases of thromboembolism in 6300 healthy women using estrogens for 5 years and no significant association between estrogen therapy and thromboembolism in healthy women aged 45–60 years. It would have been useful to know how many of the 87 of 105 women with a hospital discharge diagnosis of thromboembolism and who were excluded from the study because of hypertension, operation or obesity were taking estrogens. These conditions are not uncommon in the menopausal years. The negative association has been supported by many smaller studies (patients in some groups being followed up for many years) but some authors mention thrombosis in both control and treatment groups[1]. The difference is almost certainly in patient selection. Where a patient has had a thromboembolic episode the risk of recurrence depends on the reason for the initial episode and whether the vascular system is otherwise healthy. Many follow operation and the possibility of further operative treatment is not remote. Until it can be shown that the risks from replacement therapy and operation are lower than the risks of the contraceptive pill and operation, a previous embolic episode is a contraindication for replacement therapy.

Prominence has been given to the association between the contraceptive pill and hypertension. First mentioned by Brownrigg[12] in 1962, there have been many confirmatory reports[13]. Spellacy and Burke[14] in a prospective trial showed that ethinyl estradiol produced a significant rise in diastolic pressure but there was no change in systolic or diastolic pressure with mestranol or conjugated estrogens. They noticed that hypertensives on the combined Pill often had a history of hypertension in pregnancy. Blood pressures returned to normal within 100 days of stopping the Pill and the rises were not clinically, as opposed to statistically, significant. Professor Lauritzen states there is an acute rise in blood pressure in 66% of women within 6 to 24 months of the last period[15]. Does estrogen worsen this tendency? In a hypertensive clinic[16], five previously normotensive women developed clinically significant hypertension while taking conjugated estrogens—all showed a derangement in the renin-angiotensin 11-aldosterone system. Woods[17] considered that estrogens rarely produced this derangement. The Boston programme[10] found no correlation between estrogen therapy and hypertension in fit women but provided no information about hypertensives on antihypertensive therapy. Hypertensives if treated, need frequent blood pressure recordings. In a small personal series there have been no complications using replacement therapy.

There is a highly significant association between replacement therapy and gall bladder disease, the risk factor being 2·5[10]. Patients with previous attacks of cholecystitis should be supervised if estrogens are given. Providing liver function tests have returned to normal after infective hepatitis, estrogens are not contraindicated but with continuing damage such as cirrhosis and with a history of pregnancy cholestasis, estrogens should not be given. Estrogen also has a deleterious effect on rarities such as the Rotor, Dubin Johnson syndromes and porphyria.

No doubt, advice has already been given whether to administer estrogens to known cases of atherosclerosis or familial hyperlipidaemia. The literature gives conflicting statements. The picture in diabetes is also far from clear. Ethinyl estradiol and mestranol decrease glucose tolerance and have an anti-insulin effect[11, 18]. Maturity-onset diabetes occurs when natural estrogen is declining. Estrogen may protect against atherosclerosis more commonly found in diabetes. The conclusions are: use estrogen but check the diabetic control early.

Finally, pre-menstrual epilepsy and migraine are cited as relative contra-indications, although it has been suggested that attacks occur when estrogen levels drop pre-menstrually in the younger woman. Most of these contra-indications are relative and a balance has to be set between drug side effects and the risks of not treating. Suicide risks are easy to obtain, but did that road accident result from a sleepy depressed woman stiff from her arthralgia or was it due to her tranquillizers?

Alternative therapy

This may be required instead of, or in addition to, estrogen. Insomnia, depression and anxiety are not always relieved by estrogen. Antidepressants, tranquillizers and hypnotics are often necessary and only fall into disrepute if repeat prescriptions are issued without a review of symptoms. I am not going to offer a best buy from the 120 preparations listed, for example in MIMS. The aim is to choose a drug which will relieve several symptoms, i.e. hot flushes, muscle pains and will also have a tranquillizing effect.

Psychotherapy of a non-intensive kind, i.e. a trained listener is essential[19]. The availability of this help in some trials has resulted in a marked placebo effect. A paid job not necessarily commensurate with former skills will prevent social isolation. This is as important as the 'pin money'. In these days of sophisticated medicine, simple advice is often not mentioned. Innumerable cups of coffee or tea cause caffeine excess so worsening insomnia and hot flushes. Exercise to the point of fatigue and/or a hot bath are good hypnotics.

Dr Jaszmann has indicated that all 22 symptoms of the menopause do not have to be treated concurrently. Early complaints of irregular bleeding, a fear of pregnancy or cancer are tackled by provision of effective contraception, exclusion of carcinoma and if necessary progestogens, epsikapron or hysterectomy. Symptoms associated with the autonomic nervous system follow and various drugs have been used to control flushing and sweats. None of them is as efficient as estrogen. Clonidine hydrochloride (Dixarit) originally introduced as a migraine prophylaxis decreases the frequency of flushes by 50%[20]. Patients in three trials[21, 22] of this drug were on other medication, in one instance these included hormonal preparations. The drug has not been compared with other non-hormonal preparations. Bellergal contains belladonna alkaloids egotomine and phenobarbitone. Belladonna has been used to control flushing and sweats since 1840. Bellergal partly relieves but does not abolish nervousness 87%, fatigue 62%, irritability 87%, as well as flushing 87%[23]. Whether the combination of drugs is superior to its components used separately I cannot discover. The barbiturate would relieve mild anxiety but in some women deepens depression. Norethisterone[24] has been used to relieve flushing with a reasonable degree of success. It also improves headaches and fatigue but increases premenstrual depression. Other progestogens without inherent estrogen effect have no beneficial effect except, like androgens, they may give a non-specific feeling of 'well being'. Mainly used in conjunction with estrogen to prevent overstimulation of the endometrium it should be remembered that they too have side effects—decreased glucose tolerance, anabolic weight gain and occasional virilism. It has been suggested that they, like androgen, counteract the beneficial effects of estrogen on the cardiovascular system. A trial of diazepam and propanolol[25] for the relief of hot flushes and palpitations demonstrated that the former was superior in controlling flushing and decreasing awareness rather than frequency of palpitations. In addition there was noticeable improvement in irritability—systolic and diastolic blood pressures were lowered.

The last symptoms to be reported are those associated with atrophic changes in the vagina, the urethral syndrome and prolapse. The elimination of vaginal candida and alteration of vaginal pH to prevent its recurrence will partly relieve dyspareunia. A lubricant will help mechanically and psycho-sexual advice may be required. Dilatation of the urethra, elimination of infection and drugs such as emepronium bromide (Cetiprin) are used with varying success but are never as effective as estrogen.

The role of testosterone in treating menopausal symptoms causes most controversy. Testosterone derivatives have been and are given by tablet, injection or implant together with or instead of estrogen. Its advocates point out that it does cure symptoms and may be superior to estrogen in promoting a sense of well being and also in increasing libido. Symptoms of depression lassitude and anxiety are particularly well controlled. The risk of break-through bleeding is less and it is said to protect against osteo-porosis. Its opponents point out the risk of virilization; sensitivity to andro-gens differing widely. Some women show no virilization on 100–200 mg a month, while others develop facial hair with 10 mg a month[26].

Androgens counteract the beneficial effects of estrogen on the vascular system. Providing the risk factors are going to be evaluated as meticulously as those of estrogen they may have a place in treatment where estrogen is contraindicated.

Although we have changed the drugs, the principles of non-hormonal treatment have not altered since Tilt[27] wrote 100 years ago. From the litera-ture our success rate for relieving symptoms is no higher. Firmly believing in the quality of life the writer believes the benefits of estrogen in most cases outweigh the risks.

References

1. Coope, J., Thomson, J. M. and Poller, L. (1975). Effects of 'natural oestrogen' replacement therapy on menopausal symptoms. *Br. Med. J.*, **4**, 139
2. Jaszmann, L. (1973). Epidemiology of Climacteric and post climacteric complaints. Ageing and oestrogens. *Frontiers Hormone Res.*, **2**, 22
3. Daw, E. (1974). Luteinising hormone changes in women undergoing artificial menopause. *Curr. Med. Res. Opinion*, **2**, 256

4. Lauritzen, C. (1973). Ageing and oestrogens. *Frontiers Hormone Res.*, **2,** 7
5. Netter, A. (1973). Ageing and oestrogens. *Frontiers Hormone Res.*, **2,** 145
6. A Report from the Boston Collaborative Drμg Surveillance Program 1974. *New Engl. J. Med.*, **290,** 1, 15
7. Hauser, G. A. (1973). Ageing and oestrogens. *Frontiers Hormone Res.*, **2,** 39
8. Dewhurst, G. J. (1972). *Integrated Obstetrics and gynaecology for post graduates*, 480
9. Vessey, M. P. and Doll, R. (1968). *Br. Med. J.*, **2,** 199
10. Report from the Boston Collaborative Drug Surveillance Programe 1973. *Lancet*, **ii,** 1399
11. Gow, S. and MacGillavray, I. (1971). Mestranol in oophorectomised women. *Br. Med. J.*, **2,** 73
12. Brownrigg, G. M. (1962). Toxaemia in hormonally induced pseudo pregnancy. *Can. Med. Ass. J.*, **87,** 408
13. MacKay, E. V., Khoo, S. K. and Shan, N. A. (1973). Reproductive steroids and the circulatory system. *Obstet. Gyne. Surv.*, **28,** 3, 155
14. Spellacy, W. N. and Birk, S. A. (1970). The development of elevated blood pressure while using oral contraceptives. *Fertil. Steril.*, **21,** 301
15. Lauritzen, C. (1973). Ageing and oestrogens. *Frontiers Hormone Res.*, **2,** 5
16. Crane, M. G., Harris, J. J., and Winsor, W. (1971). *Ann. Intern. Med.*, **74,** 13
17. Woods, J. W. (1967). Oral contraceptives and hypertension. *Lancet*, **ii,** 653
18. Lauritzen, C. (1973). Ageing and oestrogens. *Frontiers Hormone Res.*, **2,** 47
19. Kerr, D. M. and Vaghan, R. N. (1975). Psychohormonal treatment during the menopause. *Amer. Family Physician*, **2,** 99
20. Clayden, J. R., Bell, J. W., Pollard, P. (1974). Menopausal flushing a double clinical trial of a non hormonal preparation. *Brit. Med. J.*, **1,** 409
21. Clayden, J. R. (1972). *Lancet*, **ii,** 1361
22. Williams, C. W. L. (1973). *Lancet*, **ii,** 298
23. Kely, M. J. A., Power, R. M. H. and Arromet, G. H. (1961). Management of the perimenopausal syndrome. *Obstet. Gynecol.*, **17,** 3, 328
24. Appleby, B. (1962). Norethisterone in the control of menopausal symptoms. *Lancet*, **i,** 407
25. Kolar, E. K., Issalo, E. and Punnonen, R. (1973). Effect of propanolol and oxazepan on some vegetative menopausal symptoms. *Ann. Clin. Res.*, **5,** 208
26. Netter, A. (1973). Ageing and oestrogens. *Frontiers Hormone Res.*, **2,** 47
27. Tilt, E. J. (1870). The change of life in health and disease

34

Hormone implants in the climacteric syndrome

J. W. W. Studd

The treatment of vasomotor instability following hysterectomy and bilateral oophorectomy with an estrogen implant was first described by Bishop[1] and many publications supporting this mode of therapy subsequently appeared[2–5] and although there are no reports of major side-effects from pellet implantation, the technique has inexplicably fallen from favour. Greenblatt[6] and Schleyer-Saunders[7] have repeatedly advocated this method of hormone replacement therapy and it is to be hoped that the work of Hunter *et al.*[8] and the renewed interest in the management of the climacteric will stimulate re-appraisal of the relative merits of oral and pellet medication. This paper consists of a discussion on the technique, but the results of the clinical and endocrinological investigations of 150 patients receiving hormone implants are awaiting completion and cannot yet be presented.

There are three principal regimens of hormone therapy for the climacteric syndrome:

(1) Oral therapy with an estrogen preparation taken daily for 3 weeks out of 4 is the simplest and most commonly used method. A small withdrawal bleed may occur within the 7 tablet-free days in three or four cycles each year. Breakthrough bleeding is uncommon but a minor problem of cyclical therapy is the recurrence of vasomotor symptoms towards the end of the week off therapy.

(2) Continuous oral estrogen therapy obviates this problem but unscheduled bleeding will occur unless a progestogen is added in the last half

of the cycle. Shedding of the endometrium occurs at a predictable time and the theoretical possibility of over-stimulation of the endometrium is avoided.

(3) Implants of ovarian hormones allow the continuous release from the pellet. This is convenient for women who have undergone hysterectomy and the claim that nausea and vomiting are less common than with oral estrogens[6] is supported by our preliminary observations.

Method

The usual site of implantation is the subcutaneous fat of the abdominal wall 2 inches above and parallel to the inguinal ligament. An area of skin 2–3 inches in diameter is cleaned with iodine solution and an intradermal injection of 2 ml of local anaesthetic inserted. The cannula method of implanatation is preferred, using the small or large trocar and cannula (Organon Laboratories) designed for the cylindrical pellets of 2·2 mm or 4·5 mm diameter respectively. The whole length of the sterilized trocar is pushed through the anaesthetized area in the subcutaneous fat, avoiding the rectus sheath and any scar tissue from previous surgery. The pellet is placed into the cannula using sterile forceps and pushed to the depths of the track by the obturator. The cannula and obturator are removed and the skin wound covered with a sterile adhesive plaster. It must be kept dry for the following 2 days. The technique is simple, painless and can be performed in the outpatient department.

Estradiol pellets of 50 mg have an approximate duration of action of 6 months and the 100 mg pellets may last for 9 months, at which time the patient usually becomes aware of return of symptoms and may need a further implant. Sometimes a combination of estradiol 50 mg and testosterone 100 mg may be necessary in patients with a severe loss of libido which has not responded to estrogen alone. The androgen should not be given to hirsute patients as a slight increase in facial hair is an occasional side effect. A potential problem of implant therapy is irregular bleeding. In the past, gynaecologists have been unwilling to use this method in patients with a uterus but such selection is unnecessary as unscheduled bleeding can be prevented by provoking a progestogen withdrawal bleed each month. Norethisterone 5 mg daily may be used or medroxyprogesterone 10 mg or ethynodiol diacetate 0·5 mg daily for 5 days each month.

A convenient regimen is for the patient to take a progestogen for the first 5 days of each calendar month and a scanty withdrawal bleed can be expected on the 7th or the 8th day of the month.

Our initial experience of hormone implant therapy has been favourable, with good patient acceptibility and response of symptoms with few side effects consisting of excessive weight gain in two patients, breast discomfort in approximately one half of the study group and no incidence of troublesome nausea or breakthrough bleeding. A detailed, long-term study is in progress and will be reported.

References

1. Bishop, P. M. F. (1938). A clinical experiment in oestrin therapy. *Br. Med. J.*, **1**, 939
2. Greenblatt, R. B. and Suran, R. R. (1949). Indications for hormonal pellets in the therapy of endocrine and gynecological disorders. *Amer. J. Obstet. Gynec.*, **57**, 294
3. Brown, M. L., Lucente, E. R., Alesbury, J. M. and Perloff, W. H. (1951). Treatment of surgical menopause with estradiol implants at the time of surgery. *Amer. J. Obstet. Gynec.*, **61**, 200
4. Soule, S. D. (1951). *J. Int. Coll. Surg.*, **16**, 622
5. Delaplaine, R. W., Bottomy, J. R., Blatt, M., Wiesbader, H. and Kupperman, H. S. (1952). Effective control of the surgical menopause by estradiol pellet implantation at the time of surgery. *Surg., Gynec. Obstet.*, **94**, 323
6. Greenblatt, R. B., Bruneteau, D. G. and Merchandani, J. (1974). *The Menopausal Syndrome*, Ed. R. B. Greenblatt, V. B. Mahesh, P. G. McDonough (New York: Medcom)
7. Schleyer-Saunders, E. (1974). '*The Menopausal Syndrome*', Ed. R. B. Greenblatt, V. B. Mahesh, P. G. McDonough (New York: Medcom)
8. Hunter, D. J. S., Akande, E. O., Carr, P. and Stallworthy, J. (1973). The clinical and endocrinological effect of oestradiol implants at the time of hysterectomy and bilateral salpingo-oophorectomy. *J. Obstet. Gynaecol. Br. Cwlth*, **80**, 287

Discussion on Section I: Therapeutic Problems

Chairman: *Professor J. C. McLure Browne*

Mr L. P. Harvey (Gynaecologist, Rugby): How will Mr Studd know when his implants have exhausted themselves, and how will he assess when they need a top up, or does he not intend to top them up?

Mr J. W. W. Studd (Gynaecologist, London): The pellets begin to work after about 7 days, but it is my experience that the patients have to wait 4 or 5 weeks before they have an increase in libido. The patients know when the effect is falling off. The time when the fall off occurs depends on the dose of the pellett. A 50-mg pellet will last about six months; a 100-mg pellet about nine months. I would stress that even after the effects of the pellet have worn off, it is important to continue giving the patients a bleed every month with progestogens, otherwise they will start to bleed all around the calendar.

Mr E. S. Saunders (Gynaecologist, London). I have used implants in the abdominal wall, but I noticed too many haematomas and expulsions, and I changed to the gluteal region.

I used to use large pellets, 50 mg or 100 mg, and I found that some of them, which were taken out for examination, were encapsulated in fibrous tissue and made inactive. I therefore prefer to use 25 mg pellets.

Mr J. W. W. Studd: I cannot really comment. I have only tried the abdominal wall. I have had one haematoma in about 160 patients, and I have not yet experienced any rejection of pellets.

Mr C. H. Naylor (Gynaecologist, London): I was interested to hear about the importance of autoimmune disease in the aetiology of the premature menopause. Could we hear about the role played by estrogens in modifying autoimmune disorders and their effect in the management of premature menopausal symptoms.

Dr H. S. Jacobs (Gynaecological Endocrinologist, London): I am not too certain about the role of estrogens in modifying autoimmune disease. One of the things that Irvine did report (Irvine, W. J. (1974). *Proc. R. Soc. Med.*, **67**, 548), however, was that one of his patients with Addison's disease who had circulating antibodies to steroid-producing cells, when put on to a slightly larger dose of prednisone than is normally used in the replacement therapy of Addison's disease, got a resumption of ovulation cycles. The implication there was that the glucocorticoid had suppressed the immune response, and that perhaps there is another form of ovarian failure in which there may be a degree of reversibility. I know of no data on the effect of estrogen on the autoimmune process that complicates some cases of Addison's disease and may go on to produce ovarian failure.

Dr H. Minhas (Gynaecologist, Leeds): With HRT is there any evidence of retroperitoneal fibrosis, as has occurred with clonidine and other drugs?

Can I also ask about the medico-legal aspect of prescribing HRT. If a patient to whom one prescribes HRT should develop one of the complications about which we have heard, what would be the doctor's legal position?

Dr Audrey Midwinter (Gynaecologist, Bristol): In answer to the first question, there is no evidence at all of this particular risk with estrogen therapy. The legal risks would be the same as for treating any patient with any drug. If the doctor thought that the drug was useful in treating a symptom, and provided that the patient had been given a reasonable estimate of the risks, the doctor would not be held liable.

Section J

MANAGEMENT OF THE MENOPAUSE

Chairman: J. W. W. STUDD

35

A European viewpoint

Ch. Lauritzen

The ovary, besides the placenta and the thymus, is the only endocrine gland which regresses fairly early in life and ceases to function long before the death of the individual occurs. In contrast, the male gonads may produce hormones within a normal range into old age. So in fact, at an age of about 50 years a primary ovarian insufficiency develops in the female. This is a time when statistically the female has still about one third of her lifetime before her. The failing of the female gonads, signalled by amenorrhea and hot flushes, makes it rather brutally clear to the woman that she is no longer young and that old age is imminent.

If we consider that it is a general principle of endocrinology that an ovarian insufficiency should be treated by substitution of the missing hormone, then the question to be answered is: should the spontaneous oophoropause at 50 be judged by the same criteria as any other endocrine insufficiency or as a castration would be at a much earlier age? Let us consider this problem:

The need for a hormone replacement can be determined by the answer to two questions:

(1) Will the failing of the hormone cause severe subjective or objective withdrawal symptoms?

(2) Will the hormonal insufficiency have a negative effect on the health, the physical and mental fitness, the capability of working, the self-reliance and the self-fulfilment of the individual? Will it even provoke diseases which might reduce life expectancy?

Some of these points are indeed a possible consequence in the majority of climacteric women. So it follows, that estrogen substitution is certainly justified in climacteric women where these criteria apply.

We frequently hear the argument that the climacteric is something natural and need not, therefore, be treated. However, it is the task and the daily role of the physician to correct nature where it is thought to fail according to human standards. Moreover, in my opinion the borderline is certainly crossed if a patient genuinely suffers from her complaints and if maladies which are absolutely unnecessary (and which are safely treatable and preventable) occur as a consequence of estrogen deprivation.

From these arguments, I think, it follows that the climacteric is not always and not exclusively a physiological process and that it may frequently contain the elements of a disease according to current modern definition. So treatment of complaints and of post-menopausal diseases caused by estrogen deficiency seems both logical and in accordance with the law of cause and effect. However, the practical problem is: who should receive estrogens? Should it be a great or a small selected number of women? What are the criteria available for this decision?

It is current practice to prescribe an estrogen preparation only if a woman comes to her doctor and complains of severe climacteric symptoms. The diagnosis is then made from the typical vasomotor symptoms the patient experiences, from her age, menstrual disturbances or the absence of bleeding. Thereafter, the diagnosis is further confirmed by the exclusion of diseases with similar symptoms. When estrogen therapy removes the symptoms complained of, it can be concluded that they were probably caused by the climacteric.

But what about the women, who do not come to the surgery because they have no complaints even though they have symptoms? Should they be located through publicity and persuaded to receive prophylactic treatment? This demand has been made repeatedly by ardent defenders of prophylactic long-term estrogen therapy. However, it is not possible at present to predict, for instance, with what frequency and severity symptoms of estrogen deficiency may occur in patients who do not suffer from severe subjective climacteric complaints. Therefore, we do not know exactly whether a prophylactic treatment with estrogens would be really necessary for all patients or not. We have to rely here on circumstantial and incomplete evidence, which admittedly is becoming increasingly in favour of a broader application of prophylactic estrogen administration in the post-menopause. But it must be pointed out, that we are really acting more on the grounds of assumption at present rather than on the basis of safe knowledge.

For the time being a temporary solution to the problem may result from purely practical considerations, because a broad application of prophylactic estrogen medication is impractical in that it would impose a very heavy burden on the medical profession. So I think there is no great danger of an indiscriminate use of estrogens. A patient who is treated with hormones has to be carefully supervised and checked regularly. This undebatable necessity would clearly exceed the capacity of the average physician considering the number of patients he has to deal with. In practice, of course, a high percentage of patients will take their estrogens only for a short time and will drop out if they no longer have menopausal symptoms.

There is another point: the physician, who prescribes a hormonal preparation, of course wants to have a proper indication for so doing. So if no complaints are present and no atrophy of the genital organs is found, what criteria has he? The proliferation index of the vaginal smear may sometimes give an indication, but the correlation with other relevant parameters is not always so good. What criterion then makes a doctor confident that estrogen treatment is really necessary? In other words how can he know whether the patient later on will reliably develop estrogen deficiency symptoms which would have required prophylaxis? There is also the point that he can never be quite sure whether an individual patient will not perhaps have side-effects from the treatment such as unwanted bleedings, gall bladder disturbances or alteration of her glucose metabolism and possibly others even more severe (e.g. deep vein thrombosis and cancer).

From this, it seems quite apparent, that the criteria for an exact diagnosis of estrogen demand are required, and also that the need for estrogen administration should be more exactly defined. Lastly, parameters for the accurate doses required and for the most suitable estrogen in the individual case have to be worked out. In addition it is important to note that a scheme is urgently needed for assessing in advance the long-term effects and of possible risk factors for an individual patient. It is quite clear, that all this is unrealizable at present. But this ideal gives scientific research on the problem of the climacteric and its future aims.

With these considerations in mind we have started to determine estrogen levels in plasma, and urine and of testosterone, dehydroepiandrosterone, FSH-LH, prolactin and LH-releasing-hormone. A functional vaginal smear and an assessment of the trophic status of the genitalia of the breasts and of the skin is also done. One group presenting with climacteric complaints (or requesting estrogen therapy) is treated. The other group is not treated with estrogens irrespective of their hormone levels.

You may think this is unnecessary and that it does not perhaps represent a course of action that some research workers might find statistically meaningful, but we hope to get some knowledge from this long-term prospective study concerning the problems discussed above. There are some other, but admittedly still vague, possibilities of a prognostic or early diagnostic judgement being available for the most important diseases of post-climacteric women. More thorough investigations should be made concerning the determination of excretion of calcium in the first morning urine and of hydroxyproline as a means of an early diagnosis of osteoporosis. Much more exact, reliable and practicable tests of this kind are indeed needed. On the other hand there is the possibility of tentatively identifying risk groups for the more severe side effects such as gall bladder diseases, deep venous thromboses, and disturbances of glucose and lipid metabolism by analysing the anamnestic data and diagnostic findings in the patient.

Estrogen treatment, especially long-term medication, can only be recommended if it bears no appreciable risk and if the benefit is much greater than any possible risk. (It might certainly be said, that there is a lack of sufficiently large and well planned prospective studies and that the papers, which have been published are of questionable quality.) The practice and experience of more than 30 years post-menopausal estrogen therapy on a large scale involving about 2 million women years published in the literature has shown, in my opinion, that even long-term cyclical therapy with natural estrogens in the usual doses causes virtually no significant increase in unwanted severe side effects and has not produced a noticeable increase of carcinoma and thromboembolism so far. This, I think, is a comforting fact

None of us accepts other authorities uncritically. However, it is always interesting to know the opinion of other scientists who have dealt with the problem of post-menopausal estrogen therapy for a long time. If one is familiar with the work of different research workers on the menopause and if one reads their papers, one will find, that virtually all the most experienced workers hold the view that the greatest possible number of post-menopausal patients should receive long-term natural estrogen substitution.

It should not be overlooked of course, that there is also a contrary view held by those opposed to estrogen administration to post-menopausal women. But in many instances one finds much uncritical generalization, hidden prejudice, rigid conservatism, sheer emotion, and sometimes an astonishing lack of basic knowledge. Most reasoning against an estrogen therapy is based on a feeling that substitution up to the old age is in some way against nature There is a mythical taboo against 'sexual' hormones in general and a mostly irrational fear of a possible syncarcinogenic action of estrogens. The attitude to adopt over estrogen treatment should be determined by knowledge and information. How well informed, therefore, on this subject are practising clinicians and indeed the population as a whole in Germany?

The investigation of this question by Dr van Keep (1973) has shown that 71% of women of 50 years of age in Germany know the definition of the climacteric, of estrogens and of the possibility of treatment of the menopausal syndrome. This high degree of knowledge is largely due to the many articles in newspapers and journals. In the other European countries knowledge of the post-menopause seems less wide-spread. More than 50% of all post-menopausal women in the Federal Republic of Germany have consulted a doctor for their menopause problems. Again the percentages in the other European countries are lower.

As far as the knowledge of the doctors about climacteric problems is concerned and their willingness to prescribe estrogens I can state from my own experience that their knowledge and interest is high in my country and that the education especially of the young doctors and students in this area is increasingly satisfactory.

In the Federal Republic of Germany between 10 and 20% of all climacteric women are on estrogen treatment. We have the following oral estrogens for a treatment. (1) Conjugated estrogens, (2) estradiol valerate, (3) ethinyl-estradiol and its cyclopentyl-enol ether, (4) stilbestrol, (5) ethinyl-estradiol-methyltestosterone, (6) estriol and estriol succinate, most of them as coated tablets. Several long acting injectable preparations are available: several esters of combined estradiol–testosterone, one of estradiol–dehydroepiandrosterone enanthate and a prolonged polyestriol phosphate are also available. Lastly, depot injections of estradiol- and stilbestrol-esters are on the market.

Oral cyclic medication is the one which is most widely used. I prefer the natural estrogens, which means those estrogens occurring naturally in humans and higher animals, in contrast to the artificial estrogens—stilbestrol, mestranol and ethinyl-estradiol. Estriol is a relatively weak estrogen. However, it has the advantage of not provoking bleeding and permits continuous therapy. Estrogen–androgen combinations, although very effective, are less frequently used because of their virilizing side effects. The testosterone has been substituted in one preparation by dehydroepiandosterone enanthate an adrenocortical steroid hormone, which has been reported to exert slightly antidepressive effects. The application of dehydroepiandrosterone in the post-menopause seems to make sense, because this adrenal steroid decreases in old age and is also diminished in obesity and in mammary carcinoma. Stilbestrol, ethinylestradiol and mestranol are no longer used in my practice because of the poor tolerance, the thromboembolism reports and the negative influence on triglycerides. Treatment should be highly individualized.

In oral treatment with the conjugated estrogens, estradiol valerate and estriol, I give rather high doses in the beginning of medication, to reach a high effective estrogen level rapidly (e.g. 1 tablet three times a day). On the fourth day I decrease the dose to the maintainance level, which is about

1·25–0·6 mg conjugated estrogens and 1–2 mg estradiol valerate. Estriol is given in doses of 3 × 1 tablet in the first week and 2 × 1 in the second week, then 1–2 tablets as a maintainance dose. Estriol is given continuously without interruption in the fourth week. This overcomes the drawback of returning symptoms in the week without medication, which is often experienced with cyclical therapy. A fixed combination of an estrogen with a sedative or tranquillizer is unnecessary and cannot be recommended. In the pre-menopause with commencement of climacteric complaints I prescribe sequential preparations such as Cyclo-Progynova, an estradiol valerate with norgestrel in the second phase or Premarin with an oral progestagen in the second half of the cycle. This provides a very good stabilization of the cycle. If contraception is needed I prefer the low estrogen sequential pill, which can be given up to 52 years or even longer. Subjective side effects of oral or parenteral medication are no problem in my practice and are very considerably less than with the pill. Most patients complaining of side-effects are neurotic or are placebo reactors. It is important to note that pain in the breasts is always the first sign of estrogen overdosage. If this complaint occurs the dose must be decreased at once. With conjugated estrogens and estradiol valerate I have unwanted uterine bleedings in about 2% of the patients treated. That is in about 0·3% of all treatment cycles. Only 0·2%–0·5% of the patients treated with estriol will show uterine bleedings. This corresponds to 0·015–0·03% of all treatment cycles and is about the same frequency as with placebo or as without therapy.

Contraindications to estrogen therapy include very severe liver diseases, recent episodes of gall bladder disease and of thromboembolism and porphyria as well as untreated mammary and endometrial carcinoma. Fully treated, non-invasive mammary and endometrial carcinoma are not contraindications.

In my 20 years experience with estrogen therapy in pre- and post-menopausal patients and in my more than 700 published cases I have not seen severe deep venous thrombosis or emboli in connection with administration of the usual doses of natural estrogens. Neither have I seen cerebrovascular accidents as a consequence of estrogen therapy. I am not aware of a single case where the origin of a cervical, endometrial or mammary carcinoma or the clinical deterioration of this disease could clearly be attributed to the medication of perimenopausal estrogen therapy. In conclusion I want to give you a summary of my personal views based on my own experience, my own scientific work, my surveys of the published literature and my discussions with a great number of laymen, practitioners and leading research workers.

In my opinion it would be desirable to give estrogens to a broader population of climacteric women than is practiced at present. Treatment of climacteric complaints is recommendable and seems even necessary to me, and prophylactic medication for a very long time up to old age would be logical and well founded in the light of our present knowledge. I see long-term prophylactic medication as a method of prophylactic medicine, capable of removing unnecessary and disagreeable symptoms, and capable of preventing the atrophic changes of the uro-genital organs with their unpleasant sequelae such as discharges, pain, bleeding, craurosis, pruritus and dispareunia. The efficiency of an estrogen therapy in the post-menopause has been adequately proved in numerous double-blind studies. The long-term medication with natural estrogens in adequate doses certainly produces a better psychic stability and a sense of well being. It may improve concentration and memory and hinder the development of depressive moods. It certainly gives many women the feeling of continuing to be youthful, attractive and efficient. Estrogen therapy is apparently capable of retarding some ageing of the skin and can prevent post-menopausal osteoporosis caused by estrogen deficiency. The risk of long-term estrogen medication for the patients seems to be small and may indeed become negligible if contraindications and risk groups are adequately considered and if regular controls are performed. These groups may indeed receive better care and show better health all round.

Many problems remain to be solved. Certainly much more has to be investigated and learned, particularly from large and well-planned prospective studies on the risks and benefits of long-term estrogen medication. I am convinced, that the endocrinology of ageing and the hormonal treatment of the ageing woman and male will certainly become an important task of research and of practical care and management in the future society.

References

1. Keep, P. van and Lauritzen, Ch., Editors: (1973). Ageing and estrogens. In: *Frontiers of Hormone Research* Vol. 2 (Basel–München–Paris–London–New York–Sidney: Karger)
2. Keep, P. van and Lauritzen, Ch., Editors: (1975). Estrogens in the postmenopause. In: *Frontiers of Hormone Research* Vol. 3 (Basel–München–Paris–London–New York–Sidney: Karger)

36

An English viewpoint

R. J. Beard

In this paper I will set out my own personal views. My interest started in this subject while I was working at the Chelsea Hospital for Women.

Since leaving there, I have maintained my interest by running a similar clinic in Brighton.

Hormone replacement therapy has been slow to become popular in this country, and has been even slower to reach the majority of post-menopausal women.

Several factors are responsible. Replacement therapy has always been available to private patients as in America and on the Continent. Some English doctors have gained great experience in this field; unfortunately their work has not been greatly publicized, either because of their reticence or more probably because the medical establishment has not been keen to listen.

In the past, undergraduates were not taught about hormone replacement therapy; they were told that replacement therapy came under the heading of monkey gland treatment, was highly suspect, caused cancer of the uterus and was only used by a few unscrupulous practitioners at the wrong end of Harley Street.

Hormone replacement therapy requires time. Unfortunately time, as well as nurses, equipment and money are rare commodities in the National Health Service today. Outside teaching hospitals, a gynaecologist can seldom spend more than 10 minutes with each new patient, a general practitioner often less. Furthermore, resources are so limited, now, more than ever before, that many practitioners consider replacement therapy social medicine, and therefore not a justifiable expense.

However, over the past few years British gynaecological practice has been reluctantly changing under pressures from two influences. Firstly, there have been an increasing number of papers appearing in our medical journals extolling the virtues of estrogen therapy. Secondly, and the more important, has been the pressure from the media. As a direct result of changing attitudes and women's liberation responsible journalists, such as Wendy Cooper, have been publicizing the advantages of hormone replacement therapy. Despite *Feminine Forever*, and *No Change* most women have gained their information from articles in magazines. I think we owe these journalists a debt, because they have forced us to look more deeply into an area of gynaecology that has been previously neglected in this country. It is these articles which have kept the queues of patients outside menopause clinics from diminishing and without these patients our research would not be possible. Women frequently get their referal letters by way of presenting their general practitioners with a sheaf of relevant articles taken from women's magazines and the address of the nearest clinic.

I recently asked student nurses in Brighton to fill in a questionnaire on the menopause. Their knowledge was often shaky to say the least. 77% thought they had not been given enough information. When asked from where their information came, women's magazines came out on top, well ahead of parents, textbooks, school teachers, nursing tutors, friends, radio and television.

As a result of this increasing demand for therapy, numerous menopause clinics have been set up. These have mostly arisen in academic settings, being partly financed from sources other than the National Health Service. I would like to take this opportunity for thanking the drug companies for making these research clinics possible.

Such a menopause clinic must have the full use of the pathological services of a general hospital. Adequate time is essential. I allocate 30 minutes to each new patient and 15 minutes for each follow-up. The equipment required is the same as in every gynaecological out-patient department. One must be able to take blood pressures, cervical smears and out patient endometrial curettages. It seems to me that the Family Planning Association are in an ideal situation to set up such clinics; they have the skill, the staff, and the resources.

These clinics will continue to do important research into hormone replacement. An example of this is the very careful study being undertaken by John Studd with implants. However, no individual clinic will see enough patients to give us good epidemiological data. The Royal College has pioneered this field with the Confidential Enquiry into Maternal Deaths. I hope that it will apply the same enthusiasm in organizing multicentre prospective studies on HRT.

Hot flushes, sweats and dryness of the vagina are the only symptoms which are always alleviated by estrogen therapy. Many other symptoms appear at the time of the menopause or a little earlier.

Women often complain that their hair and nails change. Skin becomes dryer and there is a tendency to put on weight.

About a quarter of women have very few symptoms, half have some, but are able to cope, while the remainder may have marked and incapacitating symptoms which go on for years. All sorts of personal and environmental pressures influence the way in which a woman copes. Despite what I imagine, it is often difficult to predict into which particular category an individual woman will fall when she reaches the menopause.

Any of these symptoms that occur in the absence of vasomotor disturbances and vaginal dryness should be viewed with suspicion, and not automatically attributed to falling estrogen levels. Likewise, if their symptoms do not respond to therapy, other causes may be looked for.

Loss of libido is common at this time; this symptom is not helped by estrogens, unless vaginal dryness is a problem. The biochemical cause is related to reduced androgen production and hormone therapy is not so easy, but luckily this symptom does not remain a problem for long in most happily married couples.

It is all too easy to blame estrogen deficiency for the effects of ageing on skin and hair. Normal ageing occurs without estrogens. For example, a patient with primary ovarian dysgenesis (Turner's Syndrome) gets older like everybody else. Likewise, a woman on replacement therapy will look older at 70 than she does at 50. Patients have been too easily influenced by the appearance of smart, affluent and active American women seen on television. If one removed their social and economic privileges it is possible that the effects of estrogen would not be so noticeable. One can often predict which patients are going to respond well to estrogen therapy. I have found that a thin active woman, whose chief complaint is that she finds vasomotor symptoms embarrasing at work, in their office, school or shop, responds most dramatically and is the most grateful.

One may be tempted to criticize a busy doctor for giving his menopause patient diazepam, but in my opinion it is worse if one gives hormones without full examination and adequate discussion. The menopause must be explained. It is a natural phenomenon and the symptoms usually temporary. Sympathetic support from her husband and family is a great help. She must pay attention to her appearance and keep her weight down.

Mental and physical activities should be encouraged as well as increased involvement with her family and grandchildren. Sometimes taking up a part-time job adds purpose to her life and gets her out of the house away from many of her problems. At this stage in her life, a woman is often confronted by an environment which is changing more rapidly than her own hormone status. Her children may be leaving home, grandchildren and strange in-laws enter her life, and death and illness begin to appear in her close relatives and friends. Her husband is often preoccupied by his work and his sexual interests may be on the wane or transferred to another woman. It is sometimes the case that the menopause has little significance compared with these other problems.

Loss of libido requires much reassurance. Regular intercourse should be maintained, and KY jelly used if lubrication is required. Atrophic changes should be treated with local estrogens if the systemic route is not being used. I would suggest that Dienestrol cream is inserted each night with an applicator for one month, and then 2–3 times a week for a further two months.

If menopausal symptoms require further treatment beyond explanation and reassurance then estrogens should be the first choice. I do not think there is much to choose between the different natural estrogens. In Brighton I have been using Harmogen more recently, and I am entirely satisfied with the therapeutic results. I usually start with the recommended doses which for Harmogen is 1.5 mg twice daily. The great debate as to the relative advantages and disadvantages of synthetic and natural estrogens rages about us. Suffice to say, I will continue to use the natural ones despite their great cost until it has been quite definitely proven that there is no difference between the two.

If a woman still has her uterus she must be given the estrogens cyclically: for 3 weeks out of every 4. The dosage should be changed to suit the individual. Ideally one wants to use the lowest dose of estrogen which will make her vasomotor symptoms insignificant.

At the initial visit, her breasts and pelvis are fully examined, her blood pressure and cervical smear are taken. The patient is seen again 3-monthly, on two occasions, and then every 6 months. At each visit her blood pressure is checked and once a year she should be fully examined. Many of the patients in Brighton return to their own doctors after the first follow-up visit, unless required back for research purposes. She should continue on treatment for at least one year. If the estrogen therapy is to be discontinued, it should be done so gradually, over 3 or 4 months.

Estrogen deficiency symptoms which occur before the cessation of menstruation are not so easy to treat. Small doses of estrogens may be given cyclically for 21 days each month starting on the fifth day of each period.

Unfortunately this sometimes exacerbates the common menstrual disturbances that occur at this time, and it is necessary to add a progesterone. If contraception is required then I use Microgynon 30 or Ovranette. Where contraception is not required one could use Menophase or a combination of a natural estrogen and norethisterone during the last week of treatment.

The management of long-term therapy is along similar lines; although I believe in hormones, I do not think they are anything like as important as improving the general health and welfare of the ageing post-menopausal woman. More good would be done by improving her social and economic status and encouraging increased mental and physical activities.

The same dosage of estrogen should be given. Once she has been stabilized on treatment without untoward side effects, then she need only have her blood pressure checked each year and a full examination every 3 years.

The organization of a menopause clinic is all very time consuming. As you can imagine I found it difficult to set up such a clinic in a peripheral hospital.

Side effects are not common. One must warn patients about the transient nausea, breast discomfort and pelvic fullness. Initially I used to start with half the daily dose for the first month, but now I don't bother.

Vaginal bleeding can be a nuisance. Providing it occurs during the week-off treatment, it may be ignored. If it occurs at any other time, uterine curettage is mandatory. I usually perform an out-patient suction curettage, using the Vabra or Rocket curettes. I have no experience with the Gravlee jet washer. An out-patient curettage can usually be performed in 70% of patients, the remainder will require a formal dilatation and curettage under general anaesthesia.

The irregular bleeding may be treated by adding a progesterone providing the uterus has been curetted. This can be achieved by giving the estrogen continuously and by added 5 mg of norethisterone for 7 days every 6 weeks. Alternatively the patient may be put on Menophase.

Because I do not think all women should be given estrogens, the biggest problem with which I am faced in the clinic is how to decide which patients should be treated. For those with menopausal symptoms associated with flushes, sweats and vaginal dryness, there is no problem. They respond well to treatment and are extremely grateful. In the absence of vasomotor symptoms, the decision is not so easy. In Brighton, I am frequently referred patients from psychiatrists and there is no doubt that sometimes estrogen therapy considerably helps their management. I am trying to use the double-blind cross-over technique with estrogen and placebo as a therapeutic test. Unfortunately the placebo response is so good that 2 months on each drug may not be long enough and evaluation is made difficult.

The same problems arise when trying to decide who will benefit from long-term HRT

These are my guide lines. Firstly if a woman's menopausal symptoms have been successfully treated by estrogens, and she wishes to continue then I would advise her to do so. Secondarily, if a patient has been taking the Pill successfully in her late 40s, and early 50s, providing there are no medical contraindications, then she should continue on the Pill until the age of 55 and then change to natural estrogens. Thirdly, if a woman has had her ovaries removed before the age of 50 or she has developed menopausal symptoms shortly after a gynaecological operation, even though the ovaries may have been conserved, I think she should be given replacement therapy.

The decision is not so easy, when a woman who has not had any menopausal symptoms, wants to take estrogens to prevent osteoporosis. For example, we know that some women continue to produce significant amounts of estrogen after the menopause. However, there is no simple test for assertaining this point. There is so much variation in vaginal cytology and random plasma estrogen estimations, that single investigations are of little use. However, I will agree that if a woman repeatedly has well estrogenized vaginal cytology, then it is likely that long-term estrogen therapy is not required Once it is decided to start long-term estrogen therapy, then she must stay on it for the rest of her life.

In this paper I have tried to convey to you some of the practical problems that have confronted me in the menopause clinic. Estrogen replacement therapy has recently become very popular in this country and consequently we know a little more about the problems involved. However, much more long term research is needed before treatment can be recommended to all women. Estrogens do not retard ageing nor prevent the menopause from occurring.

When short-term menopausal symptoms fail to respond to simple explanations and reassurance, then estrogens should be used in preference to tranquillizers and sedatives.

In the long term, the health of some women will be adversely affected by estrogen deficiency, and they may be considerably helped by replacement therapy without risk of serious side effects. Unfortunately, there is no simple way of selecting those people and without further evidence, it is not justifiable to recommend routine replacement therapy to every post-menopausal woman.

37

Menopause—an American view

C. B. Hammond

One of the origins of this symposium is the controversy which has arisen regarding the very nature of the menopause or climacteric. The older, traditional view has been that it is a normal, physiological state which requires only education, reassurance, and on occasion, hormonal supplementation to smooth out uncomfortable moments. In more recent years, however, many have come to view the climacteric with alarm, considering it to be a pathologic state, a deficiency disease leading to various degenerative changes and requiring intervention with prolonged, even life-long hormonal therapy for all patients. Still others point out on the contrary, postmenopausal women have enjoyed good health and progressive longevity and are even more dependable in industry with less absenteeism than women 10 to 20 years younger. The role of estrogen for prophylaxis in coronary artery disease and osteoporosis has evoked much controversy. The entire subject has provoked an extraordinary amount of discussion and debate—as evidenced by this symposium. I will attempt to explore some of these areas today.

To attempt to speak for all of my colleagues in the United States is presumptuous. I will try, however, to present a consensus opinion when it exists, or to point out more controversial areas and attempt to define the pros and cons of the arguments.

The terms that I will use in this paper include *menopause*, the physiological cessation of menses. Although this term is frequently interchanged with *climacteric*, this latter term refers to the gradual decline of gonadal function—

and therefore encompasses a wide span of years, during which time the menopause occurs. The basic physiological change which occurs is gradual senescence of the ovary and, in turn, declining estrogen production.

Male–female death rates

Figure 37.1 illustrates the annual rate of mortality per 1000 people keyed in percentiles versus age in the top graph, divided between males and females[1]. You will note the slope of regression of death rate is equal until age 38 when the rate of death among males increases sharply over that of females. These rates only begin to narrow back around age 80. The reciprocal graph shows

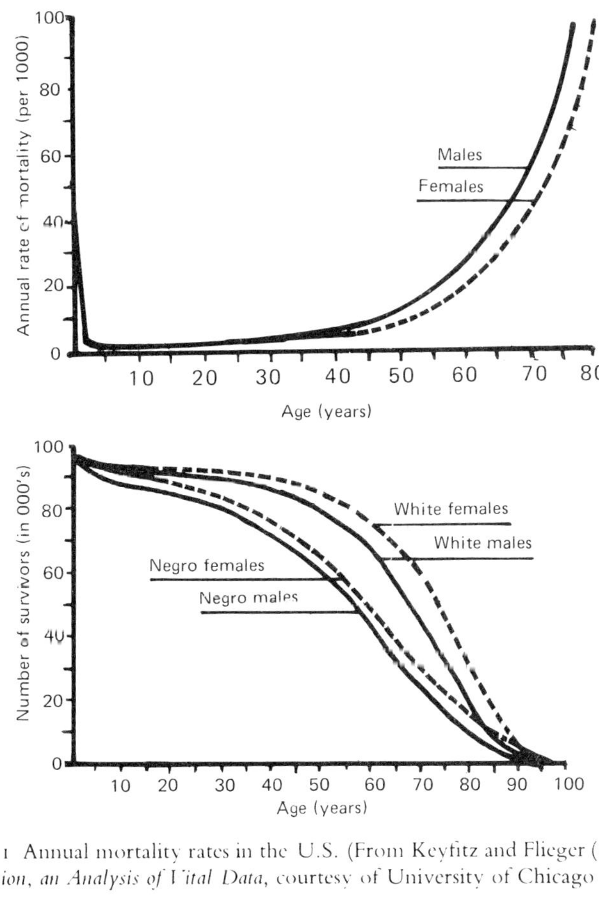

Figure 37.1 Annual mortality rates in the U.S. (From Keyfitz and Flieger (1968). *World Population, an Analysis of Vital Data*, courtesy of University of Chicago Press)

the number of survivors and likewise displays the marked disparity between males and females, again beginning around age 38–40. The primary cause of this disparity in survival is cardiovascular disease. Whether the so-called protective mechanisms operating for the female are intrinsic or whether they can be modified by exogenous hormonal therapy is unanswered.

There are three major phases in a woman's life. The *prepubescent* or growth stage is the interval from birth until menarche at age 12–13 years. During this time the secondary sex characteristics are unmatured and unstimulated but there is progressive development until puberty. During this interval gonadotropin and estrogen production are low, but increasing, and the sequential changes of pubarche, thelarche, growth spurt, and menarche are representative of this era of the pubescent process, culminating in sexual maturity at the menarche.

During the *reproductive stage* which extends from menarche until the onset of the climacteric (age 12–13 through 40–50), the secondary sex characteristics are fully developed and stimulated, and ovulatory cycles are usually present. Gonadotropins are in the adult cycling ranges and total serum estrogen values range between 50 and 300 pg/ml [2].

The age at onset of the third phase, the *climacteric*, is variable but is usually between 40 and 50 years of age. In Caucasian females with average life expectancy, a woman can now expect 26 or more years of life beyond the climacteric interval. For a black female it is 16 years. During this time there is declining maintenance of the secondary sex characteristics with atrophy of the vagina, vulva, uterus, breasts, skin and the development of osteoporosis, and cardiovascular degenerative changes. Gonadotropins are significantly elevated and work by Ross and co-authors has shown that a serum FSH in excess of 100 mIU/ml is diagnostic of ovarian failure[3]. Declining levels of estrogen are present but these declines are variable in amount. There is peripheral conversion of androstenedione which is produced from the ovary and some adrenal estrogen production. Classic symptoms of vasomotor instability, depression, emotional lability, lethargy, fatiguability, the 'androgenopause' will all be further discussed later in this paper.

Hormone patterns in the climacteric

Serum estrogen concentrations

The primary abnormality occurring in the climacteric woman is the disappearance of growing follicles in the ovary and the associated decline in estrogen secretion. Temporarily sufficient, but fluctuating amounts of estrogen are formed to produce irregular withdrawal bleeding. Eventually, however, the waves of estrogen secretion become insufficient to produce endometrial bleeding and menopause occurs.

	Estradiol (E_2)	Estrone (E_1)
A. Pre-menopausal women		
(1) Early follicular	63 ± 8	52 ± 5
(2) Late follicular	235	170 ± 13
(3) Oophorectomy	19·7 ± 5·0	26·7 ± 7·2
B. Post-menopausal women		
(1) No cancer	13·3 ± 1·1	33·8 ± 2·4
(2) Endometrial cancer	13·5 ± 2·1	28·5 ± 4·7
(3) Oophorectomized	14·1 ± 1·7	37·6 ± 7·1

(from Judd, H. L. *et al.*—*AJOG*, 118: 793, 1974)

Figure 37.2 Serum estrogen values (pg/ml ± SE)

Figure 37.2 illustrates serum concentrations of estrone and estradiol in women[4]. These data illustrate that:

(1) In pre-menopausal women, estrogen levels fluctuate in relation to the maturation and involution of the ovarian follicle and the corpus luteum.

(2) With oophorectomy there is a marked reduction of both estradiol and estrone.

(3) In post-menopausal women there is a marked reduction of circulating estradiol and estrone levels comparable to values seen in oophorectomized pre-menopausal subjects.

(4) With castration there is no discernable fall of estrogen levels in older women.

(5) In post-menopausal women with endometrial cancer estradiol and estrone levels are similar to concentrations seen in age and weight matched controls.

(6) In post-menopausal women with endometrial cancer both estrone and estradiol levels correlate directly with the patient's weight but not her age[4, 5].

Metabolic clearance rate—estrogen

If one considers the metabolic clearance rate in pre- and post-menopausal women, it is noted that there is a reduction in the metabolic clearance rate of both estrogens with the menopause (Figure 37.3)[4]. To date, the effect of oophorectomy on the clearance rate of either estradiol or estrone in pre- or post-menopausal women is not known.

Production rate—estrogen

In premenopausal women the production rate of estradiol and estrone fluctuates with the ovarian cycle (Figure 37.4). There is a marked diminution in estrogen production rate for both estrogens after menopause occurs[4, 5].

	E_2	E_1
Pre-menopausal women	1350 ± 40	2210 ± 120
Post-menopausal women	910 ± 70	1610 ± 110

Figure 37.3 Estrogen metabolic clearance rates (MCR L/24 h ± SE)

	E_2	E_1
Pre-menopausal women	80–500	110–375
Post-menopausal women	12	55

Figure 37.4 Production rates—estrogen (μg/24 h)

Sources of estrogen

If one now considers the sources of estrogen in the pre- and post-menopausal woman we note the majority of estrone is produced from direct ovarian secretion or from extraglandular conversion of androstenedione. The remainder is produced by the conversion of testosterone and estradiol. For estradiol, the majority is from direct ovarian secretion with a limited amount

Pre-menopausal women:

E_1—Majority from direct ovarian secretion or extraglandular conversion Δ. Remainder from conversion of T and E_2.

E_2—Majority from direct ovarian secretion. The remainder from peripheral conversion T, Δ, and E_1. Unknown amount by adrenal secretion.

Post-menopausal women:

E_1—Most, if not all from peripheral conversion Δ. Direct ovarian secretion is minimal.

E_2—Peripheral conversion E_1, T, and Δ. Direct ovarian secretion is minimal.

E_1—estrone T—testosterone
E_2—estradiol Δ—androstenedione

Figure 37.5 Sources of estrogen

converted in the periphery from testosterone, androstenedione and estrone. In the post-menopausal woman, most if not all estrone is produced from peripheral conversion of androstenedione while estradiol is produced by peripheral conversion of estrone, testosterone, and androstenedione. Direct ovarian secretion of either of these estrogens is minimal[4, 5].

	Testosterone	Androstenedione
A. Pre-menopausal women		
(1) Early follicular	289± 12	1689± 80
(2) Midcycle	342± 15	1932± 66
(3) Oophorectomy	129± 46	997± 324
B. Post-menopausal women		
(1) No cancer	231± 19	831± 54
(2) Endometrial cancer	230± 25	962± 64
(3) Oophorectomy	106± 14	719± 81

Figure 37.6 Serum androgen concentrations (pg/ml± SE)

Serum androgen concentrations

If we now consider androgen levels in pre- and post-menopausal women (Figure 37.6), let us first consider serum concentrations. From these data[6] we can make the following statements:

(1) In pre-menopausal women there is a small but significant rise of both androstenedione and testosterone at midcycle.

(2) With oophorectomy there is a fall of both androgens.

(3) In post-menopausal women androstenedione levels are similar but testosterone levels are distinctly higher than the quantity seen in castrated, pre-menopausal subjects.

(4) There is no difference between the testosterone and androstenedione levels found in post-menopausal women who do or do not have endometrial cancer.

(5) With oophorectomy there is a marked fall of testosterone and a distinct decrease in the androstenedione of older women.

Metabolic clearance rate—androgens

As well as the data shown in Figure 37.7 we must also add that the clearance rate of androstenedione is altered by body size while the clearance rate of testosterone is altered by several factors which include body size but also cover estrogen and androgens therapy, and oophorectomy. Menopause appears to have an effect on metabolic clearance of testosterone but not androstenedione[6].

	Testosterone	Androstenedione
Pre-menopausal		
Before oophorectomy	828 ± 45	1886 ± 228
After oophorectomy	540 ± 30	1850 ± 152
Post-menopausal	388 ± 88	1834 ± 192

Figure 37.7 Androgen—Metabolic clearance rates (MCR L/24 h ± SE)

	Testosterone	Androstenedione
Pre-menopausal women	200–300 μg/24 h	3·0 mg/24 h
Post-menopausal women	90 μg/24 h	1·5 mg/24 h

Figure 37.8 Production rates—androgen

Production rate—androgen

If one calculates the production rates of testosterone and androstenedione (Figure 37.8) we note that in pre-menopausal women there is a small fluctuation of androgen throughout the cycle[6]. There is also a marked diminution in testosterone and to a lesser extent, androstenedione, in the post-menopausal woman.

Sources of androgen

If we now attempt to determine the sources of androstenedione in pre- and post-menopausal women the following data can by summarized[6] (Figure 37.9): First, as there is no major peripheral conversion of steroids to androstenedione in women, and age and oophorectomy have no effect on metabolic clearance rate, then serum levels must reflect production. In pre-menopausal women approximately half of the circulating androstenedione is from direct adrenal secretion. The remainder is from direct ovarian secretion. In the post-menopausal woman these percentages of direct secretion are 85% adrenal, 15% ovarian.

For testosterone, two factors must be considered which influence circulating testosterone values and must be considered when studying production.

1. Androstenedione:
   (a) No major peripheral conversion to Δ in women.
   Age and oophorectomy have no effect on MCRΔ, the serum levels reflect production.
   (b) Pre-menopausal women—approximately half of circulating Δ is from direct adrenal secretion. Remainder is of direct ovarian secretion.

2. Testosterone:
   Two factors influence circulating % values and must be considered when studying production—
   (a) Menopause and oophorectomy ↓ MCR-T
   (b) 14% circulating Δ converted to T. With oophorectomy the ↓ of Δ = part of ↓ of T.

   Ovarian vein studies confirm that the post-menopausal ovary continues to produce T and Δ.

   In post-menopausal ovaries, hilus cells and luteinized stromal cells still contain enzymes specific for steroid metabolism.

   Pre-menopausal women—following oophorectomy T ↓ 185 pg/ml, Δ ↓ 815 pg/ml (↓ of Δ equals 115 pg/ml of ↓ T—Thus 70 pg/ml of T comes from ovarian secretion).

   Post-menopausal women—following oophorectomy T ↓ 130 pg/ml of Δ ↓ 245 pg/ml (↓ of Δ equals 30 pg/ml of ↓ T—Thus 100 pg/ml of T comes from ovarian secretion).

Figure 37.9 Sources of androgens

First, we know that menopause and oophorectomy both decrease the metabolic clearance rate for testosterone and second, that 14% of circulating androstenedione is converted to testosterone in the periphery. With oophorectomy the decrease of androstenedione is equal to part of the decrease of testosterone. In addition we note that ovarian vein studies confirm that post-menopausal ovaries continue to produce both testosterone and androstenedione, and hilar cells and luteinized stromal cells still contain enzymes specific for steroid metabolism.

Thus for all the calculations for testosterone in the pre-menopausal woman following oophorectomy, testosterone declines 185 pg/ml while androstenedione decreases 815 pg/ml. From these calculations 70 pg/ml of testosterone comes from direct ovarian secretion. In the post menopausal woman, following oophorectomy, testosterone decreases 130 pg/ml while androstenedione decreases 245 pg/ml. In this situation 100 pg/ml of testosterone is thought to come from ovarian secretion.

Gonadotropins

The high gonadotropin levels may be due to a decreased negative feedback of estrogen from the ovary on the hypothalamus, since implants or injections of estrogen will reduce the urinary gonadotropins. Direct evidence is lacking but frequent failure of luteal function and ovulation suggests that LH may be deficient in many women a few years before the menopause[7, 8].

Anatomical changes of the climacteric

Morphological and physiological changes associated with ageing are due to a gradual decline in the functional capacity of reproductive organs, loss of tissues, or diminished hormonal stimulation.

Organ	*Clinical and physiological changes*
Vulva	Labial folds show less prominence; skin itself becomes only a few cell layers thick; vascular and elastic fibres disappear; areas of trauma become pruritic; extreme kraurosis; hair less abundant on mons pubis and labial folds; vulvovaginal glands decrease in number and secretory activity; dermal vessels decrease; subcutaneous fat is lost; atrophic changes extend to perineal body, rectum, and anus. Loss of tone of sphincter causes mild fecal incontinence.
Vagina	Wall is shortened; thinning of wall leads to loss of rugae and less vascularity; wall is easily lacerated and irritated by bacterial or other noxious agents; vaginal secretions become scanty, with a higher pH. Lactobacilli are less frequent, bacterial flora mixed.
Uterus	Decreased in size due to fluid loss and transformation to interstitial fibrous tissues; fewer endometrial glands; attenuated myometrial fibres; myometrial blood vessels become thick and prominent.
Cervix	Reduction in size is less than that of fundus so cervical–fundal relationship reverts to that seen in the adolescent; cervical crypts atrophy; ducts stenose leading to retention cysts; cervical canal declines in size.
Oviduct	Mucosal folds become low, thin, and constricted; endosalpinx thins, flattens, and loses its cilia.
Pelvic floor	Muscle tone declines, ligaments and connective tissue lose strength and elasticity; pelvic organs relax; problems in prolapse and incontinence.

Organ	*Clinical and physiological changes*
Mammary glands	Premenopausal stage: subcutaneous fat increases; irregularities in lobules; cystic dilation; and proliferation of lobular buds; post-menopausal stage: subcutaneous fat reabsorbed and parenchymatous tissue atrophies; lobules disappear; tubules collapse; fibrous stroma condenses; nipples become smaller and less erectile; pigmentation decreases; breasts become flattened and pendulous.
Skin	Decrease elastic fibres; hyperkeratoses.

Fertility with ageing

The maternal reproductive system becomes less efficient with increasing age[9]. Studies involving the embryo transfer technique in mice and rabbits showed that the gametogenic function of the ovary outlasts the ability of the uterus to maintain pregnancy. Old ovaries grafted into young animals produce more pregnancies and neonates than did young ovaries in old mice. With ageing, the oviduct and uterus apparently become less effective in supporting young embryos. Declining fertility in aged women is partly due to less frequent ovulation. It is estimated that in women aged 40 to 45 years 75% of menstrual cycles are ovulatory; the percentages drop to 60% after age 46.

In women and higher primates, ovulation is not associated with a clearly defined period of estrus (heat). Thus spermatozoa may fertilize an ovum which has been in the oviduct for a variable length of time yet is still viable. Older women experience less frequent sexual intercourse, and the chances of an ovum becoming over-ripe prior to fertilization are increased due to the less frequent presence of viable spermatozoa. There is a possible relationship among frequency of intercourse, delayed fertilization, and the incidence of Mongolism due to trisomy of chromosome 21 in the offspring.

MENSTRUAL CYCLES

The irregularity of menstrual cycle length during the last few years of reproductive life may be due to decreased sensitivity of the hypothalamus to the feedback control of ovarian estrogen. However, there is no direct evidence to indicate that ova necessarily become 'over-ripe' prior to fertilization near the end of reproductive life.

The degree of sexual desire varies and is not directly related to the menopause. Frequently women acquire a need for sex gratification after the possibility of pregnancy has disappeared.

PREGNANCY

Attempts to ascertain the age of termination of reproductive capacity are complicated by the widespread use of contraceptive measures and the influence of socioeconomic factors. The extreme age for successful pregnancy in women is about 52, with only one out of 20 000 to 60 000 births occurring past the age of 50.

Post-menopausal pregnancies are rare. Women have conceived after 5–12 years of amenorrhea but they had not necessarily reached the menopause. It is not unusual for women to have an isolated period a year or two after the menopause, preceded by pre-menstrual molimina such as occur in ovulatory cycles.

Pregnancy in older women is generally more hazardous to both the mother and the fetus. The rates of abortion and stillbirths increase as do perinatal mortality and maternal death and complications. The problems may perhaps be partly due to the frequently high parity of these women. Mothers of nine or more children have three times as many stillbirths as women with fewer previous pregnancies. High parity also increases maternal and perinatal morbidity and the risk of thromboembolic complications.

Aborted fetuses from older mothers show higher percentage of abnormalities than from younger mothers. The cytogenic mechanisms involved are unknown; although some authors have suggested that the prolonged quiescent period of up to 50 years during the first meiotic division gives the chromosomes of oocytes ovulated in late life extensive exposure to detrimental environmental influences. There is also a high incidence of mongolism due to trisomy of chromosome 21 in the offspring of older women[10].

Future research is needed to understand the age changes in the ovum which may be responsible for the increase in congenital anomalies and intra-uterine loss characteristic of old age. It may be possible to extend the reproductive life span much beyond 60 years of age by showing the rate of atresia of oocytes. Such investigation may improve the chance of late pre-menopausal women becoming pregnant, maintaining pregnancy, and being delivered of a normal child.

Although pregnancy is unlikely, contraceptive measures are recommended until 2 years after the last menstrual period. Women taking oral contraceptives may not recognize the onset of menopause since regular menstruation usually continues while estrogen and progestagen are taken cyclically. Oral contraceptives do not seem to interfere with the normal rate of disappearance of ova or to favour pregnancies at a late age.

Common problems—climacteric

Irregular bleeding

Menopause, the final phase of female reproductive ability, refers to the cessation of menstrual periods. The manner in which menstruation ceases, however, is variable. Occasionally it may cease abruptly, but as a rule, the menstrual flow becomes gradually more scanty, and the interval between periods is increased. As ovarian function declines, the cycle may become irregular. Failure of ovulation may cause missed and shorter and less profuse periods (low estrogen production), or functional uterine bleeding with prolonged, profuse, and grossly irregular cycles (high estrogen production).

About one-half of all women experience menopause between 45 and 50, one-fourth before 45 and one-fourth after 50. The age of menopause does not seem related to the age of menarche (onset of periods), number of pregnancies, nor to prolonged anovulatory states (such as use of oral contraceptives).

Premature menopause (less than 35 or 40, depending upon sources) may occur spontaneously, or by surgical castration, ovarian irradiation, or debilitating disease. Induced menopause usually leads to more severe symptoms. Delayed menopause, after age 53, occurs in certain women and may be due to malignancy or ovarian, hormone producing tumours.

Suffice it to say that too frequent bleeding, too profuse bleeding, intermenstrual bleeding, or bleeding after 1 year without periods must always be investigated to rule out uterine malignancy; dilatation and curettage usually must be done.

Vasomotor symptoms

Perhaps the most common symptom of climacteric (40–50%) seems due to autonomic nervous instability which yields fluctuations in vascular tone and thus in blood flow. The sudden increase of blood into an area (characteristically the facies, causing redness of skin, perspiration—'hot flush'.

It is still unknown why it occurs. Recent data suggest that while estrogen is reduced and gonadotropins are elevated neither phenomena totally explains the problem[8]. Certainly, therapy with exogenous estrogen will promptly control these complaints.

Lethargy, fatiguability

Other common complaints—often difficult to evaluate—are the involutional symptoms. Frequently, the climacteric occurs at a time in life when other emotional factors are operational and yield a reactive-type depression. These include: 'loss of femininity', husband's work demands, children leaving home, 'life is nearly over'. There is an anabolic effect of steroids. Reduction of other climacteric symptoms may aid this, but at least some of the complaints are due to decreased estrogen levels.

Dyspareunia, decreased libido

Atrophy of vaginal epithelium and decreased mucus secretion in the climacteric may result in frictional dyspareunia. This, plus psychic and general metabolic changes may yield decreased libido.

Osteoporosis

Major orthopedic disorders occur in 25% of post-menopausal women. These are characterized by relatively atraumatic fractures of wrists, arm, shoulder, hip, and spine—usually occurring in women who are 2 years or more post-menopausal. There may occur a remarkable thinning of the cortex and trabeculae of bone and both increased resorption and repair occur. In general resorption is occurring more rapidly than repair.

In menopause serum calcium is normal while serum phosphorous is slightly elevated. It is obvious that normal bone density involves calcium and phosphorous metabolism, Vitamin D, thyroid and parathyroid hormones, renal function and sex steroids[11]. It is also known that premature menopause or castration is usually associated with prompt development of osteoporosis, unless estrogen is replaced. Thus—osteoporosis is a commonly seen problem in the post-menopause—and may result in major disability. While the entire mechanism is not understood, there does definitely seem to be an important role for the sex steroids.

Cardiovascular changes

There is little doubt that there are changes in the frequency, type, and severity of cardiovascular problems between pre-and post-menopausal women. There is obviously a great difference in the mortality and morbidity from coronary artery disease between men and women. After menopause the difference closes, but never quite equals that of men.

There is considerable evidence that estrogen does play a key role in protecting the female from coronary artery disease—although *how* is still being debated. Variable reports fill the literature as to cholesterol–phospholipid ratios, the presence of artheromatous plaques, and what effect estrogen therapy seems to have on coronary artery disease in both men and women.

What the role of increased ovarian androgen may be no one knows yet—but we do know in the non-estrogen replaced post-menopausal women that higher levels of androstenedione are present—perhaps exerting an effect on this process[4].

I will comment later on the possible *prophylactic* benefits of post-menopausal estrogen—but suffice it to say that replacement estrogen does seem of some aid for nearly all of these problems.

Climacteric—diagnosis

The traditional methods of documenting the climacteric are those of decreased estrogen as documented by vaginal cytologic smear[12] or by urine or serum level. The best test is elevation of gonadotropins measured in serum or urine[3]. This can also be documented by gonadal biopsy proving the absence of follicles. However, the most common diagnosis is based on the symptom complex and the cessation of menses during the appropriate interval in a woman's life.

Climacteric—therapy

What then do we know as facts about menopause from which we can base further investigation and study? First, with lengthening life women now live for more than a third of their life with reduced estrogen production, regardless of the source. Second, approximately 25% of women will consult a physician for symptoms which may be related to the menopause. Third, approximately 5–10% of women will have menopausal symptoms which will obviously be improved with replacement estrogen therapy. And finally, post-menopausal women have higher rates of coronary artery disease and osteoporosis than do pre-menopausal women.

Basically, therapy of the climacteric involves education, the consideration of the replacement of systemic estrogen or topical estrogen, and the use of tranquillizers. If estrogen replacement is to be utilized, one usually begins with a regimen of 1.25 mg of conjugated estrogen for 21 days, beginning on the fifth day post onset of menses or, beginning on the first of the calendar month if menses is not occurring or if the uterus has been removed. In addition, progestin should be added during the last 5 to 7 days of the estrogen therapy, particularly if the uterus is in place. One may have to either increase or be allowed to decrease the dosage of conjugated estrogen depending upon the improvement of the patient, eventually administering the least amount of estrogen which will alleviate her symptoms. Again, I would stress that it is my feeling that if the uterus is in place that progesterone should be added in each cycle of estrogen rather than cycling with unopposed estrogen alone.

Potential side effects of estrogen

I doubt that many readers are not aware of the increasing volume of literature about known possible side effects of estrogen therapy. Anyone who has administered these compounds has seen patients who have had complications, usually minor. Occasionally, a major problem may occur. Some of these include:

(1) Prolonged estrogen therapy may cause reactivation of endometrial growth and the occurrence of both estrogen withdrawal bleeding and endometrial hyperplasia. While neither of these problems are major, they generate considerable concern and not infrequently require diagnostic curettage.

(2) While I do not want to try to belabour the question of *de novo* carcinogenesis of estrogen, there are certain effects that we know at least cause some element of concern:

(a) There are strains of mice that, when given large doses of estrogen will develop breast cancer. These data have not, however, been confirmed in other animal strains or in man.

(b) There are higher rates of development of endometrial cancer among patients who have prolonged, high levels of estrogen—unopposed by progesterone—as in patients with granulosa-theca cell tumours or Stein-Leventhal Syndrome.

(c) There are now early reports suggesting that *de novo* endometrial adenocarcinoma may arise in patients treated with synthetic oral contraceptives. Whether this will be true for all contraceptives or replacement natural estrogen obviously requires further work. What role the addition of progesterone to the cycle of estrogen therapy has as a protective mechanism is likewise unclear at this time.

(3) Medical literature certainly supports the theory that some patients with pre-existing endometrial and breast cancers have increased growth rates if estrogens are given, or are improved by castration and estrogen deprivation. While I am not suggesting we give estrogen to patients with such *known* malignancies, one at least must wonder how many patients who have unknown tumours have been treated with these agents. Certainly the peak times of onset of these tumours are in the menopausal or post-menopausal years.

(4) Finally, both synthetic and naturally occurring estrogens have at least been incriminated in the genesis of thromboembolic disease. We must at least consider this fact prior to treating all women on these compounds.

Prophyllactic estrogen

One of the greatest areas of controversy about the climacteric revolves around the prophyllactic use of estrogens to reduce osteoporosis and coronary artery disease—problems of major frequency and consequence in the post-menopausal woman. Long-term, prospective studies regarding these areas have not yet been done. Both sides of this debate can cite studies which support or refute their claims and these questions are far from answered. Finally, the real potential hazards of estrogen therapy must also be considered.

All of this confusion has led the majority of American physicians to adopt a 'middle of the road' policy—by:

(1) Replacing estrogen in the 25% or so of the post-menopausal women who have unequivocal symptoms of estrogen deficiency.

(2) Not routinely replacing estrogen in *all* post-menopausal women.

(3) Not using replacement estrogen in any woman with a strong contra-indication to estrogen therapy—such as a breast or endometrial malignancy.

To summarize—the climacteric is a most controversial epoch in women's lives. As women live longer they seem to demonstrate the changes of estrogen deprivation, and the symptoms it causes. Only, however, with long-term, randomized studies, can we anticipate any definite answer to some of the questions which remain.

References

1. Keyfitz, N. and Flieger, W. (1968). *World Population, an Analysis of Vital Data.* (Chicago: University of Chicago Press)
2. Sherman, B. M. and Korenman, S. G. (1975). Hormonal characteristics of the menstrual cycle throughout reproductive life. *J. Clin. Invest.*, **55,** 699
3. Ross, G. T., Kohler, P. O. and Odell, W. D. (1967). Metabolic clearance and production rates of human luteinizing hormone in pre- and postmenopausal women. *J. Clin. Invest.*, **47,** 38
4. Grodin, J. M., Siiteri, P. K. and MacDonald, P. C. (1973). Source of estrogen production in postmenopausal women. *J. Clin. Endocrinol. Metab.*, **36,** 307
5. Judd, H. L., Judd, G. E., Lucas, W. E. and Yen, S. S. C. (1974). Endocrine function of the postmenopausal ovary: concentrations of androgens and estrogens in ovarian and peripheral vein blood. *J. Clin. Endocrinol. Metab.*, **39,** 1020
6. Judd, H. L., Lucas, W. E. and Yen, S. S. C. (1974). Effect of oophorectomy on circulating testosterone and androstenedione levels in patients with endometrial cancer. *Am. J. Obstet. Gynecol.*, **118,** 793
7. Ferriman, D. and Purdie, A. W. (1965). Mechanisms of menopausal 'hot flushes' indicated by the effect of a dithiocarbomoylhydrazine. *J. Endocrinol.*, **31,** 173
8. Aksel, S., Schomberg, D. W., Tyrey, L. and Hammond, C. B. (1976). Vasomotor symptoms, serum estrogens and gonadotrophin levels on surgical menopause. *Am. J. Obstet. Gynecol.* (in press)

9. Manuatov, J. M., Ramos, R. A. and Ginar, J. (1974). In: R. E. Greenblatt, V. M. Mahesh and P. G. McDonough (eds), *The Menopausal Syndrome*, pp. 162–164 (New York: Medcom)
10. Edwards, R. G. (1973). Studies on human conception. *Am. J. Obstet. Gynecol.*, **117,** 587
11. Nordin, B. E. C. (1961). The pathogenesis of osteoporosis. *Lancet*, **i,** 1011
12. Stone, S. C., Mickal, A. and Rye, P. H. (1975). Postmenopausal symptomatology, maturation index and plasma estrogen levels. *Obstet. Gynecol.*, **45,** 625

38

A dissident viewpoint

L. Goldman

There is a Danish saying to the effect that of all the things which are difficult to predict, the future is the most difficult. One of the easier things to predict is that if one is thirty-eighth on a list of thirty-nine speakers, most of the points that one wanted to make will already have been made. So I have had the somewhat doleful experience of sitting in this hall since Monday muttering to myself every now and then: 'Well, there goes another one'. I console myself by seeing my brief as taking a general perspective of the whole subject of the menopause, though inevitably I shall have to refer to data which have been repetitively mentioned by others.

Looking at the subject in a wider perspective, we realize that the quest for the elixir of youth has been going on for a very long time. Each of us, especially on the wrong side of 50, would like to have the 'gulfstream of youth', in the words of Henry Wadsworth Longfellow, flowing 'into the arctic regions of our lives'. In search of that gulfstream of youth, we have had the somewhat curious spectacle of such eminent people as Pope Pius XII, Dr Konrad Adenauer and W. Somerset Maugham—a cynic if ever there was one—queueing up to visit Dr Paul Niehans in Switzerland for an injection of embryonic cells. These cells came from the fetal ewe-lamb, although Noel Coward, I understand, found the whole proceedings distinctly non-U. Equally eminent people, at much the same time 20 years ago, sought out Dr Ana Aslan in Bucharest to obtain injections of a procaine substance known as H3.

Somewhat less eminent, but no less assiduous in their search, were the women we saw on the Horizon programme on BBC TV early this year landing at the airport at Augusta, Georgia on their way to Dr Robert Greenblatt's clinic for hormone replacement therapy. Any menopausal woman who watched that highly misleading programme, the BBC's instant guide to the menopause, could be forgiven for believing that regular estrogen administration, supplemented on occasion by a touch of testosterone, would keep her features youthful, her figure supple, her psyche outgoing and uncomplicated, and her sex life brimming with adventure.

There is obviously much more medical justification for hormone therapy than there ever was for the Niehans treatment or for injections of H3. So it is easy to understand the enthusiasm for its widespread use, particularly among the Women's Rights movement. It is still easier to understand that the enthusiasts should look upon doctors—most of us mere men—as being fundamentally unsympathetic to the plight of the middle-aged woman. They accuse the writers of some standard textbooks on gynaecology of 'sexist' beliefs, of taking too limited a view of women's problems, of being small-minded and narrow—in short, of being male chauvinist pyg - - - mies.

Why otherwise (they demand to know) is there so little concern about the problems of the climacteric—a 'disease' which seems to last for about 20 years? Why otherwise has the concept of long-term hormone therapy aroused so little interest, at least until recently? Yet, in my judgement, the need to regard hormone therapy with some reservations has less to do with male cussedness than with medical cautiousness.

I should make it clear that I do not question the value of estrogen given for a short time, a few months or so, to relieve menopausal symptoms. What troubles me is the concept of hormonal administration for a much longer time, perhaps indefinitely. If mine is the dissident view, it applies only to this long-term continuous administration of hormones.

Last year I began a study on a group of climacteric women. For various reasons this had to be abandoned, but not before it became obvious that there were all kinds of problems associated with these women—some medical, some social, and a great many which appeared to be entirely personal. Similar observations have been made by several speakers. These women were troubled by the clear signpost to old age represented by the cessation of their periods, by the loss of physical attractiveness, by their children growing up and leaving home. The woman felt that she was being left with an emptying house and a lost purpose. Dr Kerr referred to this in an evocative phrase as the 'empty nest' syndrome.

In the circumstances it was hardly surprising that such a woman would present with lack of energy, anxiety, depression, insomnia, and similar symptoms. Before one considers hormone therapy in such a patient, two considerations arise. First, she needs counselling and reassurance as much as, if not more than, she needs medicines. Second, if the spectrum of illness is partly social and personal, and only partly hormonal, then we have the perfect pharmacological setting for a very powerful placebo response, whatever we do or whatever drug we choose to give.

The paper by Jean Coope and her colleagues[1] illustrated the point beautifully. In their 30 patients, a dramatic clinical improvement occurred during the first three months of treatment, irrespective of whether estrogen or a placebo was used. Still more impressive was the fact that the placebo proved reasonably effective in controlling hot flushes, a symptom we attribute without much question to estrogen deficiency. Several other papers at the Symposium have made the same point.

Those who advocate hormonal therapy are of course concerned about a much wider benefit than merely controlling menopausal symptoms. Estrogens might prevent osteoporosis, a condition which affects women at an earlier age than men. Estrogens could protect women against coronary heart disease, which, as we have heard, is relatively rare during the reproductive years. Unfortunately, the more I study the evidence, the more I find myself baffled by an impossible therapeutic equation—for all treatment depends on striking a balance between the possible benefits and the possible hazards. I have referred briefly to the benefits. What are the hazards?

Merely to ask the question is to be brought face to face with the Four Horsemen of the Medical Apocalypse—confusion, contradiction, uncertainty and paradox. The estrogen component of the oral contraceptive pill is normally blamed for its most serious adverse effects, including thromboembolism, hypertension and gallstones. Consider only one of these adverse effects, and the evidence is enough to cause the flag of Women's Lib to droop just a little. Work at Oxford[2, 3] showed that the pill increased the risk of myocardial infarction in women older than the age of 35. But more than this, it showed that the pill acted synergistically with other risk factors, like hypertension, cigarette smoking and obesity, to cause myocardial infarction.

Here of course is the paradox. We think that the hormonal pattern of the reproductive years acts in some way to protect women against coronary heart disease; yet older women on the pill appear to be more at risk of a heart attack, presumably because of the estrogen component. Should we then consider giving post-menopausal estrogen for a very long period of time when women in their 50s and 60s may already have several potential risk factors for heart disease?

As for natural estrogens, some investigators think them safer, but both Dr Poller and Professor Bonnar showed that they affected blood-clotting mechanisms in much the same way as synthetic estrogens. Professor Oliver mentioned other evidence of possible harm from the Coronary Drug Project[4] in America. Let me emphasize that this is the only known large-scale prospective randomized trial undertaken on a natural estrogen. After 5 years, the investigators abandoned their long-term controlled trial, partly because they could find no evidence of benefit from a natural estrogen and partly—and more ominously—because of a possible increase in thrombo-embolism and malignant disease.

This study in men after a heart attack provides no direct evidence of harm to healthy women. Extrapolation of data is a popular medical pastime, but often takes us on a misdirected journey. Still, failing other direct evidence, the American data are surely enough to cause us a few indirect qualms. It may nevertheless be true that natural estrogens are safer than synthetic ones—just as it may be true that long-term estrogen therapy would significantly reduce the incidence of osteoporosis, and that the risk or price to be paid for this benefit, in terms of myocardial infarction, would be acceptable; indeed, a risk that a well-informed woman (to quote that notorious phrase about the pill) would be happy to take.

The trouble is that we simply do not have the evidence to assess the risk, to solve what I called the therapeutic equation. All we have is a benefit we cannot quantify to set against hazards we cannot predict in the management of a condition we cannot define. Or at least we cannot define it very accurately.

Ironic though that might sound, it is not a unique situation in clinical science. It is the classic therapeutic situation for the prospective, large-scale, randomized, controlled trial, as we have now heard times without number. What strikes me as almost unbelievable is that synthetic estrogens have been available for about 40 years, and natural estrogens for about 25 years, and yet no such trial has been done. I cannot help thinking, a little sardonically and siding with the feminist view, that this trial would have been undertaken years ago if only men suffered from the menopause. Of course, we have had any number of short-term studies on relatively small numbers of patients, none of which, unfortunately, resolves the practical long-term dilemma. What we need is a very large number of subjects, perhaps two or three thousand, given estrogen or a control preparation and followed for several years; something indeed like the Coronary Drug Project in design and numbers, but applied to the menopausal situation. I was indeed delighted to hear Professor Bonnar and Robert Beard, among others, call for such a trial to be undertaken by the RCOG, perhaps in association with the RCGP. I hope that the plea for such a trial does not fall on infertile ground, least of all in these surroundings.

Supporting the call for such a definitive study enables me to end my contribution on a more positive note, for I would not wish my caution about hormone replacement therapy for the rest of a woman's unnatural life to be misinterpreted as a kind of 'pharmacological Calvinism'. Not all of us, I hasten to assure supporters of menopausal women's rights, seek to deny them estrogen because of arbitrary male prejudice, or because we regard ourselves as founder-members, exclusively male, of that unpopular institution, the Royal College of Obstinate Gynaecologists.

References

1. Coope, Jean, Thomson, Jean M. and Poller, L. (1975). Effects of 'natural oestrogen' replacement therapy on menopausal symptoms and blood clotting. *Brit. med. J.*, **4**, 139
2. Mann, J. I., Vessey, M. P., Thorogood, Margaret and Doll, Sir Richard (1975). Myocardial infarction in young women with special reference to oral contraceptive practice. *Brit. med. J.*, **2**, 241
3. Mann, J. I. and Inman, W. H. W. (1975). Oral contraceptives and death from myocardial infarction. *Brit. med. J.*, **2**, 245
4. Coronary Drug Project Research Group (1973). Findings leading to discontinuation of the 2·5 mg/day estrogen group. *J. Am. Med. Ass.*, **226**, 652

39

Financial implications of hormone replacement therapy

C. J. Dewhurst

It is not easy to estimate the benefits of estrogen therapy after the menopause in strictly economic terms. It is not difficult to compute the cost to the nation but the benefit to the patient or to the state in better earning capacity and any saving in the cost of subsequent medical treatment is much more difficult to decide. It is a simple matter when the patient is consulting her doctor privately and is paying personally for the treatment she requests and receives. This is not our concern. It is, however, our concern when the cost of treatment is borne by a National Health Service.

There are approximately ten million women in Britain over 50 years of age. If this number were to be treated with estrogens the drug bill would vary with the preparation used. The cost would be £70 million or £90 million for two well-known natural estrogen preparations; the cost for two synthetic preparations commonly in use would be the order of £1·5 million or £3·5 million.

There will, however, be further costs to be considered. It is generally agreed that regular supervision is necessary for a patient on long-term estrogen therapy. It is usually suggested that she should be seen twice yearly and that at one of these examinations at least a cervical smear be carried out; and both the breasts are examined and a pelvic examination made. If the patient has vaginal bleeding she may require to be seen more often and she may need consultant advice; she may even need to go into hospital for curettage.

To estimate the cost of this is much more difficult. Here we must make some presumptions. At the moment the general practitioner receives an additional payment of £1·50 for taking a cervical smear. If we assume that he would get a similar extra-duty payment for the supervision of a patient on long-term estrogen therapy we have perhaps £3·00 per patient per year which has to be added to the bill—£30 million for ten million women. The cervical smear has to be processed, stained and reported, of course, and a figure of £3 per smear might be computed from the Report on Costing Cervical Cytology in Two Cardiff Hospitals (1970–71). Here is another £30 million. The further medical bill must be speculative. Perhaps 5% of patients might require to be referred to a gynaecological out-patients department (£4·90, Cardiff figures) which perhaps has now risen to, say, £6·00, thus adding an additional £3 million. If 10% of these patients require in-patient curettage we must add another £1·75 million. The bill for medical services, therefore, which might have to be added to the drug bill could be between £55 million and £65 million per year.

Regrettably we have very little to compare this with since, so far as I am aware, we have as yet no way of computing the loss of earning capacity or pain and disability which might result from the pathological changes which we know often follow estrogen withdrawal. It is my hope that very soon we will turn our minds to finding satisfactory data so that we can in the future compare the cost of treatment with the benefit that it is achieving.

Discussion on Section J:

Management of the Menopause

Chairman: *Mr J. W. W. Studd*

Dr Jill Dosseter (Family Planning, Cambridge): I was most interested in Mr Beard's paper, which I felt had a great practical application. However, I can see a problem and I wonder how he will overcome it. The Family Planning Association (FPA) has now been taken over by the National Health Service, and we are now only financed to prevent pregnancy. I believe, however, that the FPA has a set up in its Steering Committee that could perhaps finance hormone replacement therapy. I would be very interested in his comments on this.

Mr R. J. Beard (Gynaecologist, Brighton): Unfortunately, because the Family Planning Association has been taken over, much of its power has been taken away. I still believe, however that if menopause clinics are to meet a widespread need, the Family Planning Association has the best facilities for running them, outside of the teaching hospital research clinics.

Dr P. A. van Keep (Gynaecologist, Geneva): My experience from the Netherlands is that the menopause clinic attracts the difficult patient. They attract the typical woman who has been a complainer for a long time and who when she reaches the age of 48 and has her first hot flush is rushed off to the menopause clinic. In most continental countries, menopause clinics fill a need in those situations where there is a poor doctor–patient relationship. Ideally we feel that treatment should be given by the general practitioner and by the gynaecologist.

Dr J. W. W. Studd (Chairman): I think that we are all agreed that there is a need for the research clinics to thrash out some of the problems, but ultimately it must be the general practitioner who will prescribe the therapy for as long as is necessary.

Dr K. J. Anderton (Gynaecologist, Sheffield): In the discussions that have taken place throughout the symposium, there seems to have been something of an 'all or none' rule where treatment is concerned; in the one hand we have no treatment, or treatment for a very short period and on the other, treatment for life. Has anyone any views as to how long we should treat these patients, and should it be for either of the two extremes?

Dr C. B. Hammond (Gynaecologist, Duke University): I have a different situation in that patients purchase their own drugs, and are not in a funded programme. Frequently patients take themselves off the medication for a variety of reasons, one of which perhaps is the cost or the trouble of taking the medication. Many patients therefore probably solve the problem for us, either by that mechanism or by not returning. My personal philosophy has been to treat the individual who presents with symptoms or findings that are suggestive of estrogen deficiency for a reasonable interval of time, by which I mean 5 to 7 years depending on her age. In a case of premature ovarian failure, such as a Turner's syndrome, it will certainly be for a long interval, from the time of puberty until well after the menopause years. Then I have tended to do one of two things. If the patient still requires treatment, tolerates the compounds well, and is having no adverse effects over this 5–6 year interval, I would continue the compounds. If however her symptoms have abated properly, or she has sgnificant side effects, then I would taper the dosage and eventually terminate it.

Professor C. J. Dewhurst (Gynaecologist, London): I do not think that it is an all-or-none situation. Presented with a patient with symptoms of hot flushes, I would unquestionably treat her. It is reasonable, at least initially, in such a circumstance, unless she badly wants to continue for a long perod of time, to establish relief, and then to try to reduce the dose to see if she is no longer troubled by the particular symptom. If she is recurrently troubled by it, than an excellent case can be made out for treating her for long periods of time. If she is feeling extremely well, why not continue? If the treatment is prophylactic, and not specific to symptoms, for example to prevent osteoporosis, for which in my opinion the best case can be made out for long-term therapy, then treatment has to start soon, and has to continue indefinitely.

Mr J. W. W. Studd: Which brings us perhaps to pre-menopausal therapy. Could I ask Professor Lauritzen for his views on that? I find it easy to recognise the post-menopausal patient with symptoms, but it is the pre-menopausal patient with vague changes of mood that is difficult to assess. Is she just a psycho-neurotic woman, or does she have climacterical symptoms?

Professor C. Lauritzen (Gynaecologist, Ulm): When a woman complains to me of symptoms which are, in my opinion, clearly related to pre-climacteric estrogen deficiency, then in most cases I would treat her with estrogen–progestogen combinations, particularly where the cycle is disturbed. In cases where no cycle disturbance is present, I would prescribe small doses of estriol which do not disturb the cycle at all, and which will alleviate the milder symptoms of the pre-menopause.

Mr J. M. Emens (Gynaecologist, Birmingham): Would Professor Hammond comment on any possible racial differences in the menopausal syndrome?

Dr C. B. Hammond: The graph of death rates very clearly defines that the negro in our country has a shorter lifespan than the caucasian, probably relating to a whole variety of influences, such as higher incidence of pyelitis, recurrent urinary tract infection, hypertension and cardiovascular disease. The age of the climacteric however does not seem to be altered. I can only speak of the negro; I am unaware of any differences in regard to the oriental or any other ethnic group.

Mr S. Campbell (Gynaecologist, London): I was interested that Professor Hammond should routinely add progestogens to the treatment of his post-menopausal patients. Is this because he is particularly anxious about the possibility of unopposed estrogen causing endometrial cancer?

Dr C. B. Hammond: The question is valid. I trained in an institution and I have visited a number of other institutions where this was basic dogma. Over the years, in cyclic replacement of estrogen, we have seen a number of patients develop endometrial hyperplasia. I should not like to be so definite as to talk about a percentile chance of the progression from endometrial hyperplasia, to cystic hyperplasia, to adenomatous, to adenomatous with atypicality, to adenocarcinoma, but I personally think that it exists. It exists, as is well demonstrated by the data from patients with Stein–Leventhal syndrome or granulosa theca cell tumours having a higher rate of endometrial malignancy. We have seen the first blush of some of the commentaries about replacement therapy with synthetic sequential oral contraceptives. What the future holds for the natural estrogens in relation to the same question is up for grabs at the moment. I believe that progesterone may have a protective effect in maturing and sloughing the endometrium and if I am to err in this situation I would rather err on the side of conservatism, which to me is replacement of progesterone with the estrogen.

Dr Muriel G. Yates (General Practitioner, Liverpool): The question of hypnotics and tranquillizers has only been touched upon, and we have heard opposing views from both America and Germany. I deplore the use of tranquillizers and hypnotics on any long-term basis, and I find only too often that my patients come back from hospital with their estrogens, and with an alarming array of tranquillizers and hypnotics.

In general practice, there is a well known saying, 'the peaceful repeat prescription'. It is very easy to fall into that rather lazy habit, but I have found that a lot of my work is taken up in trying to wean patients off these very addictive drugs which are also extremely costly.

Mr R. J. Beard: This is a major problem and I had hoped that Dr Goldman would bring it up in his talk. Estrogens are slightly addictive in that once a woman has been put on them, then for psychological reasons, due to the publicity in the press, or whatever else, it is extremly difficult to get her off them again. I sidestep the situation very smartly by referring my patients back to the general practitioners, but that does not answer the problem. I believe—and the drug companies will be pleased to know this—that once a woman has been started on estrogen, providing the placebo effect and the barrage of propaganda can be kept up, she is hooked for a long time.

Dr Muriel G. Yates: I am more concerned about the tranquillizers than the estrogens. It is not generally realized that pharmacologically their action is really very short term. I think that they are only of use for the acute episode. They should not be used long term, and the menopause is not the time of life to instigate their use.

Dr C. B. Hammond: I would agree with that. The easiest thing is to write a prescription and send the patient out with it, and that is as true of the younger women as of those in the menopausal years. I would prefer to use certain drugs which are perhaps less potent for short-term usage, but primarily try to spend time in educating the patient. If the problem is more severe than that, and I think that it warrants that type of therapy, then a psychiatrist is needed.

Mr W. G. McGregor (Gynaecologist, London): I have been taught that stilbestrol is the cheapest of the estrogens. In view of the costing situation, could anybody on the panel say what is wrong with the use of the simple preparations? They are cheap.

Professor C. Lauritzen: The cheapness of stilbestrol is the only point in favour of using such a compound which is completely different in structure and in biological effects from the natural estrogens. It has some rather atypical effects on enzyme systems, which have been well demonstrated in the literature. As a compound it is rather badly tolerated, and that is one of my main arguments against its use. Many patients, especially at the beginning of the treatment, feel very unwell. It is also a compound which cannot be metabolized to any appreciable extent, by the body. Stilbestrol, especially if given orally, goes directly to the liver. It has a long half-life and binds strongly to receptors, so it can cause effects which are more than physiological. Some of its side-effects indicate that it is more active than we would wish for the treatment of climacteric complaints.

Professor C. J. Dewhurst: From the data presented at this meeting it would seem that with natural estrogens there is perhaps a smaller tendency to deep-vein thrombosis, and a less severe effect on triglyceride levels than with synthetic estrogens. The question is whether such effects are sufficiently important to justify the very large cost difference in the two. I am by no means sure.

Dr R. C. Greenberg (Community Psychiatrist, London): Some of the things that have been said in relation to the use of so-called psychotrophic drugs are quite misconceived because tranqillizers are not the same thing. Earlier on in the Symposium, we heard that monoamine oxidases are low in the serum of menopausal women. Since we know that monoamine oxidase inhibitors are a good treatment for anxiety and phobic states, what is the place of these substances in the treatment of such symptoms of the menopause?

Mr R. J. Beard: Many of my patients came from psychiatrists and from general practitioners already on monoamine oxidase inhibitors, and other psychotropic drugs. The majority of these patients feel much better when taking estrogens and therefore I conclude that as a first choice, an estrogen should be tried.

Mr J. W. W. Studd: My feeling is that there are many psychological problems of the menopause due to estrogen deficiency and it is a common event. If these are of recent onset, I should like to de-emphasize the use of 'psychiatric' drugs and initially treat these patients with estrogens. Any residual problems can then be investigated and treated.

Mr G. Christodoulacos (Gynaecologist, London): Many times we are faced with cases of menopausal women who do not like the idea of regular withdrawal bleeding. In such cases, how often should we administer progesterone? Does it have to be given every calendar month? Is three or four time a year enough to shed the endometrium?

Dr C. B. Hammond: I have no precise answer based on scientific fact. We could probably go comfortably for as long as several months between induced bleeding intervals with progesterone. I base that on the fact that a number of people will not bleed when given continuous estrogen for that length of time.

I have no solid data to show that progestogens must be given at any interval. I feel that it should be at some reasonable frequency, be it every second month, or so, and that would be about the longest I would go. Withdrawal bleeding is the price the patient pays for replacement therapy.

Mr J. McQueen (Gynaecologist, London): Even Dr Goldman has accepted that estrogens are helpful in the patient with severe menopausal symptoms in the short term. Would that be Mr Beard's experience of the general practitioners with whom he works, and does he feel, perhaps, that the message we might have to take out from here is that these patients should be treated, and not thrown out of the surgery as occasionally happens?

Mr R. J. Beard: I do think that they should be treated, and certainly in Brighton, they are already getting the treatment. The problem is the time factor. Menopausal patients need time and where the general practitioner has the time, he should treat the patient himself. Menopause clinics should exist for the difficult patients. In my clinic I do tend to see more problem patients—the neurotic woman who comes with the first flush or the patient whom the GP knows will be a problem—are often referred to the clinic, and I accept that my therapeutic role in these cases is to defuse the situation rather than anything else.

Dr D. G. May (General Practitioner, Surbiton): It is quite impracticable to carry out full HRT on the National Health because of the time factor. I do some HRT work, but I find that the first consultation usually lasts something like 45 minutes. My average National Health consultation, I regret to say, is something like 5 minutes. The two do not equate under present circumstances.

Dr L. Goldman (Medical Correspondent, London): I can only agree. The patients I saw last year with the climacteric were all patients who had been to their GPs—this is not intended as a criticism of GPs—and had been told that the time was not available. Some were perhaps more blunt about it than that. I can only re-emphasize that the management of the menopause requires time. It may require hormones as well, but unless we can give it time, we are not doing what is necessary for the patient.

Index